Oral Diseases

Edited by Gokul Sridharan,
Anil Sukumaran
and Alaa Eddin Omar Al Ostwani

Published in London, United Kingdom

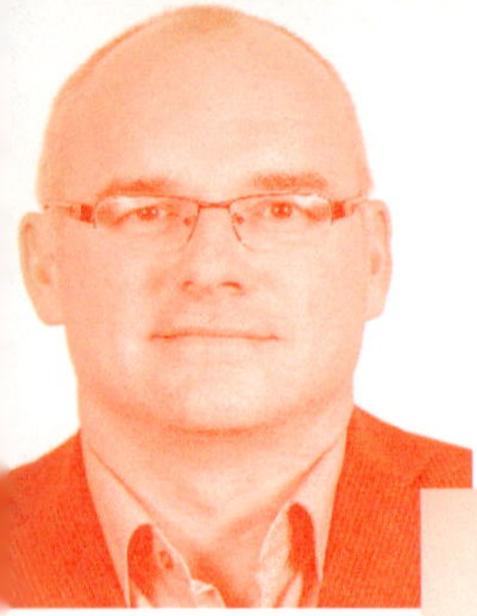
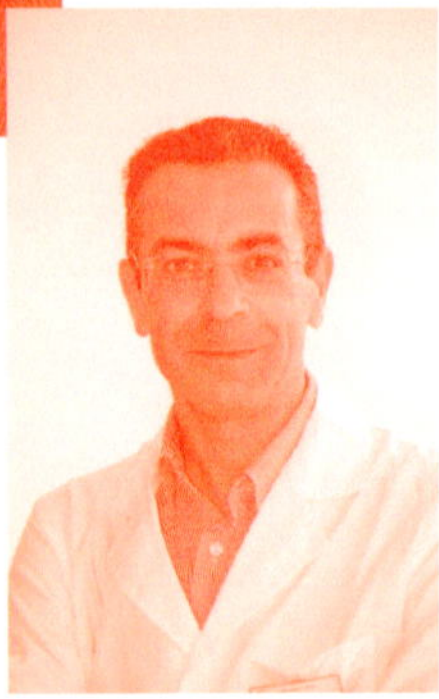
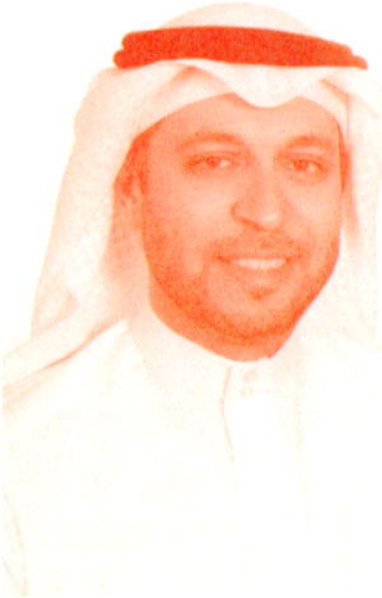
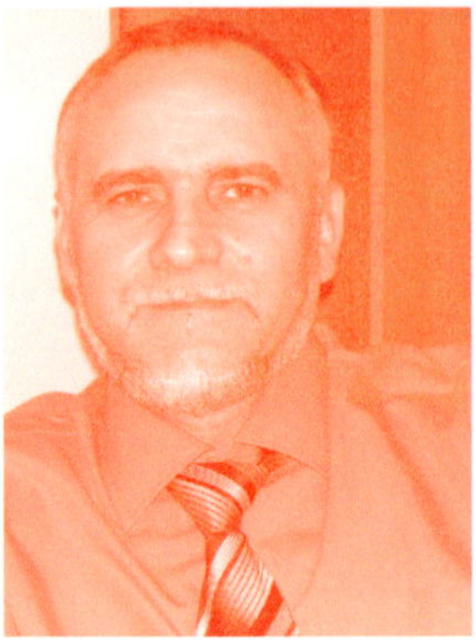
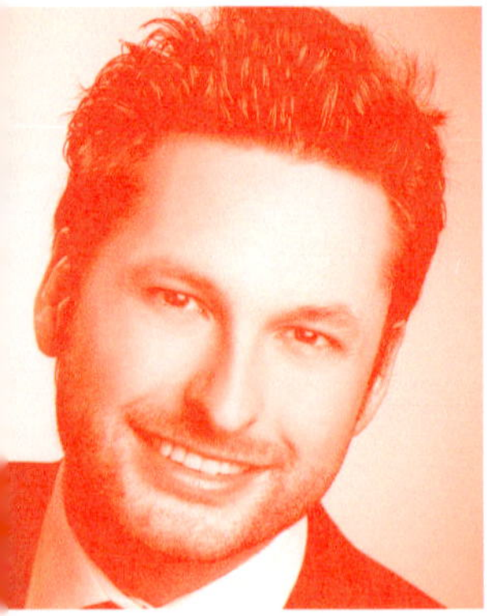
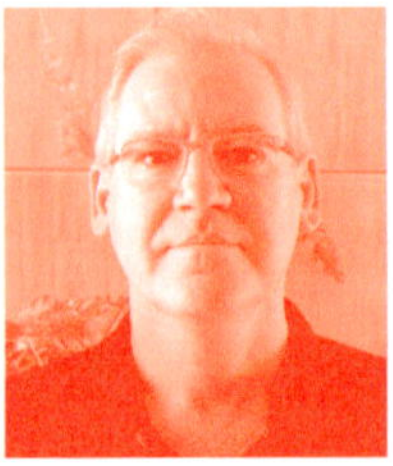
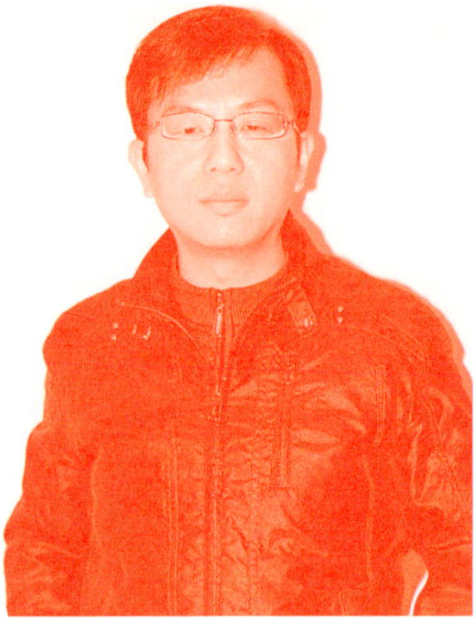

IntechOpen

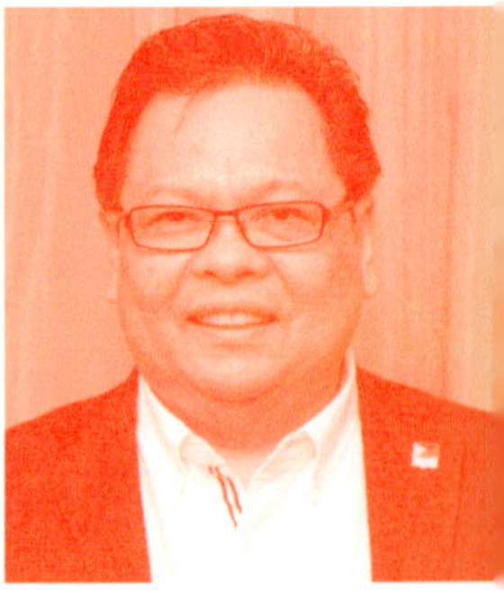
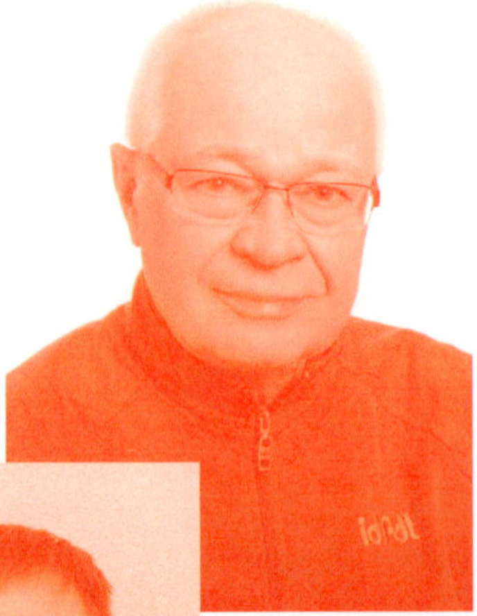
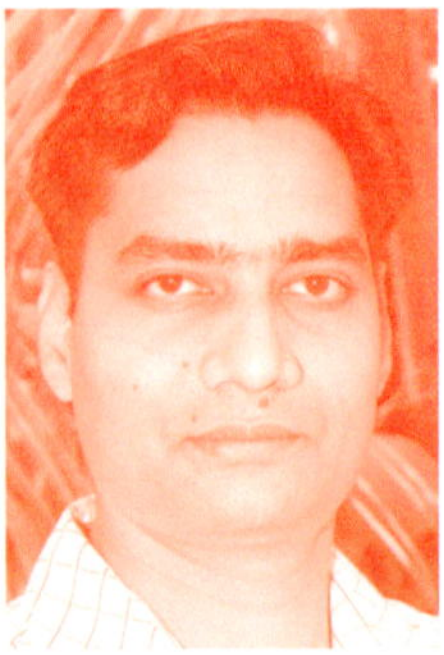
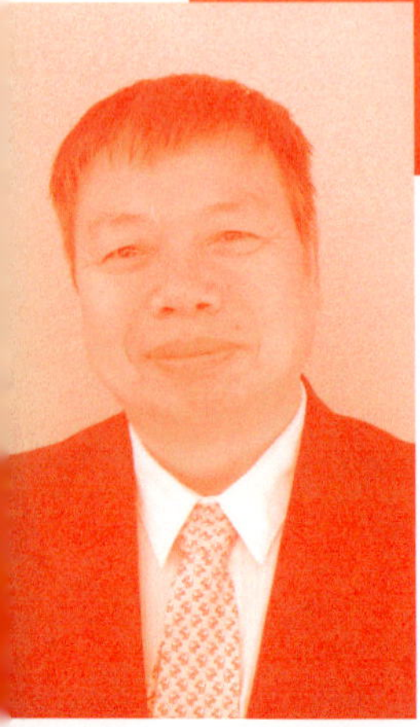
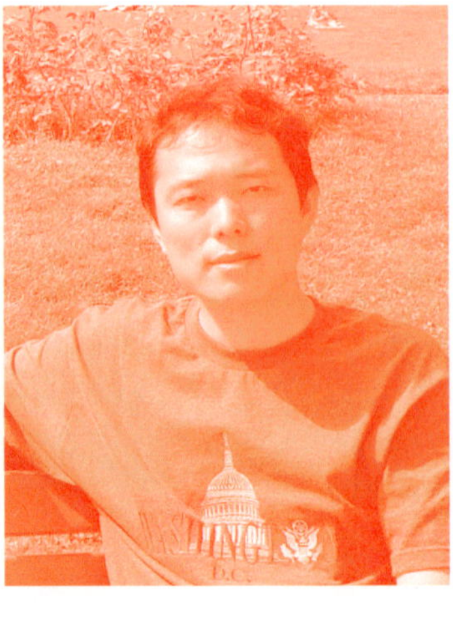
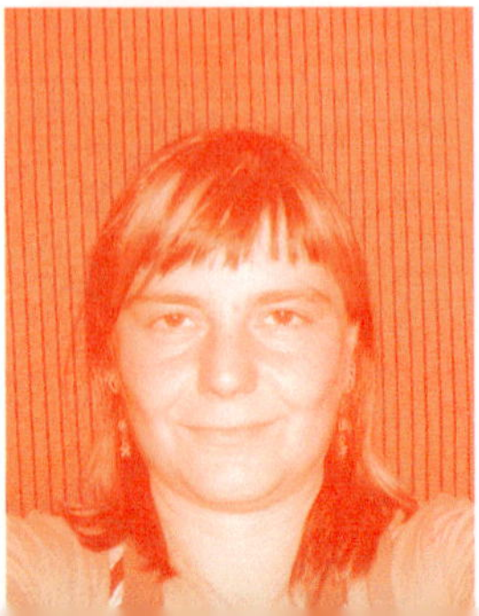

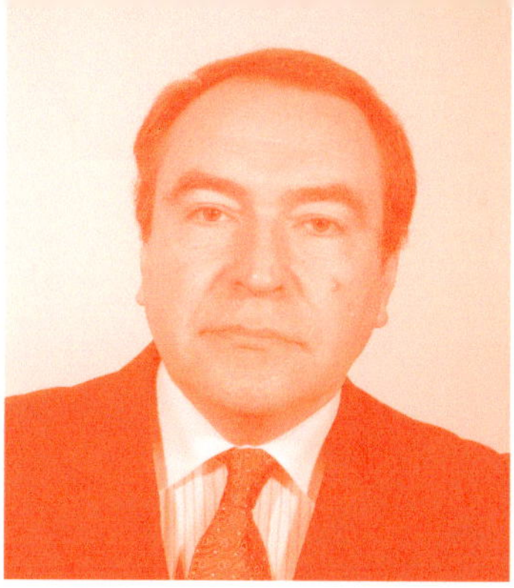
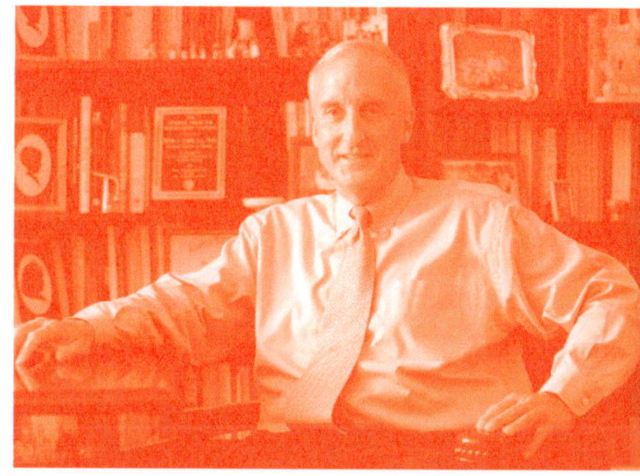
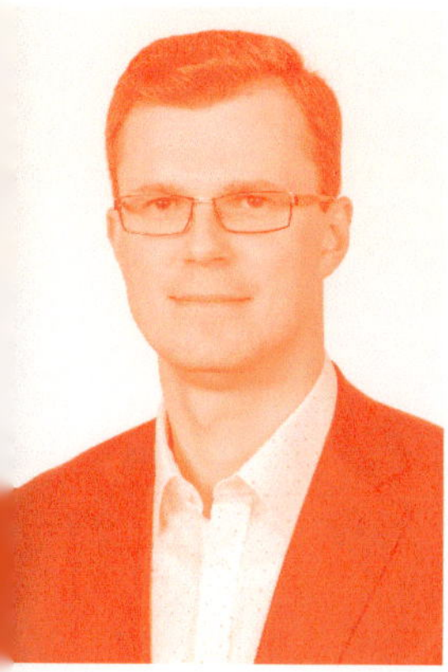
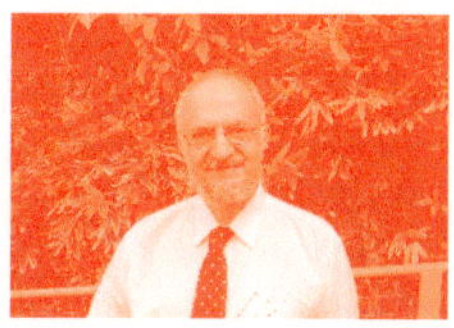
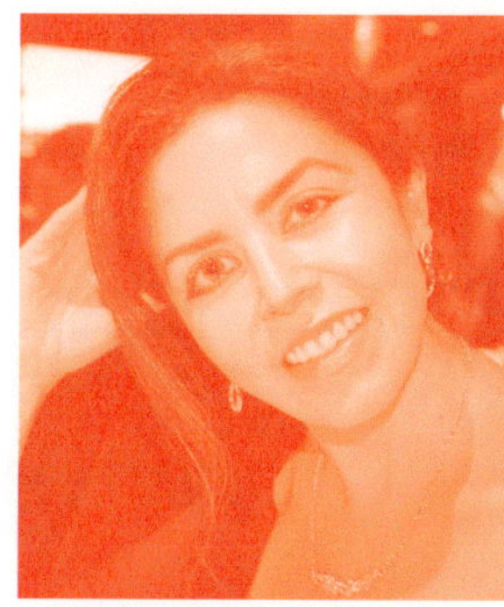

Supporting open minds since 2005

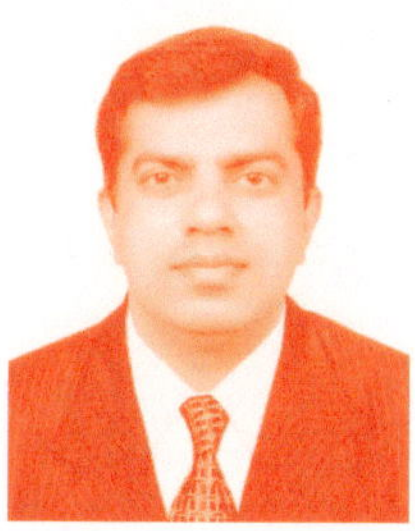
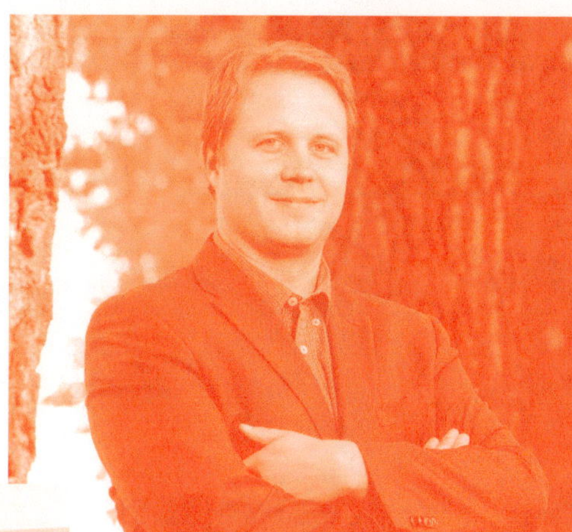
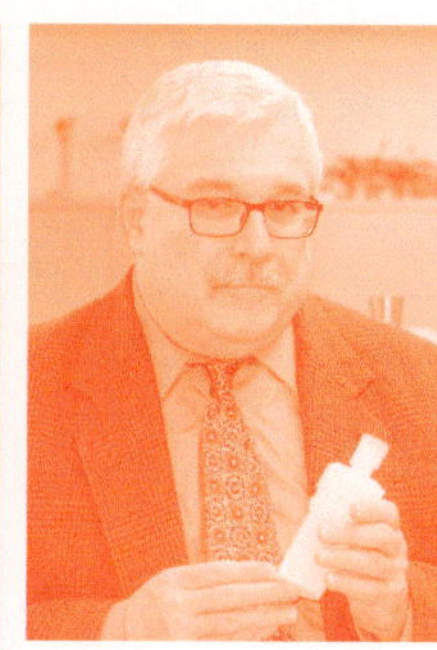
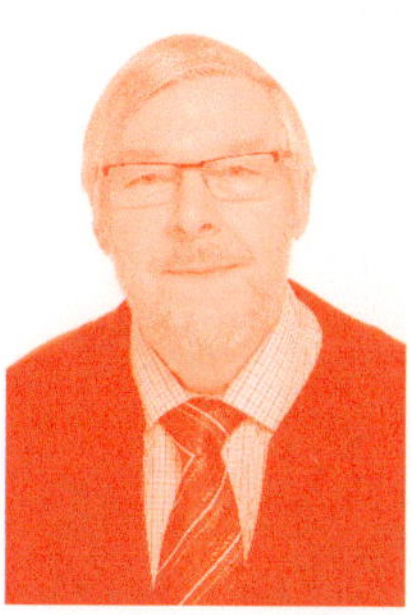
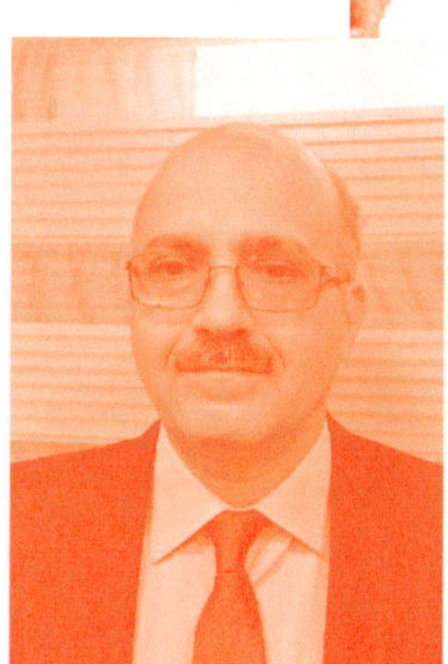
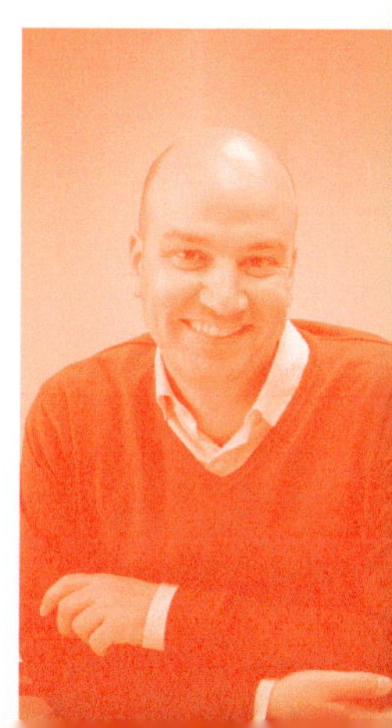
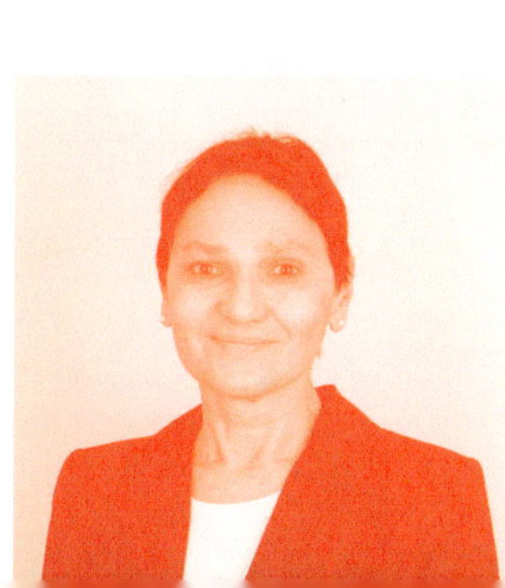

Oral Diseases
http://dx.doi.org/10.5772/intechopen.84931
Edited by Gokul Sridharan, Anil Sukumaran and Alaa Eddin Omar Al Ostwani

Contributors
Duy Quoc Ngo, Quang Le Van, Toan Tran Duc, Quy Ngo Xuan, Márcio Campos Oliveira, Igor Ferreira Borba De Almeida, Almira Oliveira Pereira, Maria Da Conceição Andrade, Viviane Ferreira Guimaraes Xavier, Luiz Moreira, Daniel Xavier, Juliana Xavier, Whyrllene Steine, Manoela Garcia Dias Da Conceição, Vera Lucia Luiza, Ana Cláudia Figueró, Randa Alfotawi, Alvaro Zubizarreta, Jesús Mena Álvarez, Reghunathan Preethanath, Wael Ibraheem, Aiswarya Anil, Andres Chala, Esra Guzeldemir-Akcakanat, Seham Alyafei, Sukumaran Anil, Elna Chalisserry, Anahita Punj, Manav Chaturvedi, Biagio Rapone, Elisabetta Ferrara, Daryl Anne Del Mundo, Alfredo Quintin Pontejos

First published in London, United Kingdom, 2020 by IntechOpen
IntechOpen is the global imprint of INTECHOPEN LIMITED, registered in England and Wales, registration number: 11086078, 7th floor, 10 Lower Thames Street, London, EC3R 6AF, United Kingdom
Printed in Croatia

British Library Cataloguing-in-Publication Data
A catalogue record for this book is available from the British Library

Additional hard and PDF copies can be obtained from orders@intechopen.com

Oral Diseases
Edited by Gokul Sridharan, Anil Sukumaran and Alaa Eddin Omar Al Ostwani
p. cm.
Print ISBN 978-1-83880-502-9
Online ISBN 978-1-83880-503-6
eBook (PDF) ISBN 978-1-83880-541-8

For EU product safety concerns:
IN TECH d.o.o., Prolaz Marije Krucifikse Kozulić 3, 51000 Rijeka, Croatia, info@intechopen.com or visit our website at intechopen.com.

Meet the editors

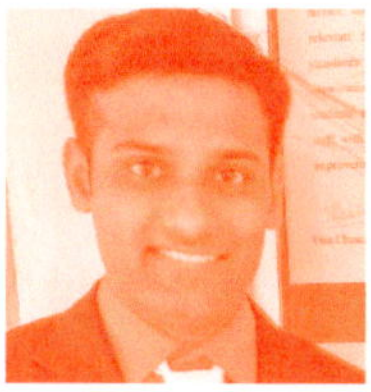

Dr. Gokul Sridharan is currently working as an associate professor in the Department of Oral Pathology and Microbiology at YMT Dental College and Hospital, Navi Mumbai. He has obtained his Doctor of Philosophy (PhD) for the work titled "Salivary and serum metabolomics in oral leukoplakia and oral squamous cell carcinoma". His field of interest includes oral pre-cancer, oral cancer, salivary diagnostics, oral and maxillofacial diseases, and advanced diagnostic aids with emphasis on bioinformatics and metabolomics. He has several scientific publications and actively contributes as a peer reviewer to numerous journals. He is an active member of the editorial board of several journals of repute. Dr. Gokul Sridharan has undergone training and is a qualified diploma holder in medial law and ethics and is also certified in tobacco cessation and control.

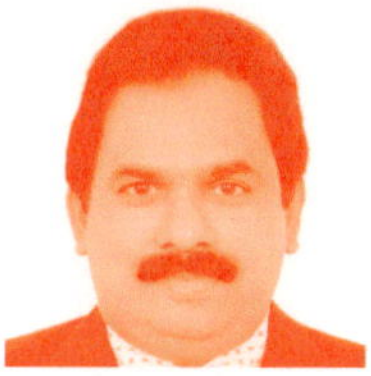

Prof. Sukumaran Anil, BDS, MDS, PhD, FDS RCPS (Glas), FDS RCS (Edin) FICD, FPFA, is currently serving as the Director of the Oral Health Institute, Hamad Medical Corporation, Doha, Qatar. He is a Professor and Senior Consultant in periodontics and implant dentistry. He received his Doctoral Degree in Dentistry (PhD) from the University of Hong Kong in 2002. Further, he underwent one year of advanced training at the UK Center for Oral HIV Research, Guys' and St. Thomas's Hospital, London. Based on his contribution to the field, Prof. Sukumaran received honorary fellowship from the Royal College of Physicians and Surgeons, Glasgow (FDS, RCPS), and Royal College of Surgeons Edinburgh (FDS RCS), International College of Dentist (FICD) and Pierre Fauchard Academy (FPFA). He has been the recipient of several awards for excellence in the field, Gold-medal winner (BDS-India), Ratan H. Doctor National Award (INDIA), Wang Gungwu Scholarship for Research Students (Hong Kong), and the Golden Quill award for research excellence from King Saud University, Riyadh. He has more than 35 years of undergraduate and postgraduate teaching experience and PhD supervision in various countries such as India, Hong Kong, Saudi Arabia, United Kingdom, The Netherlands, South Korea, and USA. Previously, he served as Full Professor at King Saud University, Riyadh for the past 12 years and worked as chairman and member of the National Accreditation (NCAAA), European and US accreditation for the courses at King Saud University. He plays a major role in developing a medical research facility (biomaterials and dental) for the medical division of the Ministry of Defense in Riyadh. He has published more than 350 research papers in high-impact journals, chapters, and books in the field.

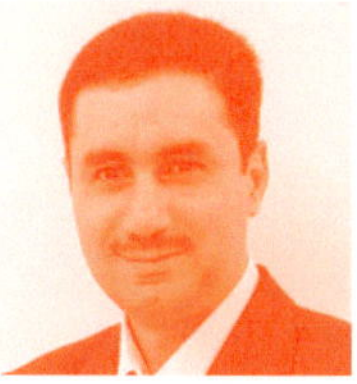

Dr. Al Ostwani Alaa Eddin Omar received a master's degree in Dentistry and a PhD in Pediatric Dentistry from Damascus University, Syria, in 2010 and 2014, respectively. He also received a fellowship diploma in Laser Dentistry and The Advanced Fellowship Postgraduate Diploma in Endodontics from the University of Genoa, Italy, in 2019 and 2020, respectively. Dr. Al Ostwani has been an assistant professor at the International University of Science and Technology (IUST) since 2014. During his academic experience he has received several awards, including the scientific research award from the Union of Arab Universities, the Syrian gold medal, and the international gold medal for invention and creativity.

He has published eight articles in international and national academic journals, and is a member of the International Association of Dental Traumatology and Syrian Society for Research and Preventive Dentistry, the editorial board for the International Journal of Dental Medicine and the reviewer board for the Indian Journal of Conservative and Endodontics.

Contents

Preface

The mouth is the mirror of the body's health.

Oral diseases are one of the most common disorders among the various communicable and non-communicable health diseases. They pose a major health burden for many countries and affect people throughout their lifetime causing pain, discomfort, disfigurement, and even death. As per WHO, it is estimated that oral diseases affect nearly 3.5 billion people globally. In developing countries, the estimate could be even higher owing to the lack of awareness among the general public, the lack of adequate infrastructure, and less accessibility to oral health care providers, especially amongst people of lower socio-economic status.

The different diseases affecting the oral cavity include dental caries, gingival and periodontal diseases, microbial infections, oral cancer, autoimmune disorders, diseases of the salivary gland, cysts and tumors of odontogenic origin etc. Additionally, the oral cavity exhibits early manifestations of systemic diseases such as diabetes, HIV, as well as metastatic cancers from other sites. In such circumstances, the role of the dental clinician assumes significance owing to their ability to diagnose the condition early and implement appropriate management strategies.

Keeping this in mind, the aim of this book project is to provide an overview of various oral diseases with emphasis on the pathogenesis, investigation, and the management protocol of different oral and maxillofacial diseases. The book has been divided into sections based on the categorisation of oral lesions into gingival and periodontal diseases, oral oncology, endodontics, and oral surgical procedures with the objective of providing a comprehensive outline of the different chapters for the readers and clinicians alike.

Dr. Gokul Sridharan MDS, PhD, PGD (Medical Law and Ethics)
Associate Professor,
Department of Oral Pathology and Microbiology,
Dr. G. D. Pol Foundation YMT Dental College and Hospital,
Kharghar, Navi Mumbai, India

Dr. Anil Sukumaran BDS, MDS, PhD, FDS RCPS (Glas), FDS RCS (Ed), FICD, FPFA
Professor, Senior Consultant,
Hamad Medical Corporation,
Doha, Qatar

Dr. Alaa Eddin Omar Al Ostwani
Assistant Professor of Pediatric Dentistry BDS, MSc, PhD,
International University for Science and Technology,
Syria

Section 1

Gingival and Periodontal Diseases

Chapter 1

Interdental Brushes in Maintaining Periodontal Health

Esra Guzeldemir-Akcakanat

Abstract

According to the World Health Organization (WHO), oral diseases are accepted as the most prevalent noncommunicable diseases. Oral hygiene and cleanliness is vital and essential to preserve and maintain oral health. Although periodontal diseases are controllable and preventable diseases, periodontal diseases are the most common type of oral disease. Mechanical plaque control is the key factor for not only in prevention but also in the treatment of periodontal diseases and maintenance of health. The primary factor for the development of gingivitis is poor oral hygiene which is microbial plaque formation. Achieving ideal plaque control may be obtained by toothbrushing together with interdental cleaning such as dental floss, interdental brushes (IDB), wood sticks, and waterjet devices. Evidence suggests that the most effective method for interdental plaque removal is the use of interdental brushes. In this chapter, while the importance of interdental brushes in oral hygiene is explained in detail, the types and use of interdental brushes will also be mentioned.

Keywords: dental hygiene, dental plaque, gingivitis, interdental brushes, interdental cleaning, oral hygiene

1. Introduction

While oral diseases are the most prevalent noncommunicable diseases, severe periodontal disease was estimated to be the 11th most prevalent human disease globally (WHO) [1]. Generally, seven oral diseases are described as follows: dental caries, periodontal diseases, oral cancers, oral manifestations of HIV, oro-dental trauma, cleft lip and palate, and noma. The Global Burden of Disease Study reported that oral diseases affected at least 3.58 billion people worldwide, and the most prevalent oral condition was caries of the permanent teeth [1].

Microbial biofilm which is a surface-associated and structurally and functionally organized multi-species biofilm [2] is the main reason of both dental caries and periodontal diseases. Microorganisms destroy not only tooth structures but also supporting structures of the tooth even though they have different microbial backgrounds. In both, the final result is losing the tooth, affecting dentition, function, esthetic, self-esteem, quality of life, and, moreover, pain, systemic infection and/or inflammation, and psychologic and physiologic discomfort. However, both diseases are preventable, and the main causes for both are poor oral hygiene and smoking which are modifiable risk factors.

Oral cleanliness, hence periodontal health, is crucial not only for maintaining the dentition but also general health, quality of life, and well-being for whole individuals [3–5]. Periodontal diseases are multifactorial in nature. While the etiology of periodontal diseases is basically associated with microbial biofilm; genetic, environmental such as smoking, alcohol consumption, unhealthy diet, stress, and immunological factors and systemic health have effects on the disease progression [6]. Current understanding is that the periodontal tissue destruction is mediated by host inflammatory mediators. Transition from gingivitis to periodontitis is still not known.

2. Prevention

Self-performed and professionally administered mechanical plaque control and removal is the pillar in prevention of dental and periodontal diseases and maintaining overall oral health. Keeping plaque accumulation around 20% would result in good periodontal health [7]. There are three stages of preventing and controlling the periodontal disease [6]. Primary prevention implies preclinical and pre-pathological stages. The aim is to prevent the onset of the disease to maintain health. Secondary prevention indicates prevention at the early stages of the disease and restoring health. The aim is to stop and reverse the progression of the disease. And tertiary prevention refers to disease conditions. The aims are to limit the sequels and regain function. In addition, supportive periodontal therapy and periodontal maintenance are crucial to maintain the oral health and prevent the recurrence, since the major risk factor for periodontal diseases is to have had the disease before.

Prevention and control of the dental and periodontal diseases rely on high standards of oral hygiene [8, 9]. Higher standards in oral hygiene can be achieved by education, teaching, motivation, risk assessment, needs-related oral hygiene instructions, and improving the individuals' skills and attitudes towards their oral health [10]. The patient has to understand the disease and its etiology. On the other side, the clinician has to be aware that every patient is unique, needing different approaches for education and clinical implementation. Moreover, there is no consensus or standard on what the proper oral cleaning or hygiene is and what the frequency and the extent of the oral hygiene are. In every situation, today, patients have an active role on their own health and responsibility, and compliance is crucial.

3. Self-administered oral care

The first step of self-administered oral care is to provide professional oral hygiene instruction. There are mechanical and chemical methods to reduce gingival inflammation by controlling the plaque biofilm. The European Federation of Periodontology recommends that "all people should brush their teeth twice a day for at least 2 min. with fluoridated dentifrice, and, periodontitis patients have to use inter-dental cleaning devices" [11].

Mechanical plaque removal may include manual or powered toothbrushes as well as interdental devices. The most common mechanical method for plaque removal is still manual toothbrushes [12]. A single, self-administered brushing with a toothbrush leads to reduction in plaque scores around 42% compared to pre-brushing scores [11]. Powered toothbrushes may increase plaque removal efficacy by 7–17% compared to manual brushes [2]. Toothbrushes do not reach the interdental areas [13].

3.1 Interdental cleaning

Interdental cleaning is essential and achieved by interdental cleaning tools such as dental floss, toothpicks (wood sticks), rubber-tip simulators, interdental brushes (IDB), single-tufted brushes, and electrically powered cleaning devices such as waterjet devices. While the adjunctive use of wood sticks, dental floss, or irrigators showed weak evidence for removal of plaque, IDB were found to be more effective than other interdental cleaning tools especially when the interdental space is not filled with gingiva [14]. Dental flossing may be a better choice for sites with intact interdental gingiva and healthy periodontium; however, self-administered flossing was found not very effective in removing interdental plaque.

3.1.1 Interdental brushes

IDB were launched in the 1960s as an alternative to wood sticks [15]. The term of IDB was used for "brushes with helical alignment of ligaments fixed to a twisted stainless steel central wire" [14]. The quality of IDB is backed by the ISO 16409 standard [16]. In ISO 16409, manual IDB is defined as "hand-powered device composed of filaments that is single strand, attached to the stem, emanating radially from a stem which is a central support structure of the manual IDB, usually of twisted wire, which secures the filaments, intended for cleaning of interdental surfaces." They may be conical or cylindrical in shape, and usually widths of IDB are ranging from 1.9 to 14 mm [4]. The ISO brush size is determined by passage hole diameter which is a minimum diameter in mm of a hole through which a manual IDB can pass without deformation of the stem. Usually, IDB tend to bend, buckle, and distort [17].

The lengths of filaments and texture of IDB vary, and they may be cylindrical, conical, or in other shapes or have hard and soft filaments and are usually available in a sealed package (**Figure 1**). Due to various interdental spaces and shapes, it is clear that various IDB shapes, sizes, and different angulations (angled or straight) are required (**Figures 2–6**).

As examples:

- **Figure 2** shows an IDB with micro ultrasoft brush-top with 1.80 mm diameter of bristle and 0.35 mm diameter of stem for narrow interdental spaces (ISO 0).

- **Figure 3** shows an IDB with extra ultrasoft brush-top with 2.00 mm diameter of bristle and 0.40 mm diameter of stem (ISO 1).

- **Figure 4** shows an IDB with super ultrasoft brush-top with 2.20 mm diameter of bristle and 0.45 mm diameter of stem. (ISO 2).

- **Figure 5** shows an IDB with conical ultrasoft brush-top with 2.50–4.50 mm diameter of bristle and 0.50 mm diameter of stem (ISO 3).

- **Figure 6** shows an IDB with middle optimized brush-top with 3.50 mm diameter of bristle and 0.60 mm diameter of stem (ISO 4).

There is a relationship between position of the tooth and interdental spaces [18]. It would be logical to use dental floss in the anterior region since the interdental spaces are narrow. However, at the premolar and molar sites, interdental spaces are larger, and IDB may even reach to dental grooves and fissures. While the clinician is searching for the most appropriate size and shape of IDB, contour and

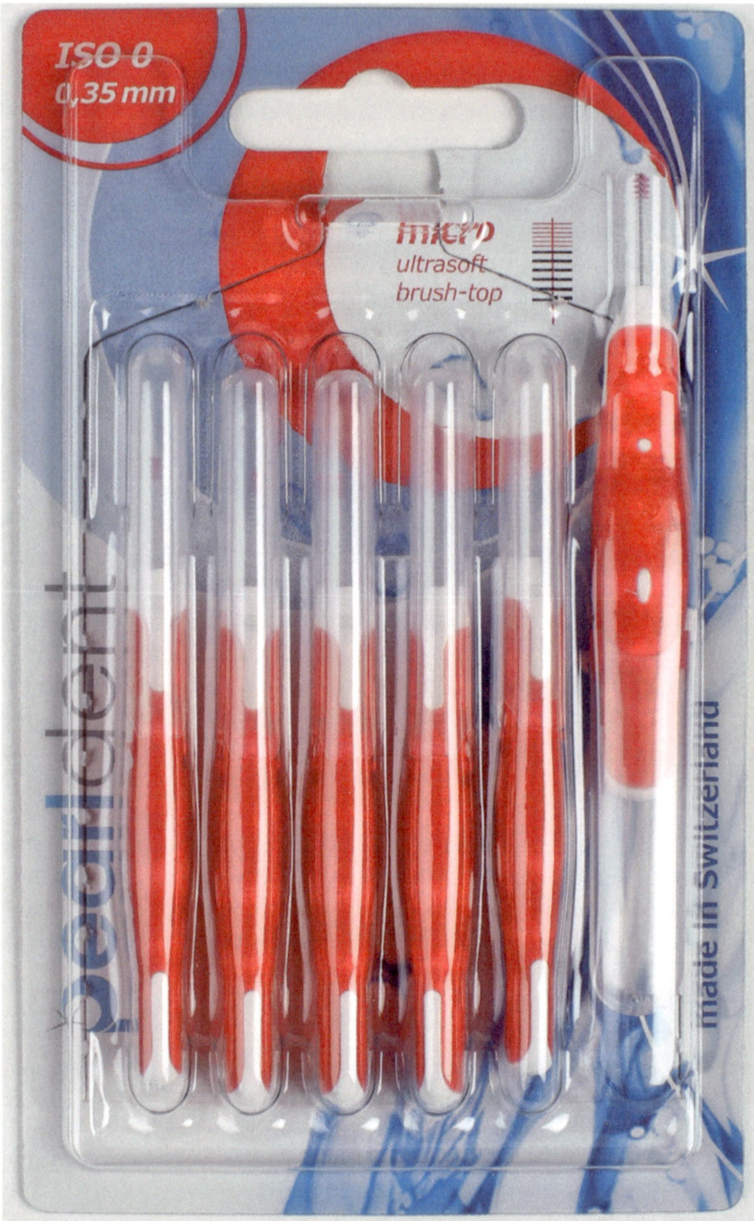

Figure 1.
A sealed package of IDB.

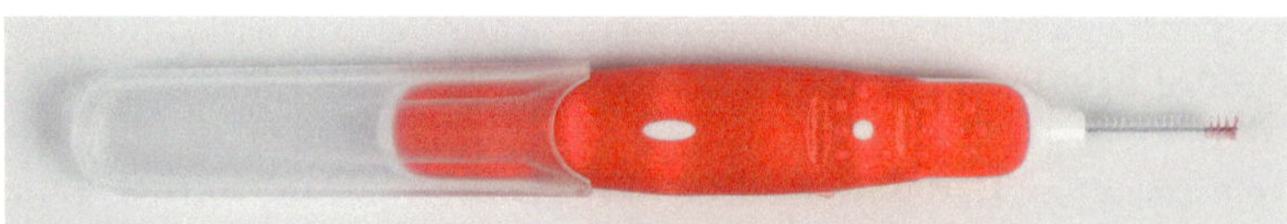

Figure 2.
ISO 0 micro IDB.

consistency of interdental tissue, and shape, alignment, and position of tooth, the size and form of embrasure have to be considered. The most appropriate interdental devices or IDB may differ between patients. In young individuals, dental floss is

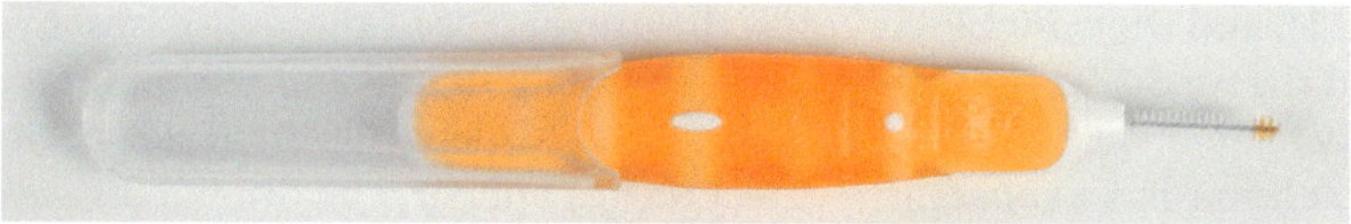

Figure 3.
ISO1 extra IDB.

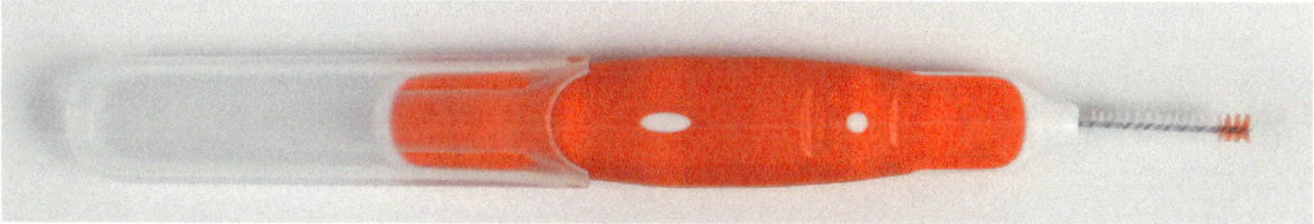

Figure 4.
ISO 2 super IDB.

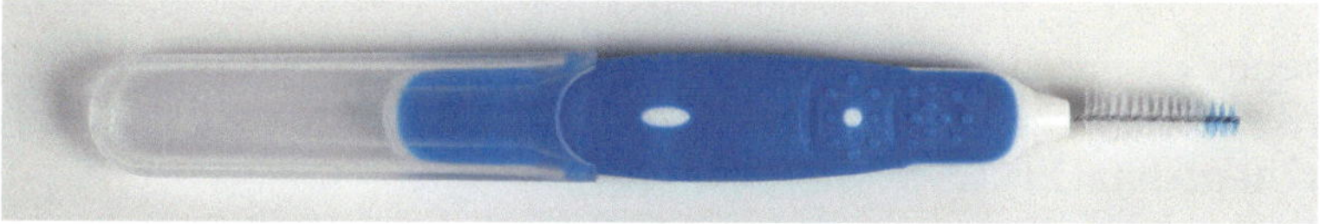

Figure 5.
ISO 3 conical IDB.

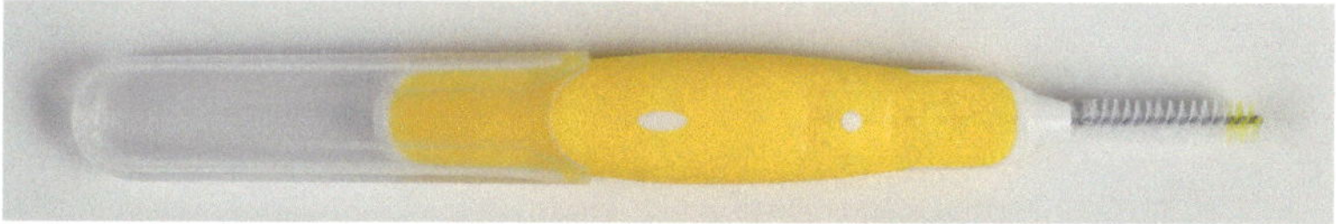

Figure 6.
ISO 4 middle IDB.

the only tool since the interdental gingival tissue fills out the interdental sites. So, the clinician should be careful when recommending IDB to periodontally healthy individuals since IDB may cause trauma at healthy sites. The European Federation of Periodontology concluded that "flossing cannot be recommended other than for sites of gingival and periodontal health, where inter-dental brushes will not pass through the interproximal area without trauma" [11].

In 1976, Waerhaug reported that IDB have an excellent effect both in the central part of the interdental space and on the embrasures; moreover, IDB may remove dental plaque as far as 2–2.5 mm below the gingival margin [19].

The use of IDB in addition to toothbrushing provides moderate evidence for higher plaque removal compared to toothbrushing alone or flossing in addition to toothbrushing [4, 20]. Although the studies which compare the efficacy of IDB with dental flossing are scarce, it was shown that IDB have a considerable effect on controlling and removal of dental plaque, and moreover, patients' perception is higher in IDB [13, 14, 21].

It was reported that interdental cleaning with IDB is the most effective method for interproximal plaque removal [7, 11, 13]. The patients' acceptance for IDB is very high, and IDB were considered as easier to use and less time-consuming than flossing [17].

4. Conclusion

Today, oral care over-the-counter products have a sizeable retail market; nevertheless, although periodontal and dental diseases are noncommunicable, controllable, and preventable diseases, the prevalence of these diseases is very high all around the world. The onset and progression of dental and periodontal diseases are mainly related with poor or inadequate oral hygiene. Optimal self-performed oral care at home has a substantial effect on not only oral health but also overall health. To prevent and control dental and periodontal diseases, toothbrushing is essential, but not enough. Based on the available data with respect to interdental plaque removal, the use of the IDB is strongly suggested.

Conflict of interest

The author declares no conflict of interest.

Notes/thanks/other declarations

The pictures are used with permission from the DentRAM Company, Istanbul, Turkey. The author would like to thank them for kindly providing pictures of Pearldent Interdental Brushes.

Author details

Esra Guzeldemir-Akcakanat
Faculty of Dentistry, Department of Periodontology, Kocaeli University, Kocaeli, Turkey

*Address all correspondence to: esragd@yahoo.com

References

[1] Vos T, Abajobir AA, Abate KH, Abbafati C, Abbas KM, et al. Global, regional, and national incidence, prevalence, and years lived with disability for 328 diseases and injuries for 195 countries, 1990-2016: A systematic analysis for the global burden of disease study 2016. Lancet. 2017;**390**(10100):1211-1259. DOI: 10.1016/S0140-6736(17)32154-2

[2] Flemmig TF, Beikler T. Control of oral biofilms. Periodontology 2000. 2011;**55**(1):9-15. DOI: 10.1111/j.1600-0757.2010.00383.x

[3] Tonetti MS, Eickholz P, Loos BG, Papapanou P, van der Velden U, Armitage G, et al. Principles in prevention of periodontal diseases: Consensus report of group 1 of the 11th European workshop on periodontology on effective prevention of periodontal and peri-implant diseases. Journal of Clinical Periodontology. 2015;**42**(Suppl 16): S5-S11. DOI: 10.1111/jcpe.12368

[4] van der Weijden F, Slot DE. Oral hygiene in the prevention of periodontal diseases: The evidence. Periodontol 2000. 2011;**55**(1):104-123. DOI: 10.1111/j.1600-0757.2009.00337.x

[5] World Health Organization. Oral health. 2018. Available from: https://www.who.int/news-room/fact-sheets/detail/oral-health [Accessed: 25 November 2019]

[6] Baehni PC. Translating science into action--prevention of periodontal disease at patient level. Periodontol 2000. 2012;**60**(1):162-172. DOI: 10.1111/j.1600-0757.2011.00428.x

[7] Drisko CL. Periodontal self-care: Evidence-based support. Periodontol 2000. 2013;**62**(1):243-255. DOI: 10.1111/prd.12012

[8] Axelsson P, Nystrom B, Lindhe J. The long-term effect of a plaque control program on tooth mortality, caries and periodontal disease in adults. Results after 30 years of maintenance. Journal of Clinical Periodontology. 2004;**31**(9):749-757. DOI: 10.1111/j.1600-051X.2004.00563.x

[9] Hujoel PP, Cunha-Cruz J, Loesche WJ, Robertson PB. Personal oral hygiene and chronic periodontitis: A systematic review. Periodontology 2000. 2005;**37**:29-34. DOI: 10.1111/j.1600-0757.2004.03795.x

[10] Dentino A, Lee S, Mailhot J, Hefti AF. Principles of periodontology. Periodontology 2000. 2013;**61**(1):16-53. DOI: 1111/j.1600-0757.2011.00397.x

[11] Chapple IL, Van der Weijden F, Doerfer C, Herrera D, Shapira L, Polak D, et al. Primary prevention of periodontitis: Managing gingivitis. Journal of Clinical Periodontology. 2015;**42**(Suppl 16):S71-S76. DOI: 10.1111/jcpe.12366

[12] Bakdash B. Current patterns of oral hygiene product use and practices. Periodontology 2000. 1995;**8**:11-14. DOI: 10.1111/j.1600-0757.1995.tb00041.x

[13] Slot DE, Dorfer CE, Van der Weijden GA. The efficacy of interdental brushes on plaque and parameters of periodontal inflammation: A systematic review. International Journal of Dental Hygiene. 2008;**6**(4):253-264. DOI: 10.1111/j.1601-5037.2008.00330.x

[14] Salzer S, Slot DE, Van der Weijden FA, Dorfer CE. Efficacy of inter-dental mechanical plaque control in managing gingivitis--a meta-review. Journal of Clinical Periodontology. 2015;**42**(Suppl 16):S92-S105. DOI: 10.1111/jcpe.12363

[15] Van der Weijden F, Slot DE. Interdental oral hygiene: The evidence. In: Bartold PM, Jin LJ, editors.

Multi-Disciplinary Management of Periodontal Disease Asian Pacific Society of Periodontology. 2012. pp. 1-18. Available from: http://www.apsperio.org/APSPProceedings2011.pdf

[16] ISO. Dentistry — Oral care products — Manual interdental brushes: ISO. 2016. Available from: https://www.iso.org/obp/ui/#iso:std:iso:16409:ed-2:v1:en [Accessed: 25 November 2019]

[17] Noorlin I, Watts TL. A comparison of the efficacy and ease of use of dental floss and interproximal brushes in a randomised split mouth trial incorporating an assessment of subgingival plaque. Oral Health & Preventive Dentistry. 2007;**5**(1):13-18. Available from: http://www.ncbi.nlm.nih.gov/pubmed/17366756

[18] Schmage P, Platzer U, Nergiz I. Comparison between manual and mechanical methods of interproximal hygiene. Quintessence International. 1999;**30**(8):535-539. Available from: http://www.ncbi.nlm.nih.gov/pubmed/10635266

[19] Waerhaug J. The interdental brush and its place in operative and crown and bridge dentistry. Journal of Oral Rehabilitation. 1976;**3**(2):107-113. DOI: 10.1111/j.1365-2842.1976.tb00934.x

[20] Worthington HV, MacDonald L, Poklepovic Pericic T, Sambunjak D, Johnson TM, Imai P, et al. Home use of interdental cleaning devices, in addition to toothbrushing, for preventing and controlling periodontal diseases and dental caries. Cochrane Database of Systematic Reviews. 2019;**4**:CD012018. DOI: 10.1002/14651858.CD012018.pub2

[21] Luz M, Klingbeil MFG, Sérgio P, Henriques G, Lewgoy HR. Comparison between interdental brush and dental floss for controlling interproximal biofilm in teeth and implants. Dental Health: Current Research. 2016;**2**(3). DOI: 10.4172/2470-0886.1000119. Available from: https://www.scitechnol.com/peerreview/comparison-between-interdental-brush-and-dental-flossfor-controlling-interproximal-biofilmin-teeth-and-implants-qT70.php?article_id=5372

Chapter 2

Pathogenesis of Gingivitis

Reghunathan S. Preethanath, Wael I. Ibraheem and Aiswarya Anil

Abstract

The 2017 World Workshop on the Classification of Periodontal and Peri-implant Diseases and Condition identified the gingivitis case by the presence of gingival inflammation at one or more sites and agreed upon bleeding on probing as the primary parameter for diagnosis of gingivitis. Clinical gingival health is generally associated with an inflammatory infiltrate and a host response consistent with homeostasis. The molecules that play a role in the pathogenesis are divided into two main groups: those derived from the subgingival microbiota (i.e., microbial virulence factors) and those derived from the host immune-inflammatory response. The immune system is essential for the maintenance of periodontal health and is categorized as innate immune system and the adaptive immune system. Innate immunity reflects the capacity of the host to defend against infectious attacks. Understanding the disease processes is important for the development of improved treatment strategies.

Keywords: pathogenesis, immune response, host susceptibility, inflammatory mediators

1. Introduction

Chronic gingivitis and periodontitis are chronic inflammatory lesions which display stages of inflammation as well as healing. The 2017 World Workshop on the Classification of Periodontal and Peri-implant Diseases and Condition identified the gingivitis case by the presence of gingival inflammation at one or more sites and agreed upon bleeding on probing as the primary parameter for diagnosis of gingivitis [1, 2]. Clinical gingival health is generally associated with an inflammatory infiltrate and a host response consistent with homeostasis.

The role of the immune response in periodontal destruction independent of bacteria was first described by Ivanyi et al. [3]. Later, Taubman et al. [4] studied the role of the immune response in a germ-free rat model of experimental periodontal disease and concluded that in order to control the disease, it would be crucial to enhance the protective "arm" of the immune response and suppress its destructive aspect [4]. The molecules that play a role in the pathogenesis are divided into two main groups: those derived from the subgingival microbiota (i.e., microbial virulence factors) and those derived from the host immune-inflammatory response. Even though "periopathogenic bacteria" are still regarded as the main initiating agents, immune-inflammatory response of the host to these pathogens plays an important role in the pathogenesis of PD [5].

2. Histopathology of gingivitis

The plaque biofilm causes most of the injury to the periodontal tissue through indirect mechanisms dependent on initiation and propagation of inflammatory host tissue reactions. The development of gingivitis is mainly the infiltration of the connective tissues by numerous defense cells, particularly neutrophils, macrophages, plasma cells, and lymphocytes. The accumulation of these defense cells and the extracellular release of their destructive enzymes cause destruction of collagen and subsequent proliferation of the junctional epithelium leading to vasodilatation, increased vascular permeability, and hyperplastic gingival tissues. Clinically it appears as erythematous and edematous gingiva: the clinical appearance of gingivitis. The classic studies of Page and Schroeder [6] described the basic understanding of histologic changes that occur in the gingival tissues as the initial, early, established, and advanced gingival lesions. These are histologic descriptions only, primarily based on findings in experimental animals.

2.1 The initial lesion

The initial lesion develops within 2–4 days of the accumulation of plaque at a site free of plaque biofilm, which is evident microscopically since the gingival tissues always have characteristics of a low-grade chronic inflammatory response as a result of the continual presence of the subgingival biofilm. In other words, the initial lesion corresponds to the histologic picture that is evident in clinically healthy gingival tissues. This low-grade inflammation characterized by vasodilatation and increased vascular permeability along with upregulation of intercellular adhesion molecule-1 (ICAM-1) and E-selectin in gingival vasculature facilitates migration of neutrophils and monocytes into the connective tissue. This influx of fluid flow from the vessels increases the hydrostatic pressure in the local microcirculation resulting in increased gingival crevicular fluid (GCF) flow.

2.2 The early lesion

The early lesion corresponds to the early clinical signs of gingivitis and characterized by erythematous clinical appearance of gingiva due to proliferation of capillaries and vasodilatation [7]. The predominant infiltrating cell types are neutrophils and T lymphocytes [7]. The basal cells of these epithelial structures proliferate apically resulting in edema of gingival tissues and deepening of gingival sulcus. The subgingival biofilm proliferates apically in this ecologic environment rendering plaque control difficult in these areas. The early gingival lesion may persist indefinitely, or it may progress further.

2.3 The established lesion

The established lesion corresponds to clinical appearance referred to as "chronic gingivitis" and depends on many factors, such as composition and quantity of the plaque biofilm, host susceptibility factors, local and systemic risk factors. A study by Page and Schroeder [6] defined established lesion as mainly dominated by plasma cells with inflammatory cell infiltrate in connective tissues and destruction of collagen fibers. Neutrophils accumulated in the tissues, which are also a major source of matrix metalloproteinase-8 (MMP-8; neutrophil collagenase) and MMP-9 (gelatinase B), release their lysosomal enzymes in the inflamed gingival tissues causing destruction of collagen bundles. This is followed by deepening of sulcus and formation of ulcerated pocket epithelium along the tooth surface resulting in bleeding on probing which is a common feature of chronic gingivitis. These inflammatory changes are still completely reversible if effective plaque control is reinstituted.

2.4 The advanced lesion

The advanced lesion, as described by Page and Schroeder [6], marks the transition from gingivitis to periodontitis which is determined by many factors, such as composition and quantity of the biofilm, the host inflammatory response, and environmental and genetic risk factors.

3. Host susceptibility

The tooth has a unique situation in the mammalian biology and presents a special challenge to the immune system [8]. The marginal gingiva includes the epithelial and connective tissue attachment apparatus that provides a biological seal between the tooth and the gingival soft tissues.

The oral cavity is a unique microenvironment where millions of bacteria live in harmony with our host defense mechanisms, with the bacterial host balance maintained by the amount of bacterial load through our regular oral hygiene practices. It is therefore important to understand the cellular and molecular elements involved in the pathways from health to disease and from disease to repair and regeneration.

3.1 Role of host susceptibility in gingivitis

Even though the development of gingivitis after plaque accumulation is a universal finding, the rate or speed of development and the degree of the clinical inflammatory response are variables between individuals, even under similar plaque accumulation conditions [9]. The studies recognizing the role of host contributing to the pathology of periodontal disease was a major breakthrough [10]. Various studies using the experimental gingivitis model showed 13% of all individuals representing a "resistant" group [9, 11, 12]. The factors modulating the appearance of gingival inflammation in response to plaque accumulation are mainly exacerbated gingival response to plaque, including metabolic factors such as puberty and pregnancy; genetic factors such as Down syndrome; nutritional factors such as vitamin C deficiency; the intake of drugs such as those leading to gingival enlargement; systemic diseases such as leukemia, immune deficiencies, and diabetes mellitus; and other conditions such as stress [9].

Gingivitis and periodontitis are the result of a coordinated action of clearly defined cellular players (proinflammatory and anti-inflammatory), which communicate with each other [13]. An inflammatory reaction can develop in two directions, either being destructive or regenerative depending on the bacterial antigen load and properties. If destructive, the innate immune reaction is followed by an adaptive or specific immune response, associated with the loss of tissue structure to create space for the immune process, and resolution of inflammation is associated with the regeneration of these structural hard and soft tissue components. It is therefore important to understand the cellular and molecular elements involved in the pathways from health to disease and from disease to repair and regeneration. The complex biological mechanisms occur in many phases from bacterial biofilm formation to periodontal regeneration and repair.

3.2 Host cells in periodontal pathogenesis

The inflammatory infiltrate of periodontal disease (gingivitis and periodontitis) is characterized by polymorphonuclear leukocytes (PMNs), macrophages, lymphocytes, plasma cells [6]. The periodontium consists of cellular elements (epithelial cells, the periodontal ligament and gingival fibroblasts, and osteoblasts and osteoclasts) and molecular elements (extracellular matrix components such as the various collagens and the noncollagenous proteins). The interactions between these components determine the nature of periodontal disease activity, whether gingivitis or periodontitis.

3.2.1 Polymorphonuclear leukocytes (PMNs/neutrophils)

PMNs are the first line of defense against bacteria, and proper PMN functionality is essential for protecting the integrity of the periodontium [14]. Neutrophils, present in clinically healthy gingival tissues, migrate through the intercellular spaces of the junctional epithelium into the sulcus [15, 16], in response to inflammatory chemotactic mediators such as IL-1, IL-8, or bacterial peptides (i.e., fMLP), and provide a "low-grade defense" against plaque bacteria [15, 17–19].

The proportion of neutrophils increases from 2% to 30% in modest inflammation causing vascular permeability which facilitates leukocyte emigration and increases the flow of GCF into the pocket [15]. At the molecular level, the interaction of adhesion molecules (e.g., ICAM-1) on endothelial and epithelial cells with β2 integrins on neutrophils facilitates neutrophil migration.

In the tissues, neutrophils phagocytose microorganisms and produce reactive oxygen species (ROS) to kill within the cells by the formation of neutrophil extracellular traps (NETs). NETs can be released by viable neutrophils and also following a form of programmed cell death called NETosis [20–24]. NETs are webs of complexed nuclear and mitochondrial chromatin/DNA and antimicrobial molecules such as histones and antimicrobial peptides (AMPs) [25, 26]. In established lesions, neutrophils release toxic superoxides, free oxygen radicals, and tissue degrading enzymes contributing to local inflammation and tissue damage [27].

3.2.2 Macrophages

Macrophages are mononuclear cells mainly participating in the early or innate defense against microorganisms and in specific immunity through their antigen-presenting function by releasing various cytokines. These cells present with varied phenotypes or subsets [28] and diverse functionality.

3.2.3 Natural killer cells

These killer cells are involved in the innate immune response by playing a vital role in host defenses against infected and malignant cells by producing cytokines such as TNF-α and interferon-g. These lymphocyte subgroup cells increase significantly from healthy human gingiva to diseased periodontal tissues [29, 30], in the immune response to plaque biofilm accumulation. Impaired lymphocyte function is also reported in various systemic conditions associated with periodontal diseases (e.g., Papillon-Lefèvre syndrome [31], Chédiak-Higashi syndrome [32], and smoking [33]).

3.2.4 Lymphocytes

Lymphocytes are one of the main types of immune cells with subsets T and B cells. When the innate or non-specific immunity is not able to cope with the bacterial challenge, it activates the adaptive immune system by a group of cells, the T cells that have specific ability to present the bacterial antigens to the immune-competent cells. T lymphocytes mainly contributes to periodontal pathogenesis by direct involvement in periodontal bone resorption [34, 35]. B cells, the second major lymphocyte subset, give rise to plasma cells that produce specific antibodies when triggered by the antigen and other regulatory cells. The number of B cells increases from health to gingivitis to periodontitis [6, 36], and its major role is in the pathogenesis of periodontitis.

4. Immune responses in periodontal pathogenesis

The immune systems are essential for the maintenance of periodontal health and are mainly categorized as innate immune system and the adaptive immune system (**Figure 1**). It is now widely studied that immune responses are complex biologic networks in which pathogen recognition, innate immunity, and adaptive immunity are integrated and mutually dependent [37]. They are also integrated with other systems, including the nervous system, hematopoiesis, and homeostasis as well as elements of tissue repair and regeneration [38] as shown in **Figure 1**.

4.1 Innate immunity

The term "innate immunity" refers to the elements of the immune response that are determined by inherited factors, that have limited specificity, and do not change or improve during an immune response or as a result of previous exposure to a pathogen. Innate immune mechanisms include a number of relatively non-specific mechanisms, including the barrier effect of an intact epithelium, saliva, and GCF (**Figure 1**). The keratinized epithelium of the sulcular and gingival epithelial tissues provides protection for the underlying periodontal tissue in addition to acting as a barrier against bacteria and their products [15, 39]. Saliva, secreted from three major salivary glands, plays an important role in preventing the attachment of bacteria to the dentition and the oral mucosal surfaces. These components include molecules that non-specifically inhibit the formation of the plaque biofilm by inhibiting adherence to oral surfaces and promoting agglutination (e.g., mucins), those that inhibit specific virulence factors (e.g., histatins that neutralize lipopolysaccharide (LPS)) and those that inhibit bacterial cell growth (e.g., lactoferrin) and

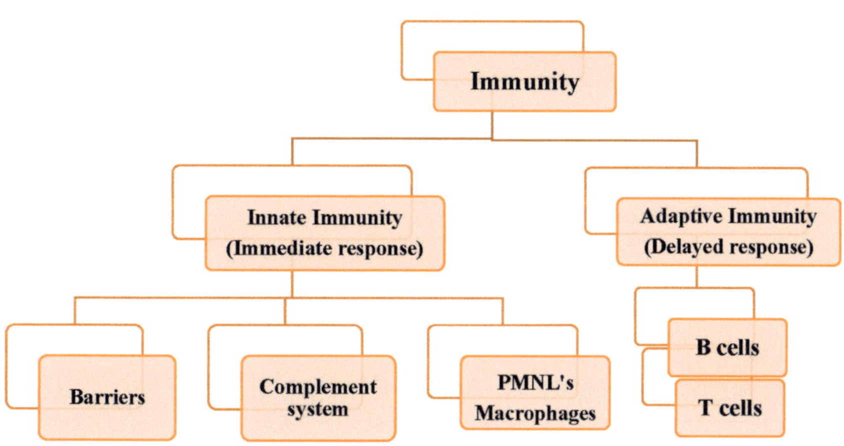

Figure 1.
Immune responses in periodontal pathogenesis.

that may induce cell death [40, 41]. GCF originating from the postcapillary venules of the gingival plexus carries blood components like neutrophils, antibodies, and complement components which help in host defense mechanism [42].

Saliva, as part of innate immune response, is a key factor in protecting dental enamel, gingiva, and mucosa by flushing microbes and foodstuffs, buffering acids, remineralizing the tooth, providing antimicrobial activity, and permitting selective adhesion of commensal microorganisms to maintain a symbiotic environment in the dental biofilm [43]. The salivary flow rate—high or low—is characteristic of each individual and [44–47] may promote salivary clearance of microbes from the oral cavity. Saliva also contains varying amounts of immunomodulatory interleukin-1β, interleukin-17, and interleukin-23, although it is not known whether they contribute to innate immunity on mucosal surfaces of the oral environment [48].

4.1.1 Pathogen recognition and activation of innate response

The recognition of pathogenic microorganisms and the recruitment of effector cells (e.g., neutrophils) and molecules (e.g., the complement system) are central to effective innate immunity. Innate immune responses are orchestrated by a broad range of cytokines, chemokines, and cell surface receptors, and the stimulation of innate immunity leads to a state of inflammation. When microbes penetrate the periodontal tissues, specialized cells of immune system, macrophages and dendritic cells, express a range of pattern recognition receptors (PRRs) which interact with specific molecular structures on microorganisms called microbe-associated molecular patterns (MAMPs) activating the innate immune responses (**Figure 2**).

4.2 Bacterial biofilm formation and development of a host response

Biofilms have been defined as "organized microbial communities characterized by a first group of colonizers being irreversibly adhered to a substrate or interphase in a wet media and the rest being embedded in a matrix composed of extracellular polysaccharides produced by the bacteria." The tooth surface provides a non-shedding hard surface where bacteria can adhere and form complex biofilms [8, 49].

The combination of natural host defense mechanisms and oral hygiene practices of individuals helps to have a balanced coexistence of oral microbiota in a healthy oral cavity which can be disturbed by either quantitative (higher bacterial load) or qualitative (growth of pathogenic species) changes in the biofilm leading to early stages of gingivitis [49].

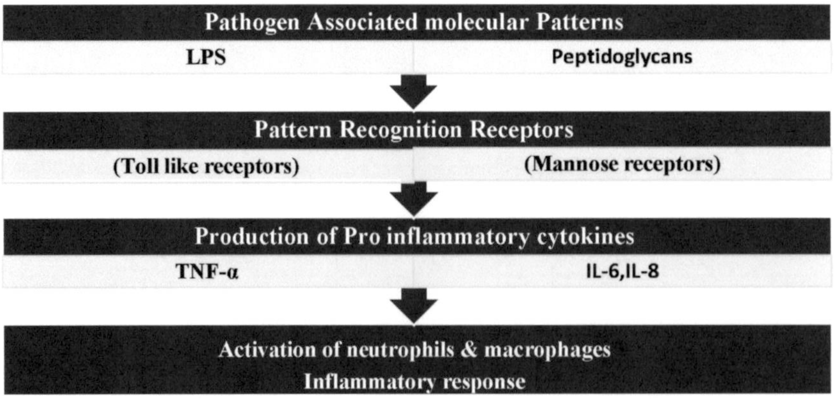

Figure 2.
Microbial- and host-associated pathogenesis of periodontal disease.

The epithelial attachment of tooth is a highly specialized structure where the junctional epithelial cells strongly attach to the tooth surface by a basal membrane, and hemidesmosomes providing the antibacterial defense mechanism by the high regeneration and desquamation rate and the continuous flow of gingival fluid through the gingival sulcus. The cells of the junctional epithelium with antibacterial proteins like human β-defensin 1 and chemokines along with intercellular adhesion molecule-1 (ICAM-1) and IL-8 help in the migration of PMN toward the gingival sulcus [8].

The protective function of the gingival epithelium is enhanced by keratinization, which helps resist abrasion. The gingival epithelium, as an innate immune barrier, is formed by interconnecting keratinocytes bridged one to another by cell adhesion molecules (CAMs) [50] which include integrins, mediating cell interactions with the extracellular matrix and basement membranes and contributing to cell-cell adhesion [51–53], as well as cadherins, which form tight contacts between cells [54]. The CAMs of the multilayered syncytium are susceptible to digestion by gingipains from *Porphyromonas gingivalis*, which could increase tissue permeability [55–58].

4.3 Innate immune response and gingivitis

Innate immunity is the first line of defense and the cells responsible for the innate immune response are mainly PMN, macrophages, and dendritic cells. Polymorphonuclear leukocytes (PMNs) are the first and predominant cells of the innate immune system in early gingivitis lesions [13].

The biofilm microbes on the tooth surfaces are recognized by the cells from the innate immunity through certain molecular patterns called pathogen-associated molecular patterns (PAMPs) which include lipopolysaccharide (LPS), peptidoglycans and lipoteichoic acids, N-formylmethionine, and lipoproteins. These molecules are recognized by pattern recognition receptors (PRRs) on the surface of PMNL and macrophages (**Figure 2**).

The two major families of PRRs that have been most extensively studied in the periodontium are the Toll-like receptor (TLRs) and the Nod-like receptors (NLRs) [59]. Toll-like receptors are unique receptors that recognize molecules that are broadly shared by microorganisms but are distinguishable from host molecules and can detect multiple pathogen-associated molecular patterns, including lipopolysaccharide, bacterial lipoproteins and lipoteichoic acids, flagellin, CpG DNA of bacteria and viruses, double-stranded RNA, and single-stranded viral RNA [60].

The TLR family currently consists of 10 known functional TLRs in humans [61, 62] in which TLR-1 through TLR-9 have been reported in the periodontium, in both health and disease [63]. When Toll-like receptors bind pathogen-associated molecular patterns, a series of intracellular events are initiated, leading to the production of cytokines, chemokines, and antimicrobial peptides (AMPs) [64]. Different Toll-like receptors induce different responses. For example, Toll-like receptors 1, 2, 4, 5, and 6 recognize products that are unique to bacteria and predominate in periodontal tissues, mainly in periodontitis [65] as shown in **Figure 2**.

4.4 Activation of adaptive immunity

If gingivitis persists without resolution, bacterial antigens are produced by lymphocytes, macrophages, and dendritic cells. Two different subgroups of lymphocytes, T lymphocytes and B lymphocytes, are released after being exposed with antigens by the innate immune cells. T cells are the effectors of cell-mediated immunity (delayed hypersensitivity), and B lymphocytes carry immunoglobulin molecules on their surface, which function as antigen receptors [66].

Adaptive immunity provides a more focused defense against infections than innate immune responses, which is slower and dependent on complex interactions between antigen-presenting cells (APCs) and T and B lymphocytes, specifically "cytotoxic T cells" and antibodies. Many histologic studies of periodontal disease [6, 67] have suggested the importance of adaptive immune responses in periodontal pathogenesis by the presence of leukocytes/neutrophils in the early stages of gingivitis and T cells in stable periodontal lesions. The T cells play a major role in maintaining tissue homeostasis against bacterial attack in plaque biofilm [68]. The transition from the established gingivitis lesion to periodontitis is mainly dominated by T and B cells.

5. Host-derived inflammatory mediators

The molecules participating in the cellular interactions are mainly categorized as proinflammatory and anti-inflammatory, and the balance between these two types of molecules determines the tissue response and the initiation or progression of disease. The key proinflammatory mediators in periodontal disease pathogenesis are as follows.

5.1 Cytokines

Cytokines are produced by resident cells, such as epithelial cells and fibroblasts, by phagocytes (neutrophils and macrophages) in the acute and early chronic phases of inflammation, and by immune cells (lymphocytes) in established and advanced lesions [69]. Interleukin-1β and interleukin-6 are the main innate cytokines and, together with tumor necrosis factor alpha, are the first to appear in the periodontal disease pathogenesis pathways [70]. Cytokines are effective in very low concentrations and have pleiotropic effects (i.e., multiple biologic activities) on a large number of cell types.

Cytokines are key inflammatory mediators in periodontal disease [71]. They are soluble proteins acting as messengers and binding to specific receptors on target cells to initiate intracellular signaling cascades resulting in cellular changes by altered gene regulation [72, 73]. The genetic regulation leading to the secretion of proinflammatory cytokines from a variety of cells is generally dependent on the activation of nuclear factor kappa-B transcription [74, 75]. The nuclear factor kappa-B-regulated pathways are activated by pathogen-associated molecular patterns, such as lipopolysaccharide, through the Toll-like receptor pathway [75].

5.1.1 Interleukin-1 family cytokines

The IL-1 family of cytokines comprises at least 11 members, including IL-1α, IL-1β, IL-1 receptor antagonist (IL-1Ra), IL-18, and IL-33 [71].

IL-1α is an intracellular protein, produced by monocytic, epithelial, osteoblastic cells found in the extracellular environment or in the circulation [76]. Studies have reported elevated IL-1α levels in GCF and gingival tissues in patients with gingivitis and periodontitis [77] and involved in the bone loss that is associated with inflammation [78]. In recent nonhuman primate experiments, the use of a specific IL-1 inhibitor resulted in significant reduction of periodontopathogen-induced attachment loss, bone resorption, and inflammation [79] suggesting that IL-1 inhibitors might be useful in the management of periodontitis.

IL-1β produced by monocytes, macrophages, and neutrophils plays a key role in inflammation and immunity and along with IL-1α induces the synthesis and secretion of other mediators that contribute to the inflammatory changes and tissue damage. IL-1β stimulates the synthesis of PGE2, platelet-activating factor, and nitrous oxide, resulting in vascular changes associated with inflammation [80]. Studies have shown increased concentration of IL-1β in GCF at sites affected by gingivitis [81] and tissue levels of IL-1β correlates with clinical periodontal disease severity [82]. IL-1β increases the expression of ICAM-1 on endothelial cells and stimulates the secretion of the chemokine CXCL8 (IL-8), thereby stimulating and facilitating the infiltration of neutrophils into the affected tissues [83]. Other members of IL family have more roles in the pathogenesis of periodontal disease.

5.1.2 Chemokines

Chemokines are chemotactic cytokines with an important role in the migration of phagocytic cells to the site of infection [84, 85]. Chemokines help in leukocyte recruitment in physiologic and pathologic conditions, which results in the chemotactic migration of neutrophils through the periodontal tissues toward the site of the bacterial challenge in the periodontal pocket [86].

Chemokines are synthesized by a variety of cells including endothelial, epithelial, and stromal cells, as well as leukocytes [87]. They are divided into two subfamilies: the CC subfamily and the CXC subfamily [88]. The chemokine CXCL8, also known as IL-8, has been found to be localized in the gingival tissues in areas of plaque biofilm accumulation and also in GCF112. Interaction between bacteria and keratinocytes results in the upregulation of IL-8 and ICAM-1 expression in the gingival epithelium, thereby stimulating neutrophil migration into the tissues and the gingival sulcus [89, 90].

Chemokines target leukocytes of the innate immune system, as well as lymphocytes of the adaptive immune system [91]. Chemokines play important roles in immune responses, repair, inflammation, and regulating osteoclast activity by influencing myeloid cell differentiation into osteoclasts, which may be of particular importance in the pathogenesis of periodontitis.

5.1.3 Tumor necrosis factor alpha

TNF-α is a molecularly distinct cytokine and a key inflammatory mediator in periodontal disease that shares many biologic activities with IL-1β [92]. Tumor necrosis factor alpha is a multi-effect cytokine that has many functions, from cell migration to tissue destruction. Tumor necrosis factor alpha impacts cell migration by inducing the upregulation of adhesion molecules and adhesion of neutrophils to the vessel wall, leading to extravasation. It also stimulates the production of chemokines involved in cell migration to infected and inflamed sites [93–96]. The proinflammatory effects of TNF-α include the stimulation of endothelial cells to express selectins that facilitate the leukocyte recruitment, the activation of macrophage IL-1β production, and the induction of PGE2 by macrophages and gingival fibroblasts [97].

5.2 Lipid mediators of inflammation-prostaglandins and thromboxanes

Prostaglandins are derived from the hydrolysis of membrane phospholipids. Prostaglandin E2 (PGE2) and thromboxane B2 are lipid molecules produced by many host cells through the cyclooxygenase pathway, one of the two major paths of arachidonic acid metabolism. Inflamed gingiva synthesizes significantly larger amounts of prostaglandins when incubated with arachidonic acid than in healthy gingiva [98]. Within gingival lesions, prostaglandin E2 is mainly localized to macrophage-like cells and is secreted when stimulated with bacterial lipopolysaccharide [99].

PGE2 induces the secretion of MMPs, as well as osteoclastic bone resorption, and it contributes significantly to the alveolar bone loss seen with all forms of periodontitis [100]. Prostaglandin E2 has biphasic actions on immune function. In high doses, it decreases the levels of IgG, but at low doses it has the potential to increase IgG. When combined with interleukin-4, low doses of prostaglandin E2 induce a synergistic rise in IgG production, suggesting an immune-regulatory role for prostaglandin E2 [101].

5.3 Matrix metalloproteinase

Matrix metalloproteinases are a family of structurally related, but genetically distinct, enzymes that degrade extracellular matrix and basement membrane components [102]. MMPs secreted by the majority of cell types in the periodontium, including fibroblasts, keratinocytes, endothelial cells, osteoclasts, neutrophils, and macrophages, are capable of degrading extracellular matrix molecules, including collagens [103, 104].

Most MMP activity in the periodontal tissues is derived from infiltrating inflammatory cells. In inflamed periodontal tissues, excessive quantities of MMPs are secreted by resident cells and neutrophils, resulting in the breakdown of the connective tissue matrix [105, 106] and leading to the development of collagen-depleted areas within the connective tissues. The predominant MMPs in periodontitis, MMP-8 and MMP-9, secreted by neutrophils [107] are effective in degrading type 1 collagen, which is the most abundant collagen type in the periodontal ligament [108].

Matrix metalloproteinase activity is controlled by changes in the delicate balance between the expression and synthesis of matrix metalloproteinases and their major endogenous inhibitors, tissue inhibitors of matrix metalloproteinases [102]. The prolonged and excessive release of large quantities of MMPs in the periodontium leads to the significant breakdown of structural components of the connective tissues, thereby contributing to the clinical signs of disease. In periodontal disease, secretion of specific matrix metalloproteinases is stimulated or downregulated by various cytokines. The main stimulatory cytokines for matrix metalloproteinases are tumor necrosis factor alpha, interleukin-1, and interleukin-6 [109].

6. Discussion

The immune and inflammatory processes that result from periodontal inflammation in response to bacterial biofilm are complex and mediated by a large number of proinflammatory and anti-inflammatory cytokines and enzymes that function as a network of mediators. Many studies have confirmed that immune cells from patients with periodontal disease secrete higher quantities of proinflammatory cytokines than do cells from persons who are periodontally healthy [72]. These findings led to the concept of the "hyperinflammatory" or "hyperresponsive" trait in which certain individuals possess a hyperinflammatory phenotype that accounts for their increased susceptibility to chronic inflammatory conditions such as periodontitis [110].

Although plaque bacteria initiate the inflammatory response, most of the tissue damage results from the host response, which is influenced by genetic factors, as well as environmental and acquired risk factors [111]. An essential goal of interventions in inflammatory disease is the return of tissue to homeostasis, by rapid elimination of invading leukocytes from a disease site [112].

Inadequate resolution of inflammation and failure to return tissue to homeostasis result in neutrophil-mediated destruction and chronic inflammation [113], with destruction of both extracellular matrix and bone [114] leading to advanced periodontitis.

Recently efforts are undergoing to control inflammation by the use of pharmacologic agents that inhibit proinflammatory mediator pathways (e.g., nonsteroidal anti-inflammatory drugs) [115] which target cyclooxygenase 1-dependent and cyclooxygenase 2-dependent pathways, inhibiting the generation of prostanoids. Accordingly, there is a need for the development of adjunctive agents for the management of periodontitis based on the current understanding of the etiology and pathobiology of periodontal disease. Host modulation therapy is an important emerging treatment strategy for managing all forms of periodontitis.

7. Conclusion

Periodontal diseases (gingivitis and periodontitis) are inflammatory diseases in which microbial etiologic factors induce a series of host responses that mediate inflammatory events. The maintenance of a healthy mucosal system is characterized by a continuous coordinated network of immune response that maintains the integrity of the tissue. Persistence of bacterial infection results in cellular and molecular modifications of the host response resulting in clinical manifestations of disease.

The presence of increased inflammation due to persistence of microbial pathogens with a failure of innate immunity systems will cause the shift of disease to a chronic state, later progressing to bone loss and periodontal tissue destruction. Even though persistent gingivitis is a risk factor for periodontal attachment loss, periodontitis is always a successor of gingivitis. However, studies in the last decade have brought significant understanding of the pathogenesis of periodontal disease by the recognition of dental plaque as a biofilm, discovery of new disease-associated bacterial species, the role of risk factors in disease susceptibility, and advanced host-derived cellular and molecular mechanisms in periodontal destruction.

Conflict of interest

None.

Notes/thanks/other declarations

Nil.

Author details

Reghunathan S. Preethanath[1*], Wael I. Ibraheem[1] and Aiswarya Anil[2]

1 College of Dentistry, Jazan University, Jazan, Kingdom of Saudi Arabia

2 Sree Mookambika Institute of Dental Sciences, Tamilnadu, India

*Address all correspondence to: drpreethanath@gmail.com

References

[1] Lang NP, Bartold PM. Periodontal health. Journal of Periodontology. 2018;**89**(Suppl 1):S9-S16

[2] Trombelli L, Farina R, Silva CO, Tatakis DN. Plaque-induced gingivitis: Case definition and diagnostic considerations. Journal of Periodontology. 2018;**89**(Suppl 1): S46-S73

[3] Ivanyi L, Wilton J, Lehner T. Cell-mediated immunity in periodontal disease; cytotoxicity, migration inhibition and lymphocyte transformation studies. Immunology. 1972;**22**(1):141-145

[4] Taubman MA, Yoshie H, Ebersole JL, Smith DJ, Olson CL. Host response in experimental periodontal disease. Journal of Dental Research. 1984;**63**(3):455-460

[5] Seymour GJ, Gemmell E. Cytokines in periodontal disease: Where to from here? Acta Odontologica. 2001;**59**(3):167-173

[6] Page RC, Schroeder HE. Pathogenesis of inflammatory periodontal disease. A summary of current work. Laboratory Investigation. 1976;**33**:235-249

[7] Payne WA, Page RC, Ogilvie AL, et al. Histopathologic features of the initial and early stages of experimental gingivitis in man. Journal of Periodontal Research. 1975;**10**:51-64

[8] Bosshardt DD, Lang NP. The junctional epithelium: From health to disease. Journal of Dental Research. 2005;**84**:9-20

[9] Tatakis DN, Trombelli L. Modulation of clinical expression of plaque-induced gingivitis. I. Background review and rationale. Journal of Clinical Periodontology. 2004;**31**:229-238

[10] Ohlrich EJ, Cullinan MP, Seymour GJ. The immunopathogenesis of periodontal disease. Australian Dental Journal. 2009;**54**(1):S2-S10

[11] Wiedemann W, Lahrsow J, Naujoks R. Über den Einflussder Parodontalen Resistenzeauf die Experimentelle Gingivitis. [The effect of periodontal resistance on experimental gingivitis.]. Dtsch Zahnarztl Z. 1979;**34**:6-9 [in German]

[12] van der Weijden GA, Timmerman MF, Danser MM, et al. Effect of pre-experimental maintenance care duration on the development of gingivitis in a partial mouth experimental gingivitis model. Journal of Periodontal Research. 1994;**29**:168-173

[13] Garlet GP, Avila-CamposMJ, Milanezi CM, Ferreira BR, Silva JS. Actinobacillus actinomycetemcomitans-induced periodontal disease in mice: Patterns of cytokine, chemokine, and chemokine receptor expression and leukocyte migration. Microbes and Infection. 2005;**7**:738-747

[14] Van Dyke TE, Levine MJ, Genco RJ. Neutrophil function and oral disease. Journal of Oral Pathology. 1985;**14**:95-120

[15] Schroeder HE, Listgarten MA. The gingival tissues: The architecture of periodontal protection. Periodontology 2000. 1997;**13**:91-120

[16] Komai-Koma M, Xu D, Li Y, et al. IL-33 is a chemoattractant for human Th2 cells. European Journal of Immunology. 2007;**37**:2779-2786

[17] Herrmann JM, Meyle J. Neutrophil activation and periodontal tissue injury. Periodontology 2000. 2015;**69**:111-127

[18] Kolaczkowska E, Kubes P. Neutrophil recruitment and function

in health and inflammation. Nature Reviews Immunology. 2013;**13**:159-175. DOI: 10.1038/nri3399

[19] Marki A, Esko JD, Pries AR, Ley K. Role of the endothelial surface layer in neutrophil recruitment. Journal of Leukocyte Biology. 2015;**98**:503-515. DOI: 10.1189/jlb.3MR0115-011R

[20] Campbell EL, Colgan SP. Neutrophils and inflammatory metabolism in antimicrobial functions of the mucosa. Journal of Leukocyte Biology. 2015;**98**:517-522. DOI: 10.1189/jlb.3MR1 114-556R

[21] Hirschfeld J. Dynamic interactions of neutrophils and biofilms. Journal of Oral Microbiology. 2014;**6**:26102. DOI: 10.3402/jom. v6.26102

[22] Hirschfeld J, Dommisch H, Skora P, Horvath G, Latz E, Hoerauf A, et al. Neutrophil extracellular trap formation in supragingival biofilms. International Journal of Medical Microbiology. 2015;**305**:453-463. DOI: 10.1016/j. ijmm.2015.04.002

[23] White P, Cooper P, Milward M, Chapple I. Differential activation of neutrophil extracellular traps by specific periodontal bacteria. Free Radical Biology and Medicine. 2014;**75**(Suppl 1):S53. DOI: 10.1016/j. freeradbiomed.2014.10.827

[24] White PC, Chicca IJ, Cooper PR, Milward MR, Chapple IL. Neutrophil extracellular traps in periodontitis: A web of intrigue. Journal of Dental Research. 2016;**95**:26-34. DOI: 10.1177/0022034515609097

[25] Brinkmann V, Reichard U, Goosmann C, Fauler B, Uhlemann Y, Weiss DS, et al. Neutrophil extracellular traps kill bacteria. Science. 2004;**303**:1532-1535. DOI: 10.1126/science.1092385

[26] Yousefi S, Mihalache C, Kozlowski E, Schmid I, Simon HU. Viable neutrophils release mitochondrial DNA to form neutrophil extracellular traps. Cell Death and Differentiation. 2009;**16**:1438-1444. DOI: 10.1038/cdd.2009.96

[27] Cortes-Vieyra R, Rosales C, Uribe-Querol E. Neutrophil functions in periodontal homeostasis. Journal of Immunology Research. 2016;**2016**:1396106. DOI: 10.1155/2016/1396106

[28] Schlegel Gomez R, Langer P, Pelka M, et al. Variational expression of functionally different macrophage markers (27E10, 25F9, RM3/1) in normal gingiva and inflammatory periodontal disease. Journal of Clinical Periodontology. 1995;**22**:341-346

[29] Wynne SE, Walsh LJ, Seymour GJ, et al. In situ demonstration of natural killer (NK) cells in human gingival tissue. Journal of Periodontology. 1986;**57**:699-702

[30] Cobb CM, Singla O, Feil PH, et al. Comparison of NK-cell (Leu-7þ and Leu-11bþ) populations in clinically healthy gingiva, chronic gingivitis and chronic adult periodontitis. Journal of Periodontal Research. 1989;**24**:1-7

[31] Lundgren T, Parhar RS, Renvert S, et al. Impaired cytotoxicity in Papillon-Lefévre syndrome. Journal of Dental Research. 2005;**84**:414-417

[32] Orange JS. Human natural killer cell deficiencies and susceptibility to infection. Microbes and Infection. 2002;**4**:1545-1558

[33] Zeidel A, Beilin B, Yardeni I, et al. Immune response in asymptomatic smokers. Acta Anaesthesiologica Scandinavica. 2002;**46**:959-964

[34] Teng YT, Nguyen H, Gao X, et al. Functional human T-cell immunity and osteoprotegerin ligand control alveolar bone destruction in periodontal infection. The Journal of Clinical Investigation. 2000;**106**:R59-R67

[35] Taubman MA, Kawai T. Involvement of T-lymphocytes in periodontal disease and in direct and indirect induction of bone resorption. Critical Reviews in Oral Biology and Medicine. 2001;**12**:125-135

[36] Seymour GJ, Powell RN, Davies WI. Conversion of a stable T-cell lesion to a progressive Bcell lesion in the pathogenesis of chronic inflammatory periodontal disease: An hypothesis. Journal of Clinical Periodontology. 1979;**6**:267-277

[37] Fraser ID, Germain RN. Navigating the network: Signaling cross-talk in hematopoietic cells. Nature Immunology. 2009;**10**:327-331

[38] Nathan C. Points of control in inflammation. Nature. 2002;**420**:846-852

[39] Bartold PM, Walsh LJ, Narayanan AS. Molecular and cell biology of the gingiva. Periodontology 2000. 2000;**24**:28-55

[40] Giannobile WV, Beikler T, Kinney JS, et al. Saliva as a diagnostic tool for periodontal disease: Current state and future directions. Periodontology 2000. 2009;**50**:52-64

[41] Lamont RJ, Jenkinson HF. Subgingival colonization by *Porphyromonas gingivalis*. Oral Microbiology and Immunology. 2000;**15**:341-349

[42] Griffiths GS. Formation, collection and significance of gingival crevice fluid. Periodontology 2000. 2003;**31**:32-42

[43] Van Nieuw Amerongen A, Bolscher JG, Veerman EC. Salivary proteins: Protective and diagnostic value in cariology? Caries Research. 2004;**38**:247-253. DOI: 10.1159/000077762

[44] Stookey GK. The effect of saliva on dental caries. Journal of the American Dental Association. 2008;**139**(Suppl):11S-17S

[45] Tenovuo J. Salivary parameters of relevance for assessing caries activity in individuals and populations. Community Dentistry and Oral Epidemiology. 1997;**25**:82-86

[46] de Almeida Pdel V, Gregio AM, Machado MA, de Lima AA, Azevedo LR. Saliva composition and functions: A comprehensive review. The Journal of Contemporary Dental Practice. 2008;**9**:72-80

[47] Leonor SP, Laura SM, Esther IC, Marco ZZ, Enrique AG, Ignacio MR. Stimulated saliva flow rate patterns in children: A six-year longitudinal study. Archives of Oral Biology. 2009;**54**:970-975. DOI: 10.1016/j.archoralbio.2009.07.007

[48] Liukkonen J, Gursoy UK, Pussinen PJ, Suominen AL, Kononen E. Salivary concentrations of interleukin (IL)-1beta, IL-17A, and IL-23 vary in relation to periodontal status. Journal of Periodontology. 2016;**87**:1484-1491. DOI: 10.1902/jop.2016.160146

[49] Marsh PD, Devine DA. How is the development of dental biofilms influenced by the host? Journal of Clinical Periodontology. 2011;**38**(Suppl. 11):28-35

[50] Groeger SE, Meyle J. Epithelial barrier and oral bacterial infection. Periodontology 2000. 2015;**69**:46-67. DOI: 10.1111/prd.12094

[51] Larjava H, Koivisto L, Hakkinen L, Heino J. Epithelial integrins with special reference to oral epithelia. Journal of Dental Research. 2011;**90**:1367-1376. DOI: 10.1177/0022034511402207

[52] Larjava H, Koivisto L, Heino J, Hakkinen L. Integrins in periodontal

disease. Experimental Cell Research. 2014;**325**:104-110. DOI: 10.1016/j.yexcr.2014.03.010

[53] Danen EH, Sonnenberg A. Integrins in regulation of tissue development and function. Journal of Pathology. 2003;**201**:632-641. DOI: 10.1002/path.1472

[54] Juliano RL. Signal transduction by cell adhesion receptors and the cytoskeleton: Functions of integrins, cadherins, selectins, and immunoglobulin-superfamily members. Annual Review of Pharmacology and Toxicology. 2002;**42**:283-323. DOI: 10.1146/annurev.pharmtox.42.090401.151133

[55] Hintermann E, Haake SK, Christen U, Sharabi A, Quaranta V. Discrete proteolysis of focal contact and adherens junction components in *Porphyromonas gingivalis*-infected oral keratinocytes: A strategy for cell adhesion and migration disabling. Infection and Immunity. 2002;**70**:5846-5856

[56] Groeger S, Doman E, Chakraborty T, Meyle J. Effects of *Porphyromonas gingivalis* infection on human gingival epithelial barrier function in vitro. European Journal of Oral Sciences. 2010;**118**:582-589

[57] Katz J, Sambandam V, Wu JH, Michalek SM, Balkovetz DF. Characterization of *Porphyromonas gingivalis*-induced degradation of epithelial cell junctional complexes. Infection and Immunity. 2000;**68**:1441-1449

[58] Nisapakultorn K, Ross KF, Herzberg MC. Calprotectin expression in vitro by oral epithelial cells confers resistance to infection by *Porphyromonas gingivalis*. Infection and Immunity. 2001;**69**:4242-4247. DOI: 10.1128/IAI.69.7.4242-4247.2001

[59] Akira S, Uematsu S, Takeuchi O. Pathogen recognition and innate immunity. Cell. 2006;**124**(4):783-801

[60] Iwasaki A, Medzhitov R. Toll-like receptor control of the adaptive immune responses. Nature Immunology. 2004;**5**:987-995

[61] O'Neill LA, Golenbock D, Bowie AG. The history of Toll-like receptors: Redefining innate immunity. Nature Reviews. Immunology. 2013;**13**(6):453-460

[62] Kawai T, Akira S. The role of pattern-recognition receptors in innate immunity: Update on Toll-like receptors. Nature Immunology. 2010;**11**(5):373-384

[63] Beklen A, Hukkanen M, RichardsonR,etal.Immunohistochemical localization of Toll-like receptors 1-10 in periodontitis. Oral Microbiology and Immunology. 2008;**23**(5):425-431

[64] Kahari VM, Saarialho-Kere U. Matrix metalloproteinases in skin. Experimental Dermatology. 1997;**6**:199-213

[65] Hatakeyama J, Tamai R, Sugiyama A, Akashi S, Sugawara S, Takada H. Contrasting responses of human gingival and periodontal ligament fibroblasts to bacterial cell-surface components through the CD14/toll-like receptor system. Oral Microbiology and Immunology. 2003;**18**:14-23

[66] Cekici A, Kantarci A, Hasturk H, Van Dyke TE. Inflammatory and immune pathways in the pathogenesis of periodontal disease. Periodontology 2000. 2014;**64**(1):57-80. DOI: 10.1111/prd.12002

[67] Kornman KS, Page RC, Tonetti MS. The host response to the microbial challenge in periodontitis: Assembling the players. Periodontology 2000. 1997;**14**:33-53

[68] Gemmell E, Yamazaki K, Seymour GJ. The role of T cells in periodontal disease: Homeostasis and autoimmunity. Periodontology 2000. 2007;**43**:14-40

[69] Ara T, Kurata K, Hirai K, Uchihashi T, Uematsu T, Imamura Y, et al. Human gingival fibroblasts are critical in sustaining inflammation in periodontal disease. Journal of Periodontal Research. 2009;**44**:21-27

[70] Garlet GP. Destructive and protective roles of cytokines in periodontitis: A re-appraisal from host defense and tissue destruction viewpoints. Journal of Dental Research. 2010;**89**:1349-1363

[71] Preshaw PM, Taylor JJ. How has research into cytokine interactions and their role in driving immune responses impacted our understanding of periodontitis? Journal of Clinical Periodontology. 2011;**38**(Suppl 11):60-84

[72] Taylor JJ, Preshaw PM, Donaldson PT. Cytokine gene polymorphism and immunoregulation in periodontal disease. Periodontology 2000. 2004;**35**:158-182

[73] Birkedal-Hansen H. Role of cytokines and inflammatory mediators in tissue destruction. Journal of Periodontal Research. 1993;**28**:500-510

[74] Baldwin AS Jr. The NF-kappa B and I kappa B proteins: New discoveries and insights. Annual Review of Immunology. 1996;**14**:649-683

[75] Hanada T, Yoshimura A. Regulation of cytokine signaling and inflammation. Cytokine & Growth Factor Reviews. 2002;**13**:413-421

[76] Dinarello CA. Immunological and inflammatory functions of the interleukin-1 family. Annual Review of Immunology. 2009;**27**:519-550

[77] Rasmussen L, Hanstrom L, Lerner UH. Characterization of bone resorbing activity in gingival crevicular fluid from patients with periodontitis. Journal of Clinical Periodontology. 2000;**27**:41-52

[78] Tanabe N, Maeno M, Suzuki N, et al. IL-1 alpha stimulates the formation of osteoclast-like cells by increasing M-CSF and PGE2 production and decreasing OPG production by osteoblasts. Life Sciences. 2005;**77**:615-626

[79] Delima AJ, Karatzas S, Amar S, et al. Inflammation and tissue loss caused by periodontal pathogens is reduced by interleukin-1 antagonists. The Journal of Infectious Diseases. 2002;**186**:511-516

[80] Delaleu N, Bickel M. Interleukin-1 beta and interleukin-18: Regulation and activity in local inflammation. Periodontology 2000. 2004;**35**:42-52

[81] Heasman PA, Collins JG, Offenbacher S. Changes in crevicular fluid levels of interleukin-1β, leukotriene B4, prostaglandin E2, thromboxane B2 and tumour necrosis factor alpha in experimental gingivitis in humans. Journal of Periodontal Research. 1993;**28**:241-247

[82] Stashenko P, Fujiyoshi P, Obernesser MS, et al. Levels of interleukin 1 beta in tissue from sites of active periodontal disease. Journal of Clinical Periodontology. 1991;**18**:548-554

[83] Ben-Sasson SZ, Hu-Li J, Quiel J, et al. IL-1 acts directly on CD4 T cells to enhance their antigen-driven expansion and differentiation. Proceedings of the National Academy of Sciences of the United States of America. 2009;**106**:7119-7124

[84] Rousset F, Garcia E, Defrance T, Peronne C, Vezzio N, Hsu DH, et al. Interleukin 10 is a potent growth and

differentiation factor for activated human B lymphocytes. Proceedings of the National Academy of Sciences of the United States of America. 1992;**89**:1890-1893

[85] Zlotnik A, Yoshie O. Chemokines: A new classification system and their role in immunity. Immunity. 2000;**12**:121-127

[86] Silva TA, Garlet GP, Fukada SY, et al. Chemokines in oral inflammatory diseases: Apical periodontitis and periodontal disease. Journal of Dental Research. 2007;**86**:306-319

[87] Takata T, Donath K. The mechanism of pocket formation: A light microscopic study on undecalcified human material. Journal of Periodontology. 1988;**59**:215-221

[88] Sharma M. Chemokines and their receptors: Orchestrating a fine balance between health and disease. Critical Reviews in Biotechnology. 2010;**30**:1-22

[89] Tonetti MS. Molecular factors associated with compartmentalization of gingival immune responses and transepithelial neutrophil migration. Journal of Periodontal Research. 1997;**32**:104-109

[90] Tonetti MS, Imboden MA, Lang NP. Neutrophil migration into the gingival sulcus is associated with transepithelial gradients of interleukin-8 and ICAM-1. Journal of Periodontology. 1998;**69**:1139-1147

[91] Terricabras E, Benjamim C, Godessart N. Drug discovery and chemokine receptor antagonists: Eppur si muove! Autoimmunity Reviews. 2004;**3**:550-556

[92] Graves DT, Cochran D. The contribution of interleukin-1 and tumor necrosis factor to periodontal tissue destruction. Journal of Periodontology. 2003;**74**:391-401

[93] Wajant H, Pfizenmaier K, Scheurich P. Tumor necrosis factor signaling. Cell Death and Differentiation. 2003;**10**:45-65

[94] Peschon JJ, Torrance DS, Stocking KL, Glaccum MB, Otten C, Willis CR, et al. TNF receptor-deficient mice reveal divergent roles for p55 and p75 in several models of inflammation. Journal of Immunology. 1998;**160**:943-952

[95] Kindle L, Rothe L, Kriss M, Osdoby P, Collin-Osdoby P. Human microvascular endothelial cell activation by IL-1 and TNF-alpha stimulates the adhesion and transendothelial migration of circulating human CD14+ monocytes that develop with RANKL into functional osteoclasts. Journal of Bone and Mineral Research. 2006;**21**:193-206

[96] Dinarello CA. Proinflammatory cytokines. Chest. 2000;**118**:503-508

[97] Page RC. The role of inflammatory mediators in the pathogenesis of periodontal disease. Journal of Periodontal Research. 1991;**26**:230-242

[98] Mendieta CF, Reeve CM, Romero JC. Biosynthesis of prostaglandins in gingiva of patients with chronic periodontitis. Journal of Periodontology. 1985;**56**:44-47

[99] Loning T, Albers HK, Lisboa BP, Burkhardt A, Caselitz J. Prostaglandin e and the local immune response in chronic periodontal disease. Immunohistochemical and radioimmunological observations. Journal of Periodontal Research. 1980;**15**:525-535

[100] Garrison SW, Nichols FC. LPS-elicited secretory responses in monocytes: Altered release of PGE2 in patients with but not IL-1 adult periodontitis. Journal of Periodontal Research. 1989;**24**:88-95

[101] Harrell JC, Stein SH. Prostaglandin E2 regulates gingival mononuclear cell immunoglobulin production. Journal of Periodontology. 1995;**66**:222-227

[102] Uitto VJ, Overall CM, McCulloch C. Proteolytic host cell enzymes in gingival crevice fluid. Periodontology 2000. 2003;**31**:77-104

[103] Kinane DF, Darby IB, Said S, et al. Changes in gingival crevicular fluid matrix metalloproteinase-8 levels during periodontal treatment and maintenance. Journal of Periodontal Research. 2003;**38**:400-404

[104] Ryan ME, Ramamurthy NS, Golub LM. Matrix metalloproteinases and their inhibition in periodontal treatment. Current Opinion in Periodontology. 1996;**3**:85-96

[105] Birkedal-Hansen H. Role of matrix metalloproteinases in human periodontal diseases. Journal of Periodontology. 1993;**64**:474-484

[106] Tervahartiala T, Pirila E, Ceponis A, et al. The in vivo expression of the collagenolytic matrix metalloproteinases (MMP-2, -8, -13, and -14) and matrilysin (MMP-7) in adult and localized juvenile periodontitis. Journal of Dental Research. 2000;**79**:1969-1977

[107] Golub LM, Sorsa T, Lee HM, et al. Doxycycline inhibits neutrophil (PMN)-type matrix metalloproteinases in human adult periodontitis gingiva. Journal of Clinical Periodontology. 1995;**22**:100-109

[108] Mariotti A. The extracellular matrix of the periodontium: Dynamic and interactive tissues. Periodontology 2000. 1993;**3**:39-63

[109] Visse R, Nagase H. Matrix metalloproteinases and tissue inhibitors of metalloproteinases: Structure, function, and biochemistry. Circulation Research. 2003;**92**:827-839

[110] Champagne CM, Buchanan W, Reddy MS, et al. Potential for gingival crevice fluid measures as predictors of risk for periodontal diseases. Periodontology 2000. 2003;**31**:167-180

[111] Johannsen A, Susin C, Gustafsson A. Smoking and inflammation: Evidence for a synergistic role in chronic disease. Periodontology 2000. 2014;**64**:111-126

[112] Van Dyke TE. Control of inflammation and periodontitis. Periodontology 2000. 2007;**45**:158-166

[113] Van Dyke TE, Serhan CN. Resolution of inflammation: A new paradigm for the pathogenesis of periodontal diseases. Journal of Dental Research. 2003;**82**:82-90

[114] Van Dyke TE. The management of inflammation in periodontal disease. Journal of Periodontology. 2008;**79**:1601-1608

[115] Serhan CN, Brain SD, Buckley CD, Gilroy DW, Haslett C, O'Neill LA, et al. Resolution of inflammation: State of the art, definitions and terms. The FASEB Journal. 2007;**21**:325-332

Chapter 3

Diagnosis and Treatment Plan for Gingival Diseases and Conditions

Anahita Punj and Manav Chaturvedi

Abstract

The prevalence of gingival and periodontal disease is manifold and has not been highlighted much due to its asymptomatic and milder symptoms. It is usually given its due importance when the gingival disease progresses to advanced periodontal disease, displays symptoms of dull pain and tooth mobility, and is associated with pus discharge. The starting point of periodontal disease is usually gingival disease which is a reversible condition. It is therefore necessary to diagnose gingival diseases at an early stage to prevent its progression to irreversible periodontal disease. The diagnosis of gingival disease becomes cumbersome due to its similarity in the presentation of signs and symptoms. Gingival diseases can occur due to microbial attack from the plaque biofilm which is usually bacterial in nature. There are other viral, fungal, and immune-mediated mechanisms which can result in gingival diseases. Some systemic conditions also influence the gingiva which allows for diagnosing systemic diseases and treating these conditions appropriately. It is said that oral cavity is the mirror of the body, and in that sense the gingiva is the biggest surface where any changes or manifestations could be observed.

Keywords: gingivitis, gingival disease, diagnosis, treatment

1. Introduction

The gingiva or commonly referred to as gums surround and protect the teeth (**Figure 1**). Gingival diseases by namesake denote to the diseases affecting the gingival tissues. These diseases have burdened the human race since the early civilization, and this is proof enough to gauge the importance of diagnosing gingival diseases and treating them. Gingival disease if left untreated can progress to periodontal tissues and result in periodontal disease which is easier to diagnose probably due to its chronic and severe nature as compared to gingival disease. No wonder periodontal disease has been mentioned in the literature of ancient Egypt and a step toward preventing it by means of oral hygiene practices deserves its mention in the ancient scriptures [1].

2. Gingival disease terminology

The gingival disease terminology and classification has undergone many changes, and the current classification given at the World Workshop in 2017

IntechOpen

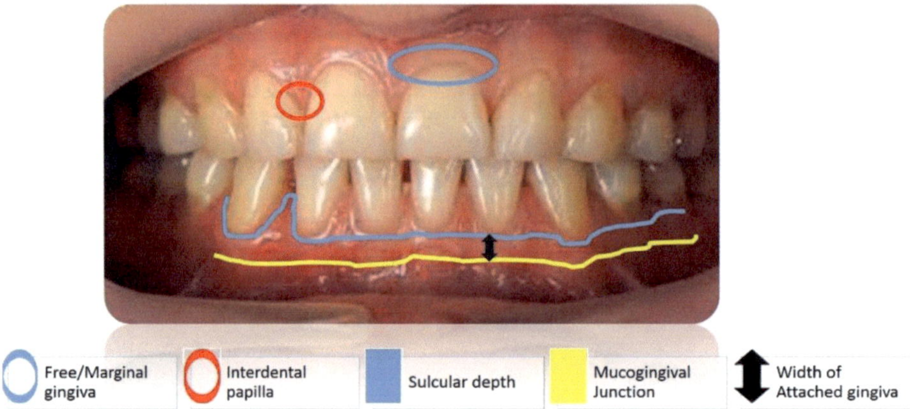

Figure 1.
The diagnosis of any disease is based on a proper documentation of case history which requires precise identification of signs and symptoms of disease and also any underlying medical disease/condition which may influence the same. The next step is to correlate clinical, pathological, laboratory and radiological findings. This sequence of steps also holds true for gingival diseases. This chapter attempts to focus on the minute differences in the diagnosis of gingival diseases which becomes cumbersome due to a simple fact that any infection or inflammation usually results in swelling up of the gingiva, bleeding, or formation of ulcers or vesicles. Such symptoms could be due to a single to multiple etiologic agents corresponding to varied diagnoses and treatment regimens [2].

classifies gingival condition in health and disease under three broad categories of health, dental biofilm-induced gingivitis, and non-dental biofilm-induced gingival disease [3] (**Table 1**).

Periodontal health and gingival health			**Dental biofilm-induced gingivitis**			**Non-dental biofilm-induced gingival disease**
Clinical gingival health on an intact periodontium	Clinical gingival health on a reduced periodontium		Associated only with dental biofilm	Mediated by systemic or local risk factors	Drug-influenced gingival enlargement	Genetic/ development disorders
	Stable periodontitis	Non-periodontitis				Specific infections and inflammatory and immune conditions
						Reactive processes
						Neoplasms
						Endocrine, nutritional, and metabolic diseases
						Traumatic lesions
						Gingival pigmentation

Table 1.
Classification of periodontal health, gingival disease, and condition [3].

2.1 Diagnosis of plaque-induced gingivitis

Gingivitis per se refers to the inflammation of the gingival tissues and is labeled with different diagnostic terms based on the etiology and clinical presentation to aid in formulation of the best-suited treatment. As mentioned above, the broad etiologic factors which result in gingival disease is the dental biofilm, which contain microbes, causing a microbial attack on the gingiva resulting in a dysbiosis amounting to a host response manifested in the form of the inflammatory disease called plaque-induced gingivitis. The plaque microbes have an influence on the gingiva depending upon its quantity and quality of pathogens present. Although the increased plaque burden is almost always associated with gingivitis, there are instances where paucity of plaque can again result in gingivitis due to the effect of modifying factors which make the host response more accentuated and exaggerated as they tend to have a more systemic affect than a local one [2, 4]. These modifying factors include few systemic conditions, factors which increase plaque accumulation and influence of drugs on gingiva. How these factors can affect gingivitis is summarized in **Table 2**.

Factor	Effect on gingiva	Signs and symptoms for diagnosis	Diagnosis	Treatment [5]
Bacterial dental biofilm only	Microbial attack mounts a host response in the form of inflammation	Mild redness with or without broken line of bleeding	Incipient gingivitis	OHI
		Mild changes in color and texture of the gingiva	Mild gingivitis	OHI +/OP
		Glazing redness, edema, enlargement, bleeding on probing	Moderate gingivitis	OHI + OP
			Overt redness and edema and bleeding on palpation rather on probing	Severe gingivitis
Potential modifying factors of plaque-induced gingivitis				
Systemic conditions				
Sex steroid hormones (estrogen and progesterone) (1) Puberty	Exaggerate the host inflammatory response in the presence of minimal plaque	Bleeding on probing or bleeding with toothbrushing, mild to moderate redness	Diagnostic term not given as not seen frequently in population and if present can be diagnosed as gingivitis associated with puberty	OHI + OP
(2) Menstrual cycle	Exaggerates the host inflammatory response in the presence of minimal plaque	Mild redness, edema based on severity of inflammation seen during the menstrual cycle	Diagnostic term not given as not seen frequently in population and if present can be diagnosed as gingivitis	

Factor	Effect on gingiva	Signs and symptoms for diagnosis	Diagnosis	Treatment [5]
			associated with menstrual cycle	
(3) Pregnancy	The hormones exaggerate the host inflammatory response in the presence of minimal plaque	Deep gingival probing depths, bleeding on probing or bleeding with toothbrushing, and elevated gingival crevicular fluid flow in pregnancy	Pregnancy-associated gingivitis	
(4) Oral contraceptives	The high-dose hormones in the pills exaggerate the host inflammatory response in the presence of minimal plaque; low dose does not have much effect	Mild redness, edema based on severity of inflammation seen after 1 to 3 months of use	Currently the dose of oral contraceptives is low; hence diagnostic terms have been removed	OHI + OP + reduction of high-dose oral contraceptive Low-dose contraceptive does not require any change
Hyperglycemia	High blood glucose levels increase the pathogenic bacteria and also form more AGE which affect collagen turnover and healing	Signs of inflammation of gingivitis + high blood glucose levels	Gingivitis associated with diabetes mellitus	OHI + OP + maintenance of blood glucose levels by diet restriction/ exercise/ medication
Leukemia	Increases number of WBCs which accumulate in the gingival tissues and decreases number of platelets which causes bleeding	Cervical lymphadenopathy, petechiae, ulcers seen in the mucosa, bleeding on slight provocation, swollen, glazed, spongy gingiva, red to deep purple color of gingival lesions	Gingivitis associated with acute/chronic leukemia	Treat leukemia + symptomatic treatment for gingivitis with careful OHI and OP to prevent excessive bleeding
Smoking	Direct smoking can cause vasoconstriction of gingival vasculature	No redness, edema, or swelling present. Color may change to blue and pale pink. No gingival changes and pocket depths increase when lesions progress to periodontitis	No gingivitis	Smoking cessation
Malnutrition	Deficiency of vitamin C affects crosslinking of collagen	Bleeding on probing, mobility, and swollen gums in severe cases with minimal plaque	Scurvy	Vitamin C supplementation + OHI + OP
Oral factors enhancing plaque accumulation				

Factor	Effect on gingiva	Signs and symptoms for diagnosis	Diagnosis	Treatment [5]
Prominent subgingival restoration margins	Roughness and closeness of these restorations to gingival tissue cause accumulation of plaque bacteria and irritation	Localized mild redness, bleeding on probing, slight edema in area of restoration	Gingivitis due to faulty restoration	Correction of restoration + OHI + SRP
Hyposalivation	Decreased saliva causes sticking of bacteria on tooth surfaces	Dental caries, taste changes, halitosis, mucosal and gingival dryness, and gingival inflammation	Gingivitis associated with hyposalivation	OHI + OP+ salivary substitutes
Drug-influenced gingival enlargements				
Phenytoin, sodium valproate	Drugs and plaque cause fibroblasts to increase production of collagen and extracellular connective tissue	Onset after 3 months of drug intake, common in anterior gingiva, gingival size increases which starts from interdental papilla and may extend to the margin and attached gingiva in severe cases. The enlarged areas are firm to soft depending upon the presence of gingival inflammation	Drug-influenced mild gingival enlargement (if only papilla is involved) Drug-influenced mild gingival enlargement (if papilla and margin is involved) Drug-influenced mild gingival enlargement (if papilla, margin, and attached gingiva is involved)	OHI + OP+ drug substitution if required, followed by gingivectomy to correct enlarged gingival tissues
Nifedipine, amlodipine, verapamil, diltiazem, felodipine				
Cyclosporine				

OHI, oral hygiene instruction, OP, oral prophylaxis.

Table 2.
Diagnosis based on etiology, modifying factors, and clinical features [2, 4].

2.2 Tools used for gingival diagnosis

The crude tools used are a questionnaire/interview to collect important aspects of the patient demographics, medical history, current medications, and habits. The next step involves patient examination starting from extraoral structures to any abnormal intraoral findings to specific examination of the gingiva. The gingival disease is visually examined for clinical signs and symptoms using a mouth mirror under ambient lighting of the dental chair, cotton/gauze to dry the tissues, and sometimes the use of three-way air water syringe to wash way the debris for better inspection. Changes in color, contour, consistency, texture, size, position, etc. are

Advanced diagnostic aid for gingival disease	Mechanism/working	Inference
Periotemp probe	Detects the difference in subgingival temperature which is reflected by red or green light	Red light indicates future periodontal breakdown and increase in periopathogens
New generation of periodontal probes	First-generation	Detects pocket depth using traditional probes
	Second-generation	Pressure-sensitive probe with uniform pressure
	Third-generation	Pressure-sensitive and captures data on computer
	Fourth-generation	Uses 3D technology to detect pocket
	Fifth-generation	Uses 3D technology and ultrasound to detect pocket
Advances in radiography	Use of charged-coupled device, complementary metal oxide semiconductor, and cone beam-computed tomography allow digital recording	These are used to detect bone loss and bone defects in 2D and 3D for periodontal defects rather than gingival diseases
Advances in microbial culturing	High-performance liquid chromatography	Can detect bacterial cell wall components
	Flow cytometry	Can detect various bacteria
	Latex agglutination test	Can detect pathogenic antigen, proteins, and antibody by agglutination reaction
	Direct and indirect immunofluorescence	Can detect pathogenic antigen, proteins, and antibody by agglutination and adding fluorescent dyes
	Enzyme-linked immunosorbent assay	Evalusite can detect *P. gingivalis*, *P. intermedia*, and *A. actinomycetemcomitans*
	Nucleic acid and DNA checkerboard hybridization techniques	Detects microbes based on matching of unknown sample with known hybridization technique of nuclei acid/DNA
	DNA probe	Omnigene can detect *P. gingivalis*, *P. intermedia*, *A. actinomycetemcomitans*, *E. corrodens*, *C. rectus*, *F. nucleatum*
	Perioscan uses BANA (N-benzoyl-DL arginine naphthylamide) hydrolysis carried out by trypsin-like protease	Detects trypsin-like protease releasing bacteria, such as *P. gingivalis*, *T. denticola*, and *T. forsythus*
	IAI Pado Test 4.5 RNA probe test kit uses oligonucleotide probes complementary to conserve fragments of the 16S rRNA gene that encodes the rRNA	Detects *A. actinomycetemcomitans*, *P. gingivalis*, *Tannerella forsythia*, and *T. denticola*
	MyPerioPath is a DNA test and uses saliva samples	To identify the type and concentration of periodontal bacteria
Advances in biochemical test kits	Perio-Check	Detects neutral proteases like collagenases in GCF (gingival crevicular fluid)

Advanced diagnostic aid for gingival disease	Mechanism/working	Inference
	Prognos-Stik: detects serine proteinase elastase in GCF	Shows active disease sites
	PocketWatch: detects aspartate aminotransferase in GCF	Differentiates active and non-active sites of disease
	PerioGard: detects aspartate aminotransferase in GCF	Differentiates active and non-active sites of disease
	Perio 2000: detects volatile sulfur compounds	To detect halitosis
	Toxicity prescreening assay (TOPAS)	Detects bacterial toxins and proteins
	Dipstick	Detects (matrix metalloproteinase) MMP-8 in GCF
	Integrated microfluidic platform for oral diagnostics (IMPOD)	Saliva-based detection of MMP-8
	Oral fluid nanosensor test (OFNASET): saliva-based detection of (interleukin) IL-1, IL-8	Used for detection of salivary biomarkers for oral cancer
	Electronic taste chip (ETC)	Detects C-reactive protein which is an important biomarker for inflammation
Genetic tests	Genetic periodontitis susceptibility trait (PST) test	Detects IL-1 polymorphism
	MyPerioID	Saliva-based detection of genetic susceptibility

Table 3.
Diagnostic tools for gingival disease [5, 6].

noted. This is followed by palpation of the gingiva for any spontaneous bleeding, pain, discharge, blanching, consistency (by checking the resiliency of tissues on applying pressure), and pitting edema. The UNC-15 or the Michigan O periodontal probe with William's marking is used to check for bleeding on probing, subgingival faulty restorative margins, and the presence of deeper than 5-mm pockets which is the critical probing depth to differentiate between gingivitis and periodontitis. Apart from these traditional tools used, advanced diagnostic aids have been introduced to further confirm the presence of gingival disease (**Table 3**) [5, 6].

2.3 Diagnosis of non-plaque-induced gingival diseases

Apart from plaque-induced gingivitis, it is imperative to diagnose and differentiate the non-plaque-induced gingival diseases and conditions to provide appropriate treatment and to avoid overtreatment. The etiology of non-plaque-associated gingival disease is usually related to some genetic defect or systemic disorder. In many instances the oral lesions precede the extraoral findings and can help in diagnosing a disease which could affect the full body. Therefore, while diagnosing these conditions, we need to look for other associated conditions to arrive at a correct diagnosis. **Table 4** attempts to highlight the clinical features to help arrive at a diagnosis [7–11].

C	Cr	Cs	T	S	P	L	Lab & H/P	Add Sym	D	Rx
G	Flat or rounded	Firm and resilient	Loss of stippling	++	Coronal to CEJ	Gingival enlargement	Excisional biopsy shows fibrous connective tissue		Hereditary gingival fibromatosis	Gingivectomy to contour the topography + OHI
P-R/B-Br	Blunted	Soft and friable	Ulcerative	−−	Varies from papillary destruction to beyond mucogingival junction	Gingival ulceration	Bacterial culture for various bacteria types such as *Treponema*, *Selenomonas*, *Fusobacterium*, and *Prevotella intermedia*. H/P Loss of the epithelium in ulcerated areas	Loss of taste, woody sensation in teeth and feeling of extruded teeth accompanied with underlying risk factors such as poor oral hygiene and systemic conditions	Necrotizing periodontal disease	Debridement of local factors + CHX+ amoxicillin and metronidazole
FR/W	No change	Soft and edematous	Ulcerative/white pseudomembranous	+	No change	Erythematous	Bacterial culture for *Neisseria gonorrhoeae*	Pharyngitis and lymphadenopathy. Other sites: urethra, anus, cervix, oral mucosa	Gonorrhea	Systemic antibiotic therapy
FR	No change	Edematous	Loss of stippling and ulceration with whitish membrane	+	No change	Chancre (rare)	Bacterial culture for *Treponema pallidum*, followed by serologic reaction tests	Genital and skin lesions	Syphilis	Systemic antibiotic therapy
R-Gy patches	No change	Firm	Nodular/papillary proliferation	+	No change	Nodular/papillary proliferation	Positive delayed hypersensitivity (tuberculin) skin reaction to purified protein derivative (ppd), isolation of mycobacterial antigen from bacterial cultures, and demonstration of acid-fast mycobacteria in clinical specimens. H/P: characteristic multinucleated giant cells	Commonly associated with lung infections. Involves floor of the mouth, extraction sites, and lymph nodes	Tuberculosis	Regimens of multiple antibiotics like isoniazid, rifampicin, pyrazinamide, or ethambutol

DOI: http://dx.doi.org/10.5772/intechopen.91726

C	Cr	Cs	T	S	P	L	Lab & H/P	Add Sym	D	Rx
							and granulomas are diagnostic features			
RP	Rounded	Soft	Erythematous patch				Culture for streptococcal strains. Biopsy	Upper respiratory infections	Streptococcal gingivitis	OHI+ antibiotics
RP	No change	Soft and ulcerative	Small vesicles/ fibrinous coated ulcer	–	Blunted papilla sometimes	Painful ulcers after vesicle rupture		Skin lesions, low-grade fever	Hand, foot and mouth disease	Supportive treatment to correct fever and pain
RP	Flat and rounded	Soft and edematous	Ulcerated, loss of stippling	+	Coronal or apical to CEJ			Lymphadenitis, fever, malaise	Primary herpetic gingivostomatitis	Acyclovir and spirin/ paracetamol, fluids. Dyclonine hydrochloride 0.5% for anesthesia
RP	Flat and rounded	Soft and edematous	Ulcerated	+	Attached gingival and hard palate		Rarely required. If needed fluorescent staining is more sensitive. HSV isolation of a virus in tissue. Culture is the most positive method of identification. Scraping made from the base of the lesion and stained with giemsa. H/P: Wright's or Papanicolaou stain and shows syncytium and ballooning. Degeneration of the nucleus	Fever	Recurrent intraoral herpes simplex	Acyclovir and aspirin/ paracetamol, fluids. Dyclonine hydrochloride 0.5% for anesthesia
BR	No change	Soft	Vesicular	+/−	Diffuse erythema and isolated small vesicles that rupture quickly leaving ulcerations	Lesions on skin and mucosa	Fluorescent-antibody staining of smears using fluorescein-conjugated monoclonal antibodies is more reliable than routine cytology	Fever, malaise, and skin rash	Chicken pox (Varicella)	Acyclovir/valacyclovir for healing and reducing acute pain. Systemic corticosteroids to prevent postherpetic neuralgia, combination of

C	Cr	Cs	T	S	P	L	Lab & H/P	Add Sym	D	Rx
										intralesional steroids and local anesthetics to decrease healing time and prevent postherpetic neuralgia and application of capsaicin
R patches +W halo	Blunt or rounded	Soft and friable	Ulcerated	—	Unilateral vesicles which rupture	Necrosis of periodontium and alveolar bone	Culture	Skin lesion	Shingles (herpes zoster)	Oral acyclovir 800 mg five times a day, famciclovir 500 mg three times a day, or valacyclovir 500 mg three times a day
Pi	No change	Soft	Papules	++	Raised nodular or popular lesions	Mucosal lesions are rare		Discrete papules on skin of face and trunk and in genital areas	*Molluscum contagiosum* virus	Cryotherapy/laser
G	No change	Firm	Exophytic and verrucous	++		Exophytic papillomatous, verrucous or flat lesions			Squamous cell papilloma, condyloma acuminatum, verruca vulgaris, focal epithelial hyperplasia	Surgical removal, laser ablation, cryotherapy, and topical application of keratinolytic agents. For smaller lesions, topical application of 25% podophyllum resin to reduce the size. Intralesional injection of interferon-α 1,000,000 iu/cm^2 once weekly and subcutaneous injections 3,000,000 iu/cm^2 twice weekly

DOI: http://dx.doi.org/10.5772/intechopen.91726

C	Cr	Cs	T	S	P	L	Lab & H/P	Add Sym	D	Rx
W-R	No change	Soft and resilient	Scrapable lesion	+/−		Pseudomembrane/ erythematous/plaque-like/ nodular	H/P: culture of infected tissues or exudates on Sabouraud's dextrose agar or other appropriate media	Oral involvement is secondary to serious systemic infection	Candidiasis	Topical antifungal medications, nystatin, and amphotericin b
BR	Rounded	Soft and friable	Chronic vegetating painful ulcer	++		Nodular, papillary, or granulomatous lesions	Biopsy of infected tissue shows small oval yeasts within macrophages and reticuloendothelial cells as well as chronic granulomas, epithelioid cells, giant cells, and occasionally caseation necrosis	Cavitation of the lung and dissemination of the organism to the liver, spleen, adrenal glands, and meninges	Histoplasmosis	Ketoconazole or itraconazole for 6–12 months
RP	Violaceous marginal gingiva in early stage	Soft and friable	Necrosis and covered with pseudomembrane in advanced cases	−−		Lesions are necrotic and covered by pseudomembrane		Systemic involvement is present. Late stage involves destruction of alveolar bone and facial muscles	Aspergillosis	Systemic antifungals
R+ W streaks	Normal	Soft	Lichenoid reaction	No change		Lichenoid-like reaction	Patch test by placing aluminum disks with known allergens for 48 hours on hairless skin and wait for any inflammation as a positive test. H/P: chronic inflammatory reaction with lichenoid infiltration of lymphocytes		Contact allergy	Topical corticosteroids

C	Cr	Cs	T	S	P	L	Lab & H/P	Add Sym	D	Rx
R			Velvety texture	+	Seen in anterior maxillary gingiva		Plasma cells in lamina propria		Plasma cell gingivitis	Topical corticosteroids
R-W		Soft and friable	Smooth or disrupted	—		Round lesion with central red area or pale pink surrounded by red periphery	Biopsy an epidermal pattern characterized by lichenoid vasculitis and intraepidermal vesicles and a dermal pattern characterized by lymphocytic vasculitis and subepidermal vesiculation	Skin lesions symmetrically present on distal extremities and moving proximally Hand, face, elbow and knees	Erythema multiforme	Anesthetic mouthwash, corticosteroids in severe cases, and acyclovir if associated with HSV
RP-W	Normal	Soft and friable	Smooth and loss of stippling	No change	Lesions on free and attached gingiva	Desquamative gingivitis with vesiculobullous lesions which rupture	ELISA to detect circulating antibody to desmoglein 1 and 3. Histopathology: suprabasilar acantholysis may be observed	Bullous lesions on skin	Pemphigus vulgaris	Prednisolone usually given in dosages of 1–2 mg/kg/d and later – –
R area	Normal	Soft	Smooth and loss of stippling	—	Positive Nikolsky sign: rubbing the gingiva forms bulla	Desquamative lesions with bulla formation	Histopathology: circulating antibodies not always found by indirect immunofluorescence	Scarring in ocular lesions	Pemphigoid	Systemic corticosteroids
R-W streaks	Normal	Soft and resilient	Smooth and ulcerative	No change		Papular, reticular, plaque type or bullous lesions	Hyperkeratosis and saw tooth-shaped rete pegs	Skin lesions	Lichen planus	Topical corticosteroids or intralesional steroids like 0.05% fluocinonide (Lidex) and 0.05% clobetasol (temovate)
R and W striae			Smooth and ulcerative	−/+		Central atrophic area with small white dots surrounded by white striae	Hyperorthokeratosis with keratotic plugs, atrophy of the rete ridges, and liquefactive	Red butterfly-shaped photosensitive, scaly, macules on	Lupus erythematosus	Systemic immunosuppressant and protection from sunlight

C	Cr	Cs	T	S	P	L	Lab & H/P	Add Sym	D	Rx
							degeneration of the basal celllayer	the nose bridge and cheeks		
Pl	Normal	Soft		++		Cobblestone appearance of mucosa and linear ulceration	Histopathology	Intestinal pain, anal fissures, diarrhea, and labial enlargement	Crohn's disease	Steroids and immunosuppressants to decrease progression
RP		Soft and friable	Loss of stippling	++	Gingival recession	Nodules and ulceration. Loosening of teeth	Hyperglobulinemia, an elevated level of serum angiotensin-converting enzyme, evidence of depressed cellular immunity. H/P: noncaseating epithelioid granulomas in more than one organ system	Swelling of salivary glands	Sarcoidosis	Systemic steroids and anti-inflammatory agents
Pi	Normal	Fibrous	Smooth	+		Exophytic smooth masses	H/P: bundles of collagen covered with the epithelium		Fibrous epulis	Excision and curettage
RP	Normal	Fibrous	Smooth	++	Start from interdental papilla	Pedunculated to sessile masses	H/P: cellular fibroblastic tissue containing rounded or lobulated masses of calcified cementum-like tissue		Calcifying fibroblastic granuloma	Excision of lesion
RP				+		Ulcerated, smooth, and pedunculated mass	H/P: discontinuous hyperplastic parakeratinized stratified squamous epithelium and endothelial cells in the connective tissue		Pyogenic granuloma	Excision of lesion

C	Cr	Cs	T	S	P	L	Lab & H/P	Add Sym	D	Rx
Pr-Bl-Br		Soft		++		Sessile or pedunculated tumor-like process	H/P: multinucleated giant cell forming granuloma		Peripheral giant cell granuloma	Surgical excision
W		Corrugated or verrucous surface		+		Non-removable white spot	Tissue biopsy. Vital staining with toluidine blue and cytobrush techniques. H/P: dysplastic cells with ++ hyperchromatic nuclei, cellular and nuclear pleomorphism, an ++ nucleo-cytoplasmic ratio, and generalized loss of cellular polarity and orientation	History of tobacco/alcohol intake	Leukoplakia	Surgical excision/cryosurgery and laser ablation
R		Velvety		+		Sharply demarcated from surrounding mucosa	Same as above	May be associated with oral lichen planus	Erythroplakia	Same as above
R- W patches	No change	Soft	Smooth	++	Involve keratinized gingiva	Painless exophytic mass with nonhealing ulceration	Dysplastic changes seen in the epithelium and extending into connective tissue and the presence of keratin pearls	History of tobacco/alcohol intake	Squamous cell carcinoma	Surgical removal, chemotherapy
RP	No change	Soft and edematous	Smooth	++		Pallor of oral mucosa, pain, petechiae, ecchymosis, gingival bleeding, deep punched out ulcers	Blood investigation. Bone marrow biopsy. Tooth mobility	Dysphagia, facial paralysis, paraesthesia of the face, lips, tongue, and chin, trismus sometimes	Leukemia	Monitoring of the patient for infection during neutropenic periods and early management of infection. Corticosteroids, adrenocorticotropin, or testosterone modulates the sharp reduction in marrow function. Granulocyte colony-

DOI: http://dx.doi.org/10.5772/intechopen.91726

C	Cr	Cs	T	S	P	L	Lab & H/P	Add Sym	D	Rx
										stimulating factor (G-CSF)
P	Rounded	Soft	Smooth	++			Histopathology will show Reed-Sternberg cells	Swollen lymph nodes	Lymphoma	Radiation and chemotherapy plus doxorubicin, bleomycin, vincristine, and dacarbazine for Hodgkin's lymphoma and cyclophosphamide, vincristine, and prednisone for non-Hodgkin's
W plaques	No change	Soft	Loss of stippling	+	Seen on facial attached gingiva	Leukoplakia-like asymptomatic plaque	H/P: dense fibrous connective tissue		Frictional keratosis	Prevention of deleterious habits
RP	No change	Soft and friable		—	Gingival recession	Superficial and horizontal gingival laceration	Not much significant		Toothbrushing-induced gingival ulceration	Changing the brushing technique
R-W				—		Surface slough or ulceration	Not much significant		Chemical insult due to etching, chlorhexidine, hydrogen peroxide, acetylsalicylic acid, dentifrice, detergent, calcium hydroxide, etc.	Removal of offending irritant
R				—		Erythematous lesion that slough a coagulated surface, vesicles and ulceration may be present	Not of much significance		Burns of mucosa	Supportive care and hydration

C	Cr	Cs	T	S	P	L	Lab & H/P	Add Sym	D	Rx
Br-Bl	No change	No change	No change	=			Pigmented deposits in the epithelium and connective tissue	Addison's disease, Albright syndrome, Peutz-Jeghers syndrome	Gingival pigmentation	Not required
Br	No change	Firm	No change	=	Mandibular facial gingiva		H/P: pigmented macules seen in section		Smoker's melanosis	Smoking cessation for 2 weeks
Bl-Gy–Br-Bl	No change	No change	No change	=		Diffuse pigmentation			Drug-induced pigmentation (antimalarial, minocycline)	Cessation of drug if required
Bl-Gy–Br-Bl	No change	No change	No change	=			H/P: discrete granules in connective tissue		Amalgam tattoo	Removal of amalgam debris and replacement of amalgam if required

C, color; Cr, contour; Cs, consistency; T, texture; S, size; P, position; L, lesion; lab and H/P, laboratory procedures and histopathology; add sym, additional symptoms; D, diagnosis; Rx, treatment; FR, fiery red; G, same as surrounding gingiva; W, white; PR, pink to reddish; B-Br, black to brown; R-Gy, red to gray; RP, reddish pink; BR, bright red; Pi, pink; Pl, pale pink; Pr, purple; Bl, blue; OHI, oral hygiene instruction; CHX, chlorhexidine; +, slightly increased; ++, increased; −, slightly decreased; −−, decreased; −/+, may increase or decrease; =, remains the same.

Table 4.
Clinical features for diagnosis and treatment of non-plaque-induced gingival diseases.

3. Treatment of gingival disease

The treatment of gingival disease is based on resolving the etiologic factors and maintaining the systemic status of the individual. In the case of plaque-induced gingivitis, the main treatment plan involves removal of plaque and calculus by scaling and root planning, followed by oral hygiene instruction which includes modified bass method of brushing and the use of chemical plaque control agents like 0.2% or 0.02% chlorhexidine gluconate or essential oil mouthwash. In cases of gingival enlargement, initial therapy is focused on removing plaque and calculus, followed by a review on the gingival condition; only if the condition does not improve the drug substitution may be considered, followed by gingivectomy to remove the enlarged gingival tissue. Plaque-induced gingival disease influenced by modifying factors is controlled by reducing the exposure of the modifying factor in addition to removal of plaque and calculus to maintain oral hygiene. The details of the treatment have been mentioned in **Table 2**. Non-plaque-induced gingival diseases are treated depending on the etiology of the gingival disease. For example, viral lesions are treated by providing antiviral medications in addition to oral hygiene instruction. The details of treatment in brief are mentioned in **Table 4**. Diagnosis is essential for providing the proper treatment plan and updating recent research which might help prevent undue treatment [8].

4. Conclusions

Gingival diseases are an initial starting point of the advanced periodontal disease and in some cases depict the manifestation of an underlying undiagnosed systemic condition. Therefore, the early diagnosis of gingival disease and its treatment are warranted.

Conflict of interest

The authors declare no conflict of interest.

Author details

Anahita Punj[1]* and Manav Chaturvedi[2]

1 Department of Periodontics, Army College of Dental Sciences, Secunderabad, India

2 Partha Dental, Hyderabad, India

*Address all correspondence to: anahitapunj@gmail.com

References

[1] Newman MG, Takei HH, Klokkevold PR, Carranza FA. Newman and Carranza's Clinical Periodontology. 13th ed. Philadelphia: Elsevier Saunders; 2019. pp. 55-79

[2] Newman MG, Takei HH, Klokkevold PR, Carranza FA. Newman and Carranza's Clinical Periodontology. 13th ed. Philadelphia: Elsevier Saunders; 2019. pp. 248-302

[3] Caton J, Armitage G, Berglundh T, et al. A new classification scheme for periodontal and periimplant diseases and conditions—Introduction and key changes from the 1999 classification. Journal of Clinical Periodontology. 2018; **45**(Suppl 20):S1-S8. DOI: 10.1111/jcpe.12935

[4] Chapple ILC. Dental plaque–induced gingival conditions. Journal of Clinical Periodontology. 2018;**45**(Suppl 20): S17-S27. DOI: 10.1111/jcpe.12937

[5] Newman MG, Takei HH, Klokkevold PR, Carranza FA. Newman and Carranza's Clinical Periodontology. 13th ed. Philadelphia: Elsevier Saunders; 2019. pp. 378-396

[6] Mani A, Anarthe R, Marawar PP, Mustilwar RG, Bhosale A. Diagnostic kits: An aid to periodontal diagnosis. Journal of Dental Research and Review. 2016;**3**:107-113

[7] Holmstrup P, Plemons J, Meyle J. Non–plaque-induced gingival diseases. Journal of Clinical Periodontology. 2018; **45**(Suppl 20):S28-S43. DOI: 10.1111/jcpe.12938

[8] Greenberg MS, Glick M. Burket's Oral Medicine Diagnosis & Treatment. 10th ed. Ontario: BC Decker Inc; 2003. pp. 50-118

[9] Greenberg MS, Glick M. Burket's Oral Medicine Diagnosis & Treatment. 10th ed. Ontario: BC Decker Inc; 2003. pp. 441-490

[10] Greenberg MS, Glick M. Burket's Oral Medicine Diagnosis & Treatment. 10th ed. Ontario: BC Decker Inc; 2003. pp. 552-555

[11] Pundir A, Farista S, Afroz SA. Calcifying fibroblastic granuloma—A rare case report. International Journal of Scientific and Research Publications. 2013;**3**:1-3

Chapter 4

Host Modulation

Wael I. Ibraheem and Reghunathan S. Preethanath

Abstract

Host modulation is considered to be new research area in dentistry. In medicine, host modulation was introduced way before dentistry in treating arthritis and osteoporosis. It is mainly focusing on the host part during host-bacteria interaction. Although there are many agents introduced for this purpose, the most well-studied host modulation therapy in dentistry is doxycycline. It shows less tissue destruction when used for few months along with periodontal therapy. It has anticollagenase properties which shows a promising effect when used to treat chronic inflammation.

Keywords: host modulation, doxycycline, anticollagenase, matrix metalloproteinases enzymes

1. Introduction

Host modulation therapy is a newly introduced term to the field of dentistry. Host refers to the body hosting the disease while modulation refers to changing the status of something in response to external modifier.

In periodontal diseases, bacteria/microbes are the main pathogen in initiating the disease while the host is the body hosting the bacteria. Host modulation therapy is the chemical agent that can be used as an adjunct to the systematized periodontal therapy to improve the diseased state and inhibit the tissue destruction. As proved in many studies, bacteria cause direct tissue destruction by releasing enzymes and other virulent factors and indirectly by letting the host tissue to release collagenases which in turn destruct the tissue. Host modulation is working on the indirect arm of this process.

Host modulation was introduced in dentistry by William [1] and Golub et al. [2] in the 1990s. Both discussed the idea of having a chemical agent that modulate the host response and improve the periodontal health. The response to the periodontal disease as well as the progression of the periodontal disease varies considerably among individuals. Some patients are susceptible to a disease more than others which make, the host modulation therapy preferable in such cases.

Host modulation can be used to reduce levels of enzymes, collagenases, and proinflammatory cytokines. Moreover, it can modify osteoclast and osteoblast activities (**Figure 1**). It has a role in modifiable risk factors (e.g., smoking, diabetes) and unmodifiable risk factors (e.g., genetic susceptibility) as it help the body to overcome those risk factors. In systemic host modulation, it has the effect on multiple sites on the oral cavity with 'sub-antimicrobial-dose doxycycline' (SDD) and locally with agents such as bone morphogenic proteins (BMP) to improve wound healing at the surgical site.

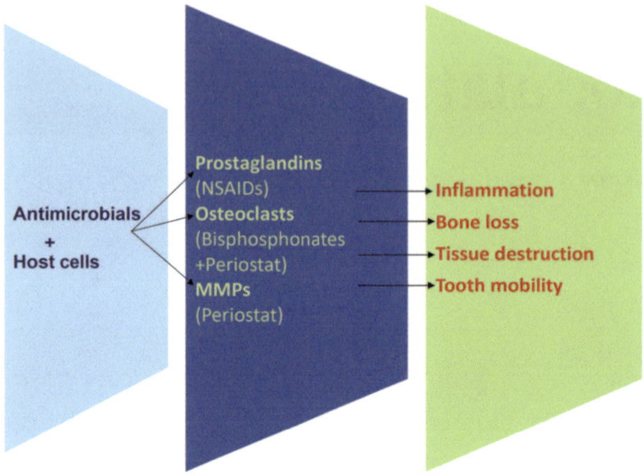

Figure 1.
The effect of different systemic host modulation therapy agents and their target during gingivitis and periodontitis.

2. Systemic host modulation

Various medications which are used for host modulation therapy are administered orally.

2.1 Bisphosphonates

Bisphosphonate is an agent that is used to inhibit bone resorption by interfering with osteoclasts. The actual mechanism of action is yet unclear. Some researches show that bisphosphonate interfere with osteoclast cellular adenosine triphosphate (ATPs) [3]. Bisphosphonate possesses anticollagenase properties [4]. Bisphosphonates is helpful in periodontal disease associated with bone loss.

In an animal study, bisphosphonate shows more bone density in beagle dogs using alendronate [5]. Complications associated with using bisphosphonate are mainly bisphosphonate-related osteonecrosis of the jaw (BRONJ). It is mainly associated with intravenous administration of bisphosphonate [6]. Bisphosphonate is not yet been approved as host modulation therapy for periodontitis.

2.2 Nonsteroidal anti-inflammatory drugs

NSAIDs decrease the production of prostaglandins (PGE). PGE_2 is produced by different cells such as neutrophils and fibroblast in response to lipo-poly saccharide. It has been shown that PGE_2 is elevated in periodontitis in response to bacteria compared to non-periodontitis cases [7]. By reducing PGE_2 production, inflammation also subsides in periodontal disease. One study showed lower levels of matrix metalloproteinase enzymes (MMP-8) at the gingival crevicular fluid (GCF) after administration of NSAIDs [8]. Some studies showed that NSAIDs such as indomethacin [9], flurbiprofen [10], and naproxen [11] show reduced bone loss when used for a period up to 3 years. These are the non-selective NSAIDs that have been investigated in research as host modulation therapy. The main side effect when NSAIDs are used for prolonged period as host modulation therapy includes gastrointestinal pain and ulcer, bleeding, and renal and hepatic impairment.

Using selective cyclooxygenase-2 (COX-2) inhibitor could be a promising solution to the side effects of non-selective NSAIDs (**Figure 2**).

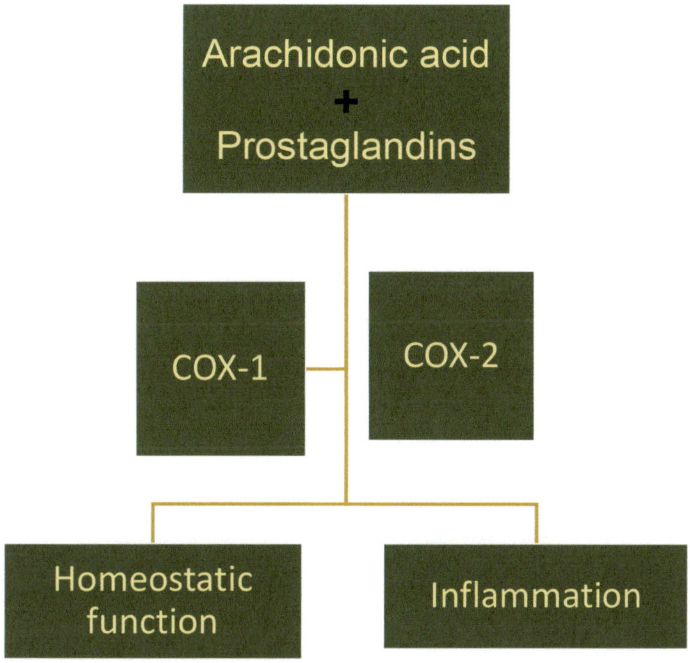

Figure 2.
Cyclooxygenase enzyme converts arachidonic acid to prostaglandins. COX-1 maintains the homeostatic functions at the body while COX-2 contributes more with the inflammation.

Some studies administering selective NSAIDs showed less PGE2 in human periodontal tissues [12]. On the other hand, selective NSAIDs reported side effects such as myocardial infarction. NSAIDs also show some rebound effects when the usage stopped which resulted in more tissue destruction afterward [13]. NSAIDs are not yet been approved as host modulation therapy for periodontitis.

2.3 Sub-antimicrobial-dose doxycycline

Sub-antimicrobial-dose doxycycline (SDD) is the only host modulation therapy approved by the U.S. Food and Drug Administration (FDA) and accepted by the American Dental Association (ADA). SDD (Periostat) is usually administered as 20 mg twice daily for a period of 3 months. Less than 3 months period was showing rebound effect of collagenase levels as the benefit of SDD is not yet been applied at the tissue [14]. In many cases, physicians are prescribing the medication for a period up to 9 months and regular follow up every 3 months to evaluate the effect of the medication.

SDD has an anticollagenase effect and inhibit osteoclast and proinflammatory cytokines. The effect of SDD is below the detection of bacteria which will not cause any resistance in the future. Moreover, there is no rebound effect registered after discontinuing the medication. The significant clinical effect of SDD compared to placebo in 266 patients when used as an adjunct to scaling and root planing (SRP) in periodontitis patients has been reported in a study [15]. Another study was showing the effect of SDD as an adjunct to SRP with smokers having periodontitis [16].

Large number of MMPs is released to the periodontal tissues during inflammation by different cells. MMP-8 and MMP-9 are major enzymes released from neutrophils during inflammation which cause tissue destruction through degrading type I collagen [17, 18]. The release of MMPs leads to progressive destruction of periodontal tissues which is related to the large number of neutrophils during inflammation.

3. Local host modulation

3.1 Enamel matrix proteins, growth factors, and bone morphogenetic proteins

The locally administered host modulation therapy is used mainly to improve wound healing, increase bone formation, and to produce new periodontal tissue including periodontal ligament and cementum. They have been applied locally along with periodontal surgery. The FDA approved local host modulatory agents includes enamel matrix proteins (Emdogain), recombinant human platelet-derived growth factor-BB (GEM 21S), and BMP-2 (rhBMP-2 [Infuse]). These materials have been proved to provide some clinical benefits when used during periodontal surgical procedures. The focus of this chapter is on the non-surgical therapy of gingivitis and periodontitis.

4. Conclusions

To summarize, patient selection and motivation to do periodontal therapy is the key to start host modulation therapy. Moreover, medical status of the patient would affect the outcome of the treatment.

Conflict of interest

None.

Author details

Wael I. Ibraheem* and Reghunathan S. Preethanath
College of Dentistry, Jazan University, Jazan, Kingdom of Saudi Arabia

*Address all correspondence to: dr.wael007@yahoo.com; wibraheem@jazanu.edu.sa

References

[1] Williams RC. Periodontal disease. The New England Journal of Medicine. 1990;**322**(6):373

[2] Golub LM, Suomalainen K, Sorsa T. Host modulation with tetracyclines and their chemically modified analogues. Current Opinion in Dentistry. 1992;**2**:80

[3] Weinreb M, Quartuccio H, Seedor JG, et al. Histomorphometrical analysis of the effects of the bisphosphonate alendronate on bone loss caused by experimental periodontitis in monkeys. Journal of Periodontal Research. 1994;**29**:35

[4] Nakaya H, Osawa G, Iwasaki N, et al. Effects of bisphosphonate on matrix metalloproteinase enzymes in human periodontal ligament cells. Journal of Periodontology. 2000;**71**:1158

[5] Reddy MS, Weatherford TW, Smith CA, et al. Alendronate treatment of naturally-occurring periodontitis in beagle dogs. Journal of Periodontology. 1995;**66**:211

[6] Carter G, Goss AN, Doecke C. Bisphosphonates and avascular necrosis of the jaw: A possible association. The Medical Journal of Australia. 2005;**182**(8):413

[7] Grenier D, Plamondon P, Sorsa T, et al. Inhibition of proteolytic, serpinolytic, and progelatinase-b activation activities of periodontopathogens by doxycycline and the non-antimicrobial chemically modified tetracycline derivatives. Journal of Periodontology. 2002;**73**:79

[8] Buduneli N, Vardar S, Atilla G, et al. Gingival crevicular fluid matrix metalloproteinase-8 levels following adjunctive use of meloxicam and initial phase of periodontal therapy. Journal of Periodontology. 2002;**73**:103-109

[9] Williams RC, Jeffcoat MK, Howell TH, et al. Indomethacin or flurbiprofen treatment of periodontitis in beagles: Comparison of effect on bone loss. Journal of Periodontal Research. 1987;**22**:403

[10] Williams RC, Jeffcoat MK, Howell TH, et al. Altering the progression of human alveolar bone loss with the non-steroidal anti-inflammatory drug flurbiprofen. Journal of Periodontology. 1989;**60**:485

[11] Howell TH, Jeffcoat MK, Goldhaber P, et al. Inhibition of alveolar bone loss in beagles with the NSAID naproxen. Journal of Periodontal Research. 1991;**26**:498

[12] Vardar S, Baylas H, Huseyinov A. Effects of selective cyclooxygenase-2 inhibition on gingival tissue levels of prostaglandin E2 and prostaglandin F2a and clinical parameters of chronic periodontitis. Journal of Periodontology. 2003;**74**:57

[13] Williams RC, Jeffcoat MK, Howell TH, et al. Three year trial of flurbiprofen treatment in humans: Post-treatment period [abstract 1617]. Journal of Dental Research. 1991;**70**:468

[14] Ashley RA. Clinical trials of a matrix metalloproteinase inhibitor in human periodontal disease. SDD Clinical Research TeamAnnals of the New York Academy of Sciences. 1999;**878**:335

[15] Preshaw PM, Novak MJ, Mellonig J, et al. Modified-release subantimicrobial dose doxycycline enhances scaling and root planing in subjects with periodontal disease. Journal of Periodontology. 2008;**79**(3):440

[16] Needleman I, Suvan J, Gilthorpe MS, et al. A randomized-controlled trial of low-dose doxycycline for periodontitis in smokers. Journal of Clinical Periodontology. 2007;**34**(4):325

[17] Golub LM, Sorsa T, Lee HM, et al. Doxycycline inhibits neutrophil (PMN)-type matrix metalloproteinases in human adult periodontitis gingiva. Journal of Clinical Periodontology. 1995;**22**:100

[18] Mariotti A. The extracellular matrix of the periodontium: Dynamic and interactive tissues. Periodontology 2000. 1993;**2000**(3):39

Chapter 5

Adverse Effects of Medications on Periodontal Tissues

Sukumaran Anil, Seham H.S.A. Alyafei, Annie Kitty George and Elna Paul Chalisserry

Abstract

Periodontal tissue is susceptible to a range of adverse effects of several medications used in daily medical practice. Phenytoin, cyclosporine, and calcium-channel blockers are the most commonly used drugs related to gingival disease. Several other medications can also have an adverse effect on the periodontium, especially in the presence of compromised oral hygiene. These medications act on periodontal tissues by triggering the inflammatory pathways involved in the pathogenesis of periodontal disease or by potentially compromising the management of patients with these conditions. Gingival overgrowth is probably the mostly widely recognized and investigated type of adverse drug reaction in the periodontal tissues. Since many patients are on such medications, dental practitioner should take a thorough medical history and be aware of medication-related problems and their potential effects on diagnosis and treatment planning. The chapter reviews the commonly prescribed medications that can affect the periodontium either in its healthy or inflamed condition.

Keywords: adverse effects, calcium channel blockers, gingival overgrowth, hypertension, anticonvulsants, immunosuppressants

1. Introduction

Medications are chemical substances used to treat, cure, prevent, or diagnose a disease or to promote well-being. An adverse drug reaction is defined by WHO as a response to a drug which is noxious and unintended, and which occurs at doses normally used in man for the prophylaxis, diagnosis, therapy of diseases or for the modification of physiological function. Several medications can cause adverse effects in the periodontium. The most common are the gingival enlargement, inflammation, pigmentations, gingival bleeding and osteonecrosis [1]. Gingival overgrowth (GO) or enlargement is a condition is characterized by an increase in the size of gingiva subsequent to the increase in extracellular tissue volume. Gingival overgrowth is a side effect of several medications used by patients have the capability to cause adverse effects in the oral cavity and periodontal tissues [2]. Though many medications have marked effects on the periodontal tissues and these adverse reactions are well documented, many have been described only as isolated case series or reports [2]. It is important for the clinician to obtain a complete record of the medications the patient takes, including prescription drugs and over-the-counter drugs. This will help the clinician to diagnose and manage the adverse effects in the periodontal tissues.

2. Drug induced gingival overgrowth (DIGO)

The main drugs associated with GO can be divided into three categories such as anticonvulsants, calcium channel blockers, and immunosuppressants. Few isolated incidences of GO associated with antibiotics and sulphonamides were also reported. Though these drugs have different pharmacologic effect and targets, all of them seem to act similarly on the gingival connective tissue as a secondary target, leading to common clinical and histopathological changes. The gingival overgrowth (GO) is consequent to the alteration of the host tissue response, resulting in an increase in collagen synthesis and cellular changes within the connective tissue. The prevalence of gingival overgrowth varies with different medications, with a reported rate of 50% for phenytoin (anticonvulsant), 25–30% for cyclosporine (immunosuppressant), 5–20% for nifedipine and 3% for amlodipine (CCBs) [2]. The drug associated gingival overgrowth is three times more prevalent among men and can be attributed to the effect of testosterone on fibroblast proliferation and collagen stimulus [3].

The GO appears normally within 1–3 months after administration of these medications (**Table 1**). The gingival enlargement may appear inflamed or more fibrotic depending on the degree of inflammation. Normally the GO is confined to the attached gingiva which might occasionally extend coronally. The enlarged gingiva produces esthetic changes and its clinical symptoms include tenderness, bleeding, interference with speech, dental occlusion problems, and enhanced susceptibility to periodontal diseases [4–6].

Histologically, the drug-induced gingival overgrowth is indistinguishable from other types of gingival enlargement. The enlargement of the gingival tissue occurs as a result of accumulation of extracellular matrix (ECM), although the pathogenesis remains multifactorial. Age, genetic predisposition, pharmacokinetic variables, drug-induced alterations in gingival connective tissue homeostasis, inflammatory changes, drug-induced action on growth factors, etc. are some of the factors that influences the occurrence and severity of the gingival overgrowth.

Genetic factors are important in the pathogenesis of drug associated gingival overgrowth. The drugs are metabolized by cytochrome p450 enzymes, which are characterized by high genetic variability. Research on genes responsible for HLA leukocyte antigen coding confirmed the theory of HLA-DR2 antigen influence, which is found much more commonly in patients with moderate or severe drug-induced gingival overgrowth than HLA-DR1 [7]. The drug variables such as dosage, duration of therapy and concentration of drug in plasma and local fluids, like gingival crevicular fluid and saliva, play an important role in DIGO [8].

2.1 Pathogenesis of DIGO

The exact mechanism behind the pathogenesis of drug-induced gingival overgrowth is not yet fully understood. Each medication has got separate impacts on the range of cytokines and growth factors involved in connective tissue metabolism. Studies revealed that the molecular markers and clinical features of gingival overgrowth differ depending on the drugs. The cytokine and growth factor balances are altered in tissues with GO, including connective tissue growth factor (CTGF), a member of the interesting CCN (cysteine-rich angiogenic protein 61) family of factors [3, 9, 10].

Cytokine dependent alterations in extracellular matrix metabolism appear to be of functional importance to gingival overgrowth. Abnormal differentiation of cells, resulting in accumulation of fibroblasts with a pathologic range of proliferative

Drugs/groups	Incidence/prevalence	References
Anticonvulsants		
Phenytoin	13%	[17]
	50.3%	[18]
	57%	[19]
	40%	[20]
	50–60%	[21]
	53%	[22]
Sodium valproate	Rare	[22]
Vigabatrin	Rare	[23, 24]
Carbamazepine	None	[22]
Immunosuppressants		
Cyclosporines	10–85%	[25]
	30%	[26]
	8–70%	[27]
	25–81%	[8]
	22.4%	[28]
Tacrolimus	14.1%	[28]
Calcium channel blockers		
Nifedipine	6.3%	[29]
	50.8%	[30]
	83%	[31]
Diltiazem	20%	[31]
Verapamil	4–19%	[32, 33]
Amlodipine	3%	[34, 35]
Felodipine	Rare	[36]

Table 1.
Medications causing drug induced gingival overgrowth (DIGO).

and synthetic phenotypes, could result from deregulated cytokines. The unique metabolic aspects of gingival extracellular matrix metabolism; and a greater understanding of interactions between and among medications, the innate and acquired immune response, cytokines and growth factors, and gingival epithelial and connective tissue cells providing more detailed molecular and mechanistic information need to be elucidated [3, 11].

2.2 Histological features

Histologically, slight to moderate hyperkeratosis, thickening of the spinous layer, fibrosis of underlying connective tissue with fibroblastic proliferation, increase in the number of capillaries with slight chronic perivascular inflammation is seen. Excessive accumulation of extracellular matrix like collagen with varying amounts of inflammatory infiltrates, predominantly plasma cells are seen. Fibroblastic proliferation may not be evident. Plasma cells are the principal type of infiltrating inflammatory cell. Parakeratinized epithelium of variable thickness covers the connective tissue stroma. The epithelial ridges may penetrate deep into the connective with columns of interspersed collagen fibers [12].

2.3 Management of drug induced DIGO

The management of medication induced gingival overgrowth depends on the degree of progression of the disease. Withdrawal or substitution of medication is one of the methods that might resolve the gingival overgrowth. However, not all patients respond to this mode of treatment especially those with long standing gingival enlargement. Professional debridement with scaling and root planning as needed has been shown to offer some remission of the gingival overgrowth in patients. Since the anterior labial gingiva is frequently involved, surgery is commonly performed for esthetic reasons. The classical surgical approach has been the external bevel gingivectomy. However, a total or partial internal gingivectomy approach has been suggested as an alternative. This approach has the benefit of limiting the large denuded connective tissue wound and thereby minimizing postoperative pain and bleeding [13].

The surgical methods include traditional scalpel gingivectomy and periodontal flap surgery. Electrocautery may be used in difficult cases, children, or where the gingiva is fragile and likely to bleed. Excision using laser provides a superior incision margin and improved wound healing due to a coagulated layer along the incision, as well as a reduced incidence of scarring. CO_2 laser is very effective in surgery of soft tissues with high water content like the gingiva. Blood vessels up to a diameter of 0.5 mm can be sealed effectively and provides a dry field for better visibility of the surgical field. A laser is preferred over the scalpel as it has strong bactericidal and hemostatic effects [14, 15]. A combined non-surgical and surgical therapy with drug substitution is the most common treatment approach in the management of medication induced gingival overgrowth [16]. In most cases, conservative methods such as professional oral hygiene maintenance, topical anti-inflammatory and antibacterial drugs and a meticulous oral hygiene measures by the patient. Surgical excision is used in cases of where the gingival overgrowth interferes with food intake, causing difficulties in speech and maintaining oral hygiene. Surgical excision is more reliable as it eliminates the hyperplastic tissue and promotes plaque control as well as improves the esthetics.

2.4 Phenytoin

Phenytoin is an anticonvulsant prescribed for the control of epilepsy and neuralgias. In the present day, phenytoin is not usually prescribed as a first line drug for the management of epilepsy due to the availability of a wide range of newer, more effective anticonvulsant drugs with fewer side effects. The prevalence of drug-induced gingival overgrowth in patients taking phenytoin is reportedly between 15% and 60% [17]. Phenytoin, or its metabolites, probably acts directly on high activity fibroblasts leading to the high levels of production of collagen in the presence of inflammation. This results in gingival enlargement, characteristically originating principally from the interdental papillae (**Figure 1**). The amount or degree of severity of the overgrowth is not related to the dose of the drug. Presence of plaque and gingival inflammation, serum concentrations of the drug are factors which increases the risk of phenytoin-induced gingival overgrowth [37].

The management of this overgrowth is based on obtaining optimal control of plaque. Where the enlargement is unsightly and disfiguring, or even interfering

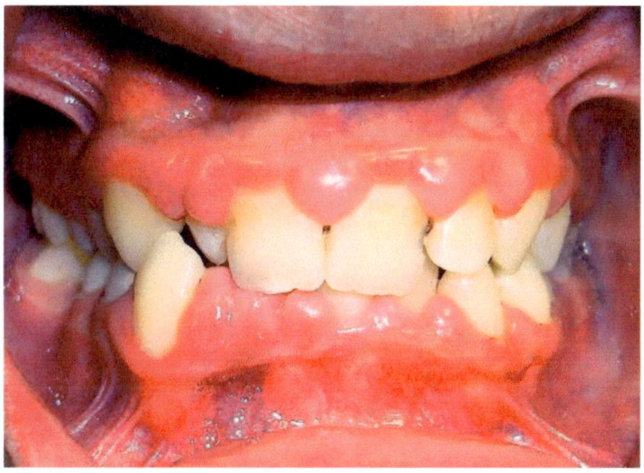

Figure 1.
A case of phenytoin induced gingival overgrowth.

with chewing, the over-growths should be removed. Gingivectomy appears to be the simplest and best way of achieving good gingival contour as a post-operative result. But optimal plaque control post-operatively is the most important determinant of success. Recent research work suggests that the use of chlorhexidine, especially brushing daily using the gel, can be of valuable assistance in controlling plaque and hence in controlling the overgrowths in the post-surgical phase.

2.5 Cyclosporin

Cyclosporin (CsA) is a cyclic polypeptide with potent immunosuppressive activity used widely to prevent organ transplant rejection and also in the treatment of autoimmune diseases [38, 39]. CsA selectively suppresses helper T-cell function and modulates the network of inflammatory cytokines. However, cyclosporin is associated with several untoward effects like nephrotoxicity, hepatotoxicity, hirsutism and gingival overgrowth [40, 41]. Gingival overgrowth is one of the common side effects of CsA treatment, observed in 13–81% of the patients [6, 39]. The prevalence of gingival overgrowth associated with CsA averages around 30%, with reported rates ranging from 10 to 85% [25]. Studies have shown certain degree of association between GO and potential risk factors, such as age, genetic susceptibility, pharmacokinetic variables, plaque-related inflammation and immunological changes [42–44]. Epidemiological studies have reported wide variation of its occurrence and it accounts for more than 70% of the transplant recipients [4, 45]. The severity of gingival overgrowth is often associated with its prolonged use and further influenced by bacterial plaque and local irritants (**Figure 2**) [46]. The use of other medication, such as calcium channel blockers along with CsA increases the prevalence of gingival overgrowth and subsequently the risks [11]. The condition can interfere with the mastication, speech and oral hygiene maintenance and has a psychological impact in the affected individual [5].

The most prominent pathologic manifestation of the gingival overgrowth is an excessive accumulation of extracellular matrix, predominantly type I collagen. Many studies have shown increased transcriptional and translational levels of type I collagen in both tissue and fibroblast cultures derived from CsA-induced gingival overgrowth [9, 10, 47]. Though the exact mechanism is not clearly understood, studies also have shown increased expression of specific cytokines, especially transforming growth factor-beta (TGF-β), in drug-induced gingival overgrowth. This suggests that TGF-β, an inflammatory mediator that regulates cell proliferation and differentiation, plays a role in enlarging the extracellular matrix in hyperplastic gingival tissue [48].

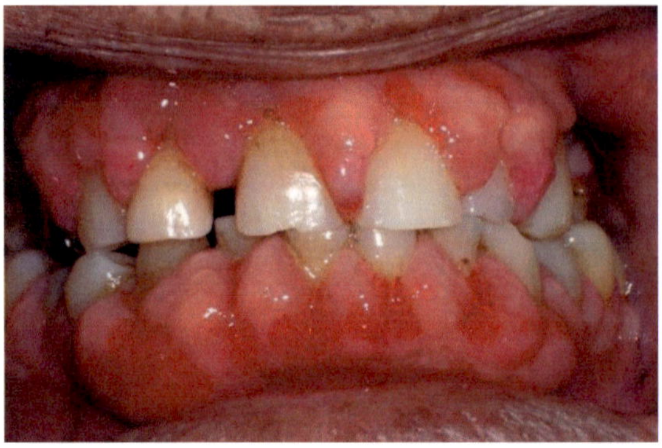

Figure 2.
A case of cyclosporin A induced gingival overgrowth.

The management of cyclosporin associated gingival overgrowth includes removal of local irritants and plaque and maintenance of adequate oral hygiene. Invasive procedures, such as gingivectomy is done in severe cases [49]. Currently the use of antibiotics has shown reduction in the GO associated with the drug usage. Azithromycin, a semi synthetic antibiotic, derived from the macrolide erythromycin has shown reduction in gingival overgrowth [50]. Roxithromycin, a macrolide antibiotic with similar characteristics of azithromycin, is also found to be effective in the reduction of gingival overgrowth in renal transplant recipients on CsA [25]. Gingival overgrowth can be prevented by intensive plaque-control practices including meticulous brushing, although critically ill patients receiving CsA may not be the ideal candidates for such intensive procedures. A combination of chlorhexidine or normal saline mouth rinses and mechanical cleaning was found to be effective in controlling the management of such patients [51, 52].

2.6 Calcium channel blockers

Drugs including diuretics, alpha and beta blockers, angiotensin converting enzyme inhibitors, angiotensin II type 1 receptor blockers and calcium channel blockers (CCBs) have been used to manage hypertension [53]. They are administered either alone or in combination, depending on the needs of the patient. The calcium channel blockers are the most frequently prescribed antihypertensive agents which is comprised of two subclasses, dihydropyridines and non-dihydropyridines. Although their mechanism of action is the same, they have varied pharmacological effects. While the dihydropyridines are potent vasodilators, the non-dihydropyridines produce more negative inotropic effects. The dihydropyridines such as nifedipine, amlodipine and felodipine are significantly associated with gingival overgrowth. The non-dihydropyridines such as diltiazem and verapamil are less commonly associated with gingival enlargement [54].

2.6.1 Nifedipine

Nifedipine, a drug that belongs to a pharmacological agent group known as calcium channel blocker was introduced in 1972 and has been used widely in the management of hypertension and angina pectoris. Lederman et al. [55] was the first to describe nifedipine-induced gingival overgrowth in patients treated with this drug. The prevalence of nifedipine-induced gingival overgrowth is between 30 and 50% and was found to be 3 times likely to develop in males [29]. The overgrowth appears 1–9 months after administration of the drug and the most common sites affected included the labial anterior gingiva of both jaws [56, 57]. A multifactorial pathogenesis has been suggested including environmental, genetic, immunological and inflammatory factors [58]. The interdental papilla becomes more grossly enlarged followed by the marginal and the attached gingiva (**Figure 3**). Presence of gingival periodontal disease and dental plaque has been reported as significant risk factors in the development of gingival enlargement. Several hypotheses have been put forward to explain the phenomena of the gingival overgrowth. The interaction between nifedipine and gingival fibroblasts contain increased sulfated mucopolysaccharides which are precursors of ground substance, leading to the overproduction of collagen and extracellular ground substance [59]. A genetically specific predetermined subpopulations of fibroblasts are identified which are sensitive to nifedipine and cause an increase in the production of collagen [60]. The dose of nifedipine is important and it was found that its presence in gingival crevicular fluid is 15–316 times higher than plasma. The higher concentration of nifedipine in the gingival crevicular fluid could increase the severity of gingival enlargement.

2.6.2 Amlodipine

Amlodipine is a third-generation dihydropyridine calcium channel blockers (CCB) that is used in the management of both hypertension and angina. The prevalence of gingival overgrowth associated with amlodipine is between 1.7% and 3.3% [35]. Though the etiopathology of this adverse reaction is not clearly understood, mechanisms such as inflammatory and non-inflammatory pathways have already been hypothesized. The non-inflammatory mechanisms involves a defective collagenase activity due to decreased uptake of folic acid, blockage of aldosterone synthesis in the adrenal cortex and consequent increase in Adrenocorticotropic hormone level, and up-regulation of keratinocyte growth factor [61]. The inflammatory pathway develops as a result of direct toxic effects of concentrated drug in gingival crevicular fluid and bacterial plaques leading to the up-regulation of several cytokine factors such as transforming growth factor-beta (TGF-β) [62].

The gingival overgrowth normally begins at the interdental papillae and is more frequently found in the anterior segment of the labial surfaces. Subsequently gingival lobulations that develop might appear as inflamed or fibrotic in nature depending on the degree of contributing factors (**Figure 4**). Normally the fibrotic enlargement is confined to the attached gingiva which might advance coronally and

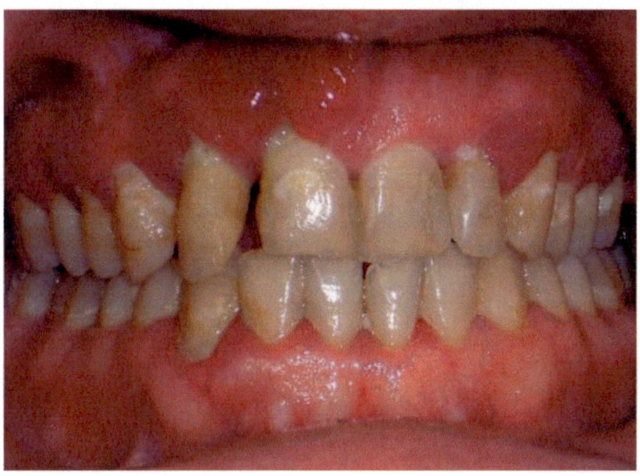

Figure 3.
A case of nifedipine induced gingival overgrowth.

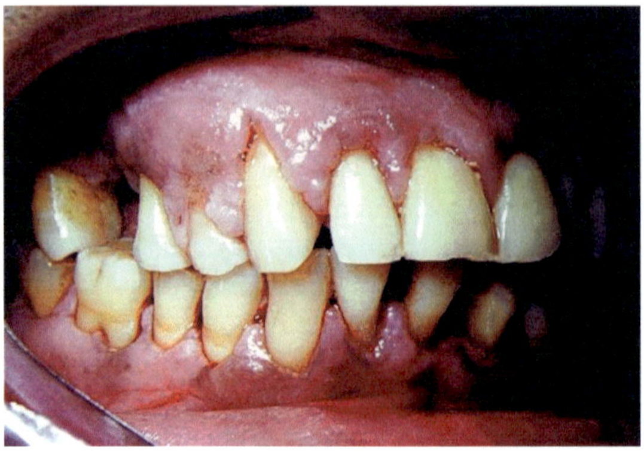

Figure 4.
A case of gingival overgrowth in a patient on amlodipine.

interfere with esthetics, mastication, or speech [63]. Management of amlodipine induced gingival overgrowth includes substitution of the drug and controlling the other risk factors with meticulous mechanical and chemical plaque control. Surgical management of the overgrowth is advised in cases to accomplish an esthetic and functional outcome [64].

2.6.3 Verapamil

Verapamil is an effective preventive agent in both episodic and chronic cluster headache. Gingival overgrowth is an infrequent adverse effect of Verapamil and a prevalence rate of around 4.2% has been reported [33]. Histologically, verapamil induced gingival enlargement shows a highly vascular connective tissue, acanthotic and thickened epithelium with long rete pegs containing dyskeratotic pearls, and varying amounts of subepithelial inflammatory infiltrate which is similar to other group of drugs [65]. The histological appearance is similar to that caused by phenytoin, cyclosporin, and other calcium channel antagonists. Discontinuation of the drug usually results in complete regression of the gingival overgrowth.

3. Other effects of medications on periodontal tissues

3.1 Minocycline

Minocycline, a semi-synthetic broad-spectrum antimicrobial agent, is mainly used for the treatment of acne, chronic respiratory diseases, and rheumatoid arthritis. It is lipid soluble and therefore can easily penetrate into body fluids, such as saliva and gingival crevicular fluid, and into various body tissues including bone and soft tissues [66]. Minocycline-induced pigmentation of oral mucous membranes including the buccal mucosa, gingiva, palatal area, lips and tongue has been reported [67–69]. The pathophysiology of minocycline staining is not clearly understood. It has been suggested that either a minocycline-metabolite complex or melanin, iron and calcium-containing granules are the source of the pigment [70]. The pigmentation of oral soft tissues appears as distinctive blue-gray or brown in color and occurs as a result of pigmented black bone visible through the thin overlying mucosa without any actual involvement of the soft tissue itself (**Figure** 5) [71]. The pigmentation appears to be related to the duration of minocycline therapy or the cumulative dose, and resolves once the drug is discontinued [69, 72]. Intraoral pigmentation can be managed with lasers [71].

3.2 Oral contraceptives

A higher prevalence of gingival inflammation, loss of attachment and gingival enlargement in woman taking hormone based oral contraceptives [73, 74]. The gingival inflammation seems to be associated to high concentrations of sex hormones present in oral contraceptives (**Figure 6**) [75]. Oral contraceptives (OCs) enhance periodontal breakdown by reducing the resistance to dental plaque and can induce gingival enlargement in otherwise healthy females [76, 77]. Oral contraceptives have pronounced effects on gingival microvasculature and it has been shown that human gingiva contains receptors for progesterone and estrogen. The dosage and duration of intake are the possible factors which influence the effect of oral contraceptives on the periodontal condition. A continued exposure of oral contraceptives for longer duration results in higher risk of periodontal disease development due to increased production of pro-inflammatory cytokines and prostaglandins as a result of elevated levels of the hormones [78, 79]. However, the currently used combined oral contraceptives showed little influence on the periodontal health, possibly related to their lower concentration of progesterone and estrogen compared to the earlier formulations [74, 80]. A critical review supports the conclusion that there is no impact of modern oral contraceptives on the periodontal and gingival tissues.

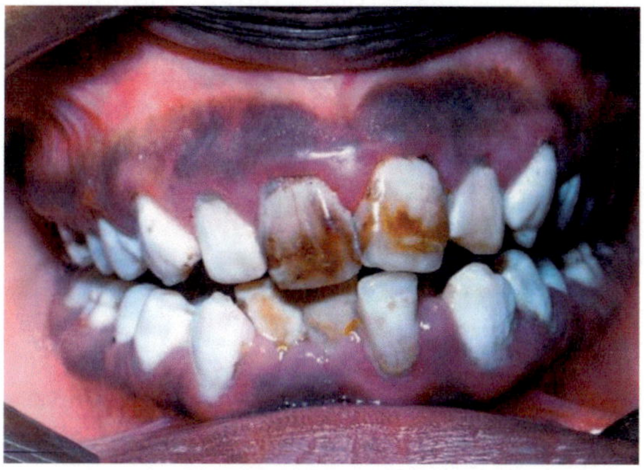

Figure 5.
Discoloration of the gingiva and teeth in a patient on minocycline therapy.

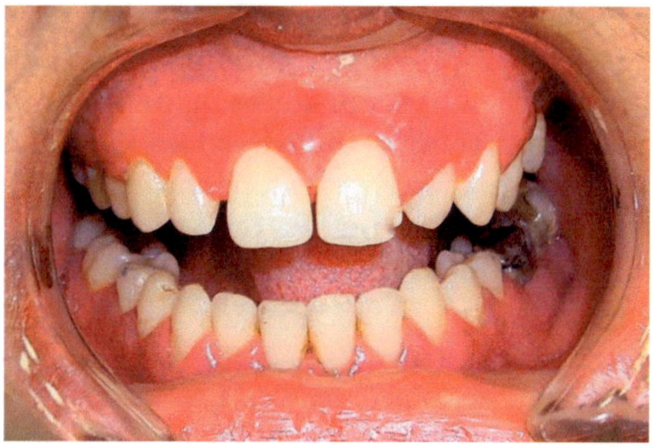

Figure 6.
Gingival changes in a patient on oral contraceptives.

Hence, it is concluded that oral contraceptives can no longer be considered to constitute a risk factor for gingivitis or periodontitis [81].

3.3 Bisphosphonates

Bisphosphonates are used widely in the management of primary and metastatic bone cancer, as well as osteoporosis. Bisphosphonates improve bone mineral density, reduce fracture risk, and reduce hypercalcemia of malignancy. Incidents of osteonecrosis of the jaw have been reported in people on bisphosphonates and undergoing invasive dental treatment procedures, including tooth extractions, dental implants, and surgical and nonsurgical periodontal treatment [82]. The risk for bisphosphonate-induced osteonecrosis may be influenced by the route of administration of the drug, the potency and the duration of use. Jaw osteonecrosis appears more associated with the intravenous use of bisphosphonates. A review showed that 94% of the published cases of osteonecrosis correlated with administration of intravenous, nitrogen-containing bisphosphonates [83].

Bisphosphonates inhibit bone resorption by acting on osteoclasts to reduce their activity or to increase the rate of apoptosis [84]. The inhibitory effect on osteoclast function, bone formation coupled with resorption results in an overall reduction in the rate of bone remodeling [85]. Moreover, bisphosphonates may antagonize the action of several matrix metalloproteinase involved in breakdown of structural components of periodontal connective tissue [86]. In view of the antiresorptive properties of bisphosphonates and the ability to inhibit cytokines of periodontal tissue destruction, there has been interest in the possible use of bisphosphonates as an adjunct to scaling and root planning in the management of periodontitis [87, 88]. Although bisphosphonates claim its effectiveness in controlling periodontal destruction, clinical use warrants further evidence. A systematic review concluded that bisphosphonates may be used topically as an adjunct to scaling and root planing [89].

3.4 Statins

Statins, or inhibitors of 3-hydroxy-3-methylglutaryl coenzyme A reductase (HMG-CoA reductase), are a group of drugs, used mainly to treat hyperlipidemia. In addition to their cholesterol lowering properties they also have strong anti-inflammatory properties and may stimulate bone growth [90]. Statins have anabolic effects on the bone by augmenting bone morphogenetic protein-2 expression and thereby contributing towards the differentiation and activity of osteoblasts [91]. Due to their activity on bone formation statins have been considered as potential agents in improving periodontal treatment outcomes [92]. Limited data is available on the impact of stains on periodontal tissues suggesting a reduction in periodontal destruction and tooth loss [93]. Experimental studies on rats support the potential protective effect of statins on periodontal bone loss. Although these basic data are interesting, further research could extrapolate the use of statins as a potential adjunctive therapeutic agent in periodontal disease and bone regeneration.

3.5 Anti-platelet drugs

Anti-platelet drugs are widely used for the treatment of established cardiovascular disease, the prevention of atherothrombotic events and the treatment of myocardial infarction. The most commonly prescribed antiplatelets drugs are aspirin and clopidogrel which are often used in combination. Both of these drugs have been reported to cause increased gingival bleeding. Patients on these medications carry a risk of an increased tendency to bleeding during or following periodontal surgery and this risk is far greater when the drugs are used in combination [94].

4. Conclusion

Several systemic factors are known to contribute to periodontal diseases or conditions and among those are the intake of drugs. The gingival overgrowth associated with medications occur as a side effect of systemic medications. These medications include the anti-seizure drug phenytoin, the immune suppressor cyclosporin A, and certain anti-hypertensive dihydropyridine calcium-channel-blockers, most notably nifedipine. It is crucial that health professionals understand the complications that medications can have on the oral health of their patients. In order to properly diagnose and treat patients, a complete medical history including prescription medications, over the counter drugs and dietary supplements must be recorded which will enable the healthcare team to identify the causative agents.

Conflict of interest

None declared.

Author details

Sukumaran Anil[1]*, Seham H.S.A. Alyafei[1], Annie Kitty George[2] and Elna Paul Chalisserry[3]

1 Department of Dentistry, Hamad Medical Corporation, Doha, Qatar

2 Department of Periodontology and Implantology, Pushpagiri College of Dental Sciences, Thiruvalla, Kerala

3 Interdisciplinary Program of Biomedical, Electrical and Mechanical Engineering, Pukyong National University, Busan, South Korea

*Address all correspondence to: drsanil@gmail.com

References

[1] Bascones-Martinez A, Munoz-Corcuera M, Bascones-Ilundain C. Side effects of drugs on the oral cavity. Medicina Clínica (Barcelona). 2015;**144**:126-131. DOI: 10.1016/j.medcli.2014.01.025

[2] Heasman PA, Hughes FJ. Drugs, medications and periodontal disease. British Dental Journal. 2014;**217**:411-419. DOI: 10.1038/sj.bdj.2014.905

[3] Ramirez-Ramiz A, Brunet LL, Lahor-Soler E, Miranda-Rius J. On the cellular and molecular mechanisms of drug-induced gingival overgrowth. The Open Dentistry Journal. 2017;**11**:420-435. DOI: 10.2174/1874210601711010420

[4] Al Sayed AA, Al Sulaiman MH, Mishriky A, Anil S. The role of androgen receptor gene in cyclosporine induced gingival overgrowth. Journal of Periodontal Research. 2014;**49**:609-614. DOI: 10.1111/jre.12141

[5] Chabria D, Weintraub RG, Kilpatrick NM. Mechanisms and management of gingival overgrowth in paediatric transplant recipients: A review. International Journal of Paediatric Dentistry. 2003;**13**:220-229. DOI: 10.1046/j.1365-263x.2003.00465.x

[6] Marshall RI, Bartold PM. Medication induced gingival overgrowth. Oral Diseases. 1998;**4**:130-151. DOI: 10.1111/j.1601-0825.1998.tb00269.x

[7] Margiotta V, Pizzo I, Pizzo G, Barbaro A. Cyclosporin- and nifedipine-induced gingival overgrowth in renal transplant patients: Correlations with periodontal and pharmacological parameters, and HLA-antigens. Journal of Oral Pathology & Medicine. 1996;**25**:128-134. DOI: 10.1111/j.1600-0714.1996.tb00207.x

[8] Seymour RA, Ellis JS, Thomason JM. Risk factors for drug-induced gingival overgrowth. Journal of Clinical Periodontology. 2000;**27**:217-223. DOI: 10.1034/j.1600-051x.2000.027004217.x

[9] Dannewitz B, Edrich C, Tomakidi P, Kohl A, Gabbert O, Eickholz P, et al. Elevated gene expression of MMP-1, MMP-10, and TIMP-1 reveal changes of molecules involved in turn-over of extracellular matrix in cyclosporine-induced gingival overgrowth. Cell and Tissue Research. 2006;**325**:513-522. DOI: 10.1007/s00441-006-0200-x

[10] Gagliano N, Moscheni C, Dellavia C, Torri C, Stabellini G, Ferrario VF, et al. Effect of cyclosporin A on human gingival fibroblast collagen turnover in relation to the development of gingival overgrowth: An in vitro study. Biomedicine & Pharmacotherapy. 2004;**58**:231-238. DOI: 10.1016/j.biopha.2003.12.011

[11] O'Valle F, Mesa F, Aneiros J, Gomez-Morales M, Lucena MA, Ramirez C, et al. Gingival overgrowth induced by nifedipine and cyclosporin A. clinical and morphometric study with image analysis. Journal of Clinical Periodontology. 1995;**22**:591-597. DOI: 10.1111/j.1600-051x.1995.tb00810.x

[12] Dongari-Bagtzoglou A, Research, Science and Therapy Committee, American Academy of Periodontology. Drug-associated gingival enlargement. Journal of Periodontology. 2004;**75**:1424-1431. DOI: 10.1902/jop.2004.75.10.1424

[13] Camargo PM, Melnick PR, Pirih FQ, Lagos R, Takei HH. Treatment of drug-induced gingival enlargement: Aesthetic and functional considerations. Periodontology 2000. 2001;**27**:131-138. DOI: 10.1034/j.1600-0757.2001.027001131.x

[14] Muralikrishna T, Kalakonda B, Gunupati S, Koppolu P. Laser-assisted

periodontal management of drug-induced gingival overgrowth under general anesthesia: A viable option. Case Reports in Dentistry. 2013;**2013**:387453. DOI: 10.1155/2013/387453

[15] Fornaini C, Rocca JP. CO_2 laser treatment of drug-induced gingival overgrowth—Case report. Laser Therapy. 2012;**21**:39-42. DOI: 10.5978/islsm.12-CR-01

[16] Tejnani A, Gandevivala A, Bhanushali D, Gourkhede S. Combined treatment for a combined enlargement. Journal of Indian Society of Periodontology. 2014;**18**:516-519. DOI: 10.4103/0972-124X.138747

[17] Thomason JM, Seymour RA, Rawlins MD. Incidence and severity of phenytoin-induced gingival overgrowth in epileptic patients in general medical practice. Community Dentistry and Oral Epidemiology. 1992;**20**:288-291. DOI: 10.1111/j.1600-0528.1992.tb01701.x

[18] Angelopoulos AP, Goaz PW. Incidence of diphenylhydantoin gingival hyperplasia. Oral Surgery, Oral Medicine, and Oral Pathology. 1972;**34**:898-906. DOI: 10.1016/0030-4220(72)90228-9

[19] Prasad VN, Chawla HS, Goyal A, Gauba K, Singhi P. Incidence of phenytoin induced gingival overgrowth in epileptic children: A six month evaluation. Journal of the Indian Society of Pedodontics and Preventive Dentistry. 2002;**20**:73-80

[20] Casetta I, Granieri E, Desidera M, Monetti VC, Tola MR, Paolino E, et al. Phenytoin-induced gingival overgrowth: A community-based cross-sectional study in Ferrara, Italy. Neuroepidemiology. 1997;**16**:296-303. DOI: 10.1159/000109700

[21] Pick L, Bauer J. Dentistry and epilepsy. Nervenarzt. 2001;**72**:946-949. DOI: 10.1007/s001150170008

[22] Suneja B, Chopra S, Thomas AM, Pandian J. A clinical evaluation of gingival overgrowth in children on antiepileptic drug therapy. Journal of Clinical and Diagnostic Research. 2016;**10**:ZC32-ZC36. DOI: 10.7860/JCDR/2016/16443.7069

[23] Katz J, Givol N, Chaushu G, Taicher S, Shemer J. Vigabatrin-induced gingival overgrowth. Journal of Clinical Periodontology. 1997;**24**:180-182. DOI: 10.1111/j.1600-051x.1997.tb00488.x

[24] Mesa F, Aguilar M, Gonzalez-Moles MA, Guerrero A, Sanchez-Alvarez JC, Del Moral RG, et al. Vigabatrin-induced modification of Ki-67 expression in gingival epithelium: Immunohistochemical study of a short series. Journal of Periodontal Research. 2004;**39**:66-71. DOI: 10.1111/j.1600-0765.2004.00711.x

[25] Conde SA, Aarestrup FM, Vieira BJ, Bastos MG. Roxithromycin reduces cyclosporine-induced gingival hyperplasia in renal transplant patients. Transplantation Proceedings. 2008;**40**:1435-1438. DOI: 10.1016/j.transproceed.2008.04.012

[26] Cebeci I, Kantarci A, Firatli E, Aygun S, Tanyeri H, Aydin AE, et al. Evaluation of the frequency of HLA determinants in patients with gingival overgrowth induced by cyclosporine-A. Journal of Clinical Periodontology. 1996;**23**:737-742. DOI: 10.1111/j.1600-051x.1996.tb00603.x

[27] Kataoka M, Kido J, Shinohara Y, Nagata T. Drug-induced gingival overgrowth—A review. Biological and Pharmaceutical Bulletin. 2005;**28**:1817-1821. DOI: 10.1248/bpb.28.1817

[28] Ellis JS, Seymour RA, Taylor JJ, Thomason JM. Prevalence of

gingival overgrowth in transplant patients immunosuppressed with tacrolimus. Journal of Clinical Periodontology. 2004;**31**:126-131. DOI: 10.1111/j.0303-6979.2004.00459.x

[29] Ellis JS, Seymour RA, Steele JG, Robertson P, Butler TJ, Thomason JM. Prevalence of gingival overgrowth induced by calcium channel blockers: A community-based study. Journal of Periodontology. 1999;**70**:63-67. DOI: 10.1902/jop.1999.70.1.63

[30] Miranda J, Brunet L, Roset P, Berini L, Farre M, Mendieta C. Prevalence and risk of gingival enlargement in patients treated with nifedipine. Journal of Periodontology. 2001;**72**:605-611. DOI: 10.1902/jop.2001.72.5.605

[31] Fattore L, Stablein M, Bredfeldt G, Semla T, Moran M, Doherty-Greenberg JM. Gingival hyperplasia: A side effect of nifedipine and diltiazem. Special Care in Dentistry. 1991;**11**:107-109. DOI: 10.1111/j.1754-4505.1991.tb00828.x

[32] Steele RM, Schuna AA, Schreiber RT. Calcium antagonist-induced gingival hyperplasia. Annals of Internal Medicine. 1994;**120**:663-664. DOI: 10.7326/0003-4819-120-8-199404150-00006

[33] Miller CS, Damm DD. Incidence of verapamil-induced gingival hyperplasia in a dental population. Journal of Periodontology. 1992;**63**:453-456. DOI: 10.1902/jop.1992.63.5.453

[34] Jorgensen MG. Prevalence of amlodipine-related gingival hyperplasia. Journal of Periodontology. 1997;**68**:676-678. DOI: 10.1902/jop.1997.68.7.676

[35] Sucu M, Yuce M, Davutoglu V. Amlodipine-induced massive gingival hypertrophy Canadian family physician. Medecin de Famille Canadien. 2011;**57**:436-437

[36] Lombardi T, Fiore-Donno G, Belser U, Di Felice R. Felodipine-induced gingival hyperplasia: A clinical and histologic study. Journal of Oral Pathology & Medicine. 1991;**20**:89-92. DOI: 10.1111/j.1600-0714.1991.tb00896.x

[37] Majola MP, McFadyen ML, Connolly C, Nair YP, Govender M, LaherMH.Factorsinfluencingphenytoin-induced gingival enlargement. Journal of Clinical Periodontology. 2000;**27**:506-512. DOI: 10.1034/j.1600-051x.2000.027007506.x

[38] Faulds D, Goa KL, Benfield P. Cyclosporin. A review of its pharmacodynamic and pharmacokinetic properties, and therapeutic use in immunoregulatory disorders. Drugs. 1993;**45**:953-1040. DOI: 10.2165/00003495-199345060-00007

[39] Ting LS, Villeneuve E, Ensom MH. Beyond cyclosporine: A systematic review of limited sampling strategies for other immunosuppressants. Therapeutic Drug Monitoring. 2006;**28**:419-430. DOI: 10.1097/01.ftd.0000211810.19935.44

[40] Seymour RA, Jacobs DJ. Cyclosporin and the gingival tissues. Journal of Clinical Periodontology. 1992;**19**:1-11. DOI: 10.1111/j.1600-051x.1992.tb01140.x

[41] Fahr A. Cyclosporin clinical pharmacokinetics. Clinical Pharmacokinetics. 1993;**24**:472-495. DOI: 10.2165/00003088-199324060-00004

[42] de Oliveira Costa F, Diniz Ferreira S, de Miranda Cota LO, da Costa JE, Aguiar MA. Prevalence, severity, and risk variables associated with gingival overgrowth in renal transplant subjects treated under tacrolimus or cyclosporin regimens. Journal of Periodontology. 2006;**77**:969-975. DOI: 10.1902/jop.2006.050327

[43] Oliveira Costa F, Ferreira SD, Lages EJ, Costa JE, Oliveira AM, Cota LO. Demographic, pharmacologic, and periodontal variables for gingival overgrowth in subjects medicated with cyclosporin in the absence of calcium channel blockers. Journal of Periodontology. 2007;**78**:254-261. DOI: 10.1902/jop.2007.050445

[44] Cota LO, Aquino DR, Franco GC, Cortelli JR, Cortelli SC, Costa FO. Gingival overgrowth in subjects under immunosuppressive regimens based on cyclosporine, tacrolimus, or sirolimus. Journal of Clinical Periodontology. 2010;**37**:894-902. DOI: 10.1111/j.1600-051X.2010.01601.x

[45] Daley TD, Wysocki GP, Day C. Clinical and pharmacologic correlations in cyclosporine-induced gingival hyperplasia. Oral Surgery, Oral Medicine, and Oral Pathology. 1986;**62**:417-421. DOI: 10.1016/0030-4220(86)90291-4

[46] Pernu HE, Pernu LM, Huttunen KR, Nieminen PA, Knuuttila ML. Gingival overgrowth among renal transplant recipients related to immunosuppressive medication and possible local background factors. Journal of Periodontology. 1992;**63**:548-553. DOI: 10.1902/jop.1992.63.6.548

[47] Schincaglia GP, Forniti F, Cavallini R, Piva R, Calura G, del Senno L. Cyclosporin-A increases type I procollagen production and mRNA level in human gingival fibroblasts in vitro. Journal of Oral Pathology & Medicine. 1992;**21**:181-185. DOI: 10.1111/j.1600-0714.1992.tb00098.x

[48] Fu MM, Chin YT, Fu E, Chiu HC, Wang LY, Chiang CY, et al. Role of transforming growth factor-beta1 in cyclosporine-induced epithelial-to-mesenchymal transition in gingival epithelium. Journal of Periodontology. 2015;**86**:120-128. DOI: 10.1902/jop.2014.130285

[49] Malek R, El Houari B, Kissa J. Periodontal management of cyclosporin A-induced gingival overgrowth: A nonsurgical approach. Case Reports in Dentistry. 2019;**2019**:8609547. DOI: 10.1155/2019/8609547

[50] Ramalho VL, Ramalho HJ, Cipullo JP, Azoubel R, Burdmann EA. Comparison of azithromycin and oral hygiene program in the treatment of cyclosporine-induced gingival hyperplasia. Renal Failure. 2007;**29**:265-270. DOI: 10.1080/08860220701263580

[51] Gau CH, Tu HP, Chin YT, Chen RY, Fu MM, Fu E. Can chlorhexidine mouthwash twice daily ameliorate cyclosporine-induced gingival overgrowth? Journal of the Formosan Medical Association = Taiwan yi zhi. 2013;**112**:131-137. DOI: 10.1016/j.jfma.2011.12.004

[52] Pilatti GL, Sampaio JE. The influence of chlorhexidine on the severity of cyclosporin A-induced gingival overgrowth. Journal of Periodontology. 1997;**68**:900-904. DOI: 10.1902/jop.1997.68.9.900

[53] Morgan TO, Anderson AI, MacInnis RJ. ACE inhibitors, beta-blockers, calcium blockers, and diuretics for the control of systolic hypertension. American Journal of Hypertension. 2001;**14**:241-247. DOI: 10.1016/s0895-7061(00)01266-8

[54] Seymour RA. Effects of medications on the periodontal tissues in health and disease. Periodontology 2000. 2006;**40**:120-129. DOI: 10.1111/j.1600-0757.2005.00137.x

[55] Lederman D, Lumerman H, Reuben S, Freedman PD. Gingival hyperplasia associated with nifedipine therapy. Report of a case. Oral Surgery, Oral Medicine, and Oral Pathology. 1984;**57**:620-622. DOI: 10.1016/0030-4220(84)90283-4

[56] Ramon Y, Behar S, Kishon Y, Engelberg IS. Gingival hyperplasia caused by nifedipine—A preliminary report. International Journal of Cardiology. 1984;**5**:195-206. DOI: 10.1016/0167-5273(84)90145-1

[57] Lucas RM, Howell LP, Wall BA. Nifedipine-induced gingival hyperplasia. A histochemical and ultrastructural study. Journal of Periodontology. 1985;**56**:211-215. DOI: 10.1902/jop.1985.56.4.211

[58] Trackman PC, Kantarci A. Molecular and clinical aspects of drug-induced gingival overgrowth. Journal of Dental Research. 2015;**94**:540-546. DOI: 10.1177/0022034515571265

[59] Mishra MB, Khan ZY, Mishra S. Gingival overgrowth and drug association: A review. Indian Journal of Medical Science. 2011;**65**:73-82. DOI: 10.4103/0019-5359.103971

[60] Barak S, Engelberg IS, Hiss J. Gingival hyperplasia caused by nifedipine. Histopathologic findings. Journal of Periodontology. 1987;**58**:639-642. DOI: 10.1902/jop.1987.58.9.639

[61] Lauritano D, Lucchese A, Di Stasio D, Della Vella F, Cura F, Palmieri A, et al. Molecular aspects of drug-induced gingival overgrowth: An in vitro study on amlodipine and gingival fibroblasts. International Journal of Molecular Sciences. 2019;**20**:2047. DOI: 10.3390/ijms20082047

[62] Lafzi A, Farahani RM, Shoja MA. Amlodipine-induced gingival hyperplasia. Medicina Oral, Patologia Oral y Cirugia Bucal. 2006;**11**:E480-E482

[63] Gaur S, Agnihotri R. Is dental plaque the only etiological factor in amlodipine induced gingival overgrowth? A systematic review of evidence. Journal of Clinical and Experimental Dentistry. 2018;**10**:e610-e6e9. DOI: 10.4317/jced.54715

[64] Nanda T, Singh B, Sharma P, Arora KS. Cyclosporine A and amlodipine induced gingival overgrowth in a kidney transplant recipient: Case presentation with literature review. BMJ Case Report. 2019;**12**. DOI: 10.1136/bcr-2019-229587

[65] Pernu HE, Oikarinen K, Hietanen J, Knuuttila M. Verapamil-induced gingival overgrowth: A clinical, histologic, and biochemic approach. Journal of Oral Pathology & Medicine. 1989;**18**:422-425. DOI: 10.1111/j.1600-0714.1989.tb01576.x

[66] Saivin S, Houin G. Clinical pharmacokinetics of doxycycline and minocycline. Clinical Pharmacokinetics. 1988;**15**:355-366. DOI: 10.2165/00003088-198815060-00001

[67] Berger RS, Mandel EB, Hayes TJ, Grimwood RR. Minocycline staining of the oral cavity. Journal of the American Academy of Dermatology. 1989;**21**:1300-1301. DOI: 10.1016/s0190-9622(89)80309-3

[68] Noonan VL, Kabani S, Wu J. Minocycline-induced staining of the oral cavity. Journal of the Massachusetts Dental Society. 2009;**57**:42

[69] LaPorta VN, Nikitakis NG, Sindler AJ, Reynolds MA. Minocycline-associated intra-oral soft-tissue pigmentation: Clinicopathologic correlations and review. Journal of Clinical Periodontology. 2005;**32**:119-122. DOI: 10.1111/j.1600-051X.2005.00646.x

[70] Siller GM, Tod MA, Savage NW. Minocycline-induced oral pigmentation. Journal of the American Academy of Dermatology.

1994;**30**:350-354. DOI: 10.1016/s0190-9622(94)70038-9

[71] Friedman IS, Shelton RM, Phelps RG. Minocycline-induced hyperpigmentation of the tongue: Successful treatment with the Q-switched ruby laser. Dermatologic Surgery. 2002;**28**:205-209. DOI: 10.1046/j.1524-4725.2002.01083.x

[72] Eisen D, Hakim MD. Minocycline-induced pigmentation. Incidence, prevention and management. Drug Safety. 1998;**18**:431-440. DOI: 10.2165/00002018-199818060-00004

[73] Domingues R S, Ferraz B F, Greghi SL, Rezende M L, Passanezi E, Sant'Ana AC. Influence of combined oral contraceptives on the periodontal condition. Journal of Applied Oral Science: Revista FOB 2012;**20**:253-259. DOI: 10.1590/s1678-77572012000200022

[74] Mullally BH, Coulter WA, Hutchinson JD, Clarke HA. Current oral contraceptive status and periodontitis in young adults. Journal of Periodontology. 2007;**78**:1031-1036. DOI: 10.1902/jop.2007.060163

[75] Pankhurst CL, Waite IM, Hicks KA, Allen Y, Harkness RD. The influence of oral contraceptive therapy on the periodontium—Duration of drug therapy. Journal of Periodontology. 1981;**52**:617-620. DOI: 10.1902/jop.1981.52.10.617

[76] Mariotti A. Sex steroid hormones and cell dynamics in the periodontium. Critical Reviews in Oral Biology & Medicine. 1994;**5**:27-53. DOI: 10.1177/10454411940050010201

[77] Prachi S, Jitender S, Rahul C, Jitendra K, Priyanka M, Disha S. Impact of oral contraceptives on periodontal health. African Health Sciences. 2019;**19**:1795-1800. DOI: 10.4314/ahs.v19i1.56

[78] Mealey BL, Moritz AJ. Hormonal influences: Effects of diabetes mellitus and endogenous female sex steroid hormones on the periodontium. Periodontology 2000. 2003;**32**:59-81. DOI: 10.1046/j.0906-6713.2002.03206.x

[79] Mistry S, Bhowmick D. Oral contraceptive pill induced periodontal endocrinopathies and its management: A case report. European Journal of Dentistry. 2012;**6**:324-329

[80] Haerian-Ardakani A, Moeintaghavi A, Talebi-Ardakani MR, Sohrabi K, Bahmani S, Dargahi M. The association between current low-dose oral contraceptive pills and periodontal health: A matched-case-control study. The Journal of Contemporary Dental Practice. 2010;**11**:033-040

[81] Preshaw PM. Oral contraceptives and the periodontium. Periodontology 2000. 2013;**61**:125-159. DOI: 10.1111/j.1600-0757.2011.00399.x

[82] AnilS, PreethanathRS, AlMoharibHS, Kamath KP, Anand PS. Impact of osteoporosis and its treatment on oral health. American Journal of Medical Science. 2013;**346**:396-401. DOI: 10.1097/MAJ.0b013e31828983da

[83] Mucke T, Krestan CR, Mitchell DA, Kirschke JS, Wutzl A. Bisphosphonate and medication-related osteonecrosis of the jaw: A review. Seminars in Musculoskeletal Radiology. 2016;**20**:305-314. DOI: 10.1055/s-0036-1592367

[84] Rogers MJ. From molds and macrophages to mevalonate: A decade of progress in understanding the molecular mode of action of bisphosphonates. Calcified Tissue International. 2004;**75**:451-461. DOI: 10.1007/s00223-004-0024-1

[85] Bellido T, Plotkin LI. Novel actions of bisphosphonates in bone: Preservation of osteoblast and osteocyte

viability. Bone. 2011;**49**:50-55. DOI: 10.1016/j.bone.2010.08.008

[86] Franco C, Patricia HR, Timo S, Claudia B, Marcela H. Matrix metalloproteinases as regulators of periodontal inflammation. International Journal of Molecular Science. 2017;**18**:440. DOI: 10.3390/ijms18020440

[87] Pradeep AR, Kumari M, Rao NS, Naik SB. 1% alendronate gel as local drug delivery in the treatment of Class II furcation defects: A randomized controlled clinical trial. Journal of Periodontology. 2013;**84**:307-315. DOI: 10.1902/jop.2012.110729

[88] Bhavsar NV, Trivedi SR, Dulani K, Brahmbhatt N, Shah S, Chaudhri D. Clinical and radiographic evaluation of effect of risedronate 5 mg as an adjunct to treatment of chronic periodontitis in postmenopausal women (12-month study). Osteoporosis International. 2016;**27**:2611-2619. DOI: 10.1007/s00198-016-3577-8

[89] Akram Z, Abduljabbar T, Kellesarian SV, Abu Hassan MI, Javed F, Vohra F. Efficacy of bisphosphonate as an adjunct to nonsurgical periodontal therapy in the management of periodontal disease: A systematic review. British Journal of Clinical Pharmacology. 2017;**83**:444-454. DOI: 10.1111/bcp.13147

[90] Lindy O, Suomalainen K, Makela M, Lindy S. Statin use is associated with fewer periodontal lesions: A retrospective study. BMC Oral Health. 2008;**8**:16. DOI: 10.1186/1472-6831-8-16

[91] Zhou H, Xie Y, Baloch Z, Shi Q, Huo Q, Ma T. The effect of atorvastatin, 3-hydroxy-3-methylglutaryl coenzyme A reductase inhibitor (HMG-CoA), on the prevention of osteoporosis in ovariectomized rabbits. Journal of Bone and Mineral Metabolism. 2017;**35**:245-254. DOI: 10.1007/s00774-016-0750-2

[92] Pradeep AR, Garg V, Kanoriya D, Singhal S. 1.2% rosuvastatin versus 1.2% atorvastatin gel local drug delivery and redelivery in treatment of intrabony defects in chronic periodontitis: A randomized placebo-controlled clinical trial. Journal of Periodontology. 2016;**87**:756-762. DOI: 10.1902/jop.2016.150706

[93] Santos BF, Souza EQ, Brigagao MR, Lima DC, Fernandes LA. Local application of statins in the treatment of experimental periodontal disease in rats. Journal of Applied Oral Science: Revista FOB. 2017;**25**:168-176. DOI: 10.1590/1678-77572016-0149

[94] Graziani F, Cei S, Guerrero A, La Ferla F, Vano M, Tonetti M, et al. Lack of short-term adjunctive effect of systemic neridronate in non-surgical periodontal therapy of advanced generalized chronic periodontitis: An open label-randomized clinical trial. Journal of Clinical Periodontology. 2009;**36**:419-427. DOI: 10.1111/j.1600-051X.2009.01388.x

Section 2

Oral Oncology

Chapter 6

Potentially Malignant Oral Disorders

Márcio Campos Oliveira, Igor Ferreira Borba de Almeida, Almira Oliveira Pereira and Maria da Conceição Andrade

Abstract

Most cancerous lesions are derived from potentially malignant oral disorders (PMOD). The World Health Organization (WHO) points out the following lesions as the main PMOD: leukoplakia, erythroplakia, actinic cheilitis, submucous fibrosis, and lichen planus. Leukoplakias are white plaques or spots that cannot be removed by scraping, and these lesions aren't characterized clinically or pathologically like any other diseases. Erythroplakias are red lesions of the oral mucosa that also cannot be characterized clinically or pathologically as another definable disease. Actinic cheilitis is an injury that affects the vermilion of the lower lip and has this anatomical location due to its etiological factor, which is the progressive and excessive exposure to ultraviolet rays of sunlight. Submucous fibrosis is a chronic disease of the mouth that presents as an inflammatory subepithelial reaction, followed by an alteration in the submucous fibroelastic tissue. Lichen planus is a dermatological disease characterized by white patches or striations, symmetrical and bilateral, and its treatment is basically done with topical corticosteroids.

Keywords: potentially malignant oral disorders, leukoplakia, erythroplasia, actinic cheilitis, lichen planus

1. Introduction

Head and neck cancer is a worldwide public health problem, and according to the International Agency for Research on Cancer (IARC) in 2018, 1,454,892 new cases of head and neck cancer worldwide have been estimated. When all the sites involving the head and neck region added, these tumors occupy the third place, behind only the lung tumors (2,093,876) and the breast (2,088,849) [1]. By analyzing the sexes separately, head and neck tumors are the fourth most common cause of cancer in men (796,946 cases), behind lung, prostate, and colorectal cancer. In women, they are also the fourth most common cause (657,966 cases), behind breast, colorectal, and lung cancer, and thyroid tumors are the most frequent in this population (436,344 cases). In Brazil, according to the National Cancer Institute (INCA), there is an estimated 11,200 new cases of cancer of the oral cavity in men and 3,500 in women for each year of the 2018–2019 biennium, placing this neoplasm in fifth place in the prevalence [2].

The incidence can change by region of the world. In developing countries, in men, lip and oral cavity cancer alone is the third in incidence, partly because of the high disease rate in India, which accounts for 36% of the population of countries with low human development index (IDH) [2].

 IntechOpen

Understanding the world statistics on cancer, more specifically on head and neck cancer, is essential in order to propose measures of prevention and early diagnosis, such as anti-smoking policies, HPV vaccination, and improvement of the oral health and diet of the population. Such measures would have a significant impact on the incidence and mortality of this disease [2].

Among the risk factors, potentially malignant oral disorders have a prominence, since they are generally the first indication of the disease [3]. The World Health Organization (WHO), in its latest publication, has defined PMSD as clinical presentations that carry a risk of developing oral cavity cancer, a clinically defined precursor lesion or clinically normal oral mucosa [4]. The WHO identifies as PMOD the following disorders: erythroplakia, erythroleukoplakia, leukoplakia, oral submucous fibrosis (OSF), congenital dyskeratosis, smokeless tobacco keratosis, palatine lesions associated with reverse smoking, chronic candidiasis, lichen planus, discoid lupus erythematosus, glossitis syphilitic, and actinic cheilitis. In this chapter, we will discuss the most common PMODs with the highest potential for malignant transformation, which are leukoplakias, erythroplasias, oral lichen planus, actinic cheilitis and oral submucous fibrosis [1, 4].

2. Leukoplakia

According to the WHO, leukoplakia is defined as a white, variable-risk plaque, excluding (other) known diseases or disorders that do not carry an increased risk of cancer; therefore, the nomenclature is restricted only to the clinical aspect and histological changes. Due to the fact that its clinical diagnosis is basically made by exclusion, this disorder makes a differential diagnosis with other well-known lesions and with very similar clinical characteristics such as pseudomembranous candidiasis, Lichen planus, leukoedema, and lupus erythematosus [5]. The specific causative factors of leukoplakia are still unknown; however, it is known that the smoking habit is closely linked to the progression of leukoplakia. In addition, other risk factors have been associated with the development of this disorder, the consumption of alcohol that would act synergistically with tobacco, trauma, as well as infestations of microorganisms such as human papillomavirus (HPV) [6].

Oral leukoplakia is the most common PMOD, presenting a prevalence of 1% and an annual malignant transformation risk of 2%. It is found in equal proportion between men and women, rarely occurs in the first two decades of life, and is more prevalent among individuals, and this is their main etiological factor. The anatomical sites in which about 70% of the leukoplakia are found are jugal mucosa, gingiva, and vermillion of the lip; however, lesions located on the tongue and floor of the mouth contribute to over 90% of the cases that present some level of dysplasia or even a carcinoma [6–8].

Clinically the leukoplakias are subdivided into homogeneous and nonhomogeneous. Homogeneous leukoplakias are characterized as uniformly flat and thin lesions that have a low percentage of malignant transformation, as well as spontaneous regression after elimination of risk factors, especially smoking habit (**Figure 1**) [3, 9]. Nonhomogeneous leukoplakias are described as white and red lesions (erythroleukoplakias), which may appear irregularly flat or nodular, and are subdivided into a variety of subtypes, such as erythematous or speckled, nodular and verrucous (**Figure 2**). Verrucous leukoplakia, one of the most misdiagnosed subtypes of nonhomogeneous leukoplakia because of its challenging clinical appearance, although presenting as a uniform white lesion, its verrucous texture is the characteristic that differentiates it from homogeneous leukoplakia (**Figure 3**) [10]. Proliferative

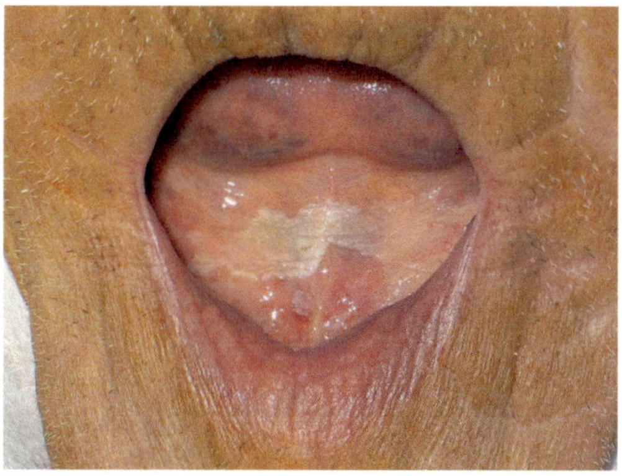

Figure 1.
Homogeneous leucoplakia on the floor of the mouth. Source: author's file.

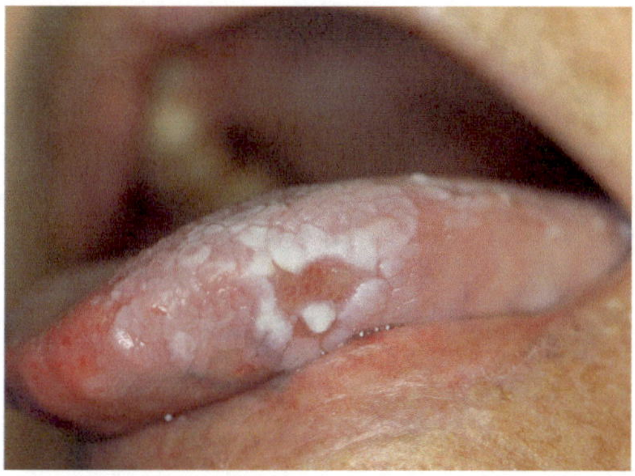

Figure 2.
Nonhomogeneous leucoplakia on the back and lateral edge of the tongue. Source: author's file.

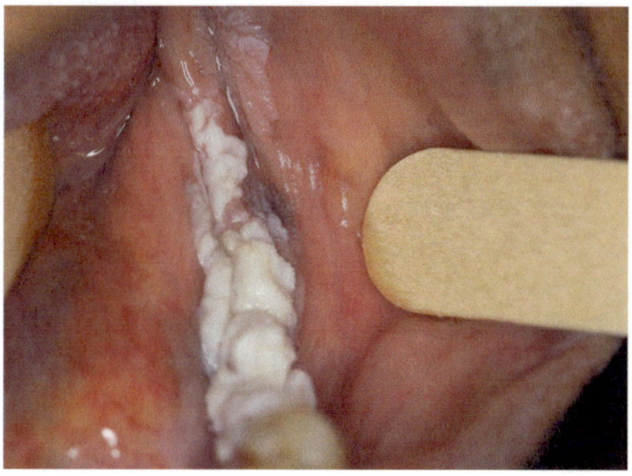

Figure 3.
Exuberant verrucous leukoplakia in the alveolar ridge. Source: author's file.

verrucous leukoplakia (PVL) is a very rare form and falls between nonhomogeneous leukoplakias and is a subtype of verrucous leukoplakia. It's a distinct, multifocal, progressive course associated with high rates of recurrence and malignant transformation [4]. PVL mainly affects middle-aged women with no harmful habits such as smoking and presents clinically as a diffuse and homogeneous white

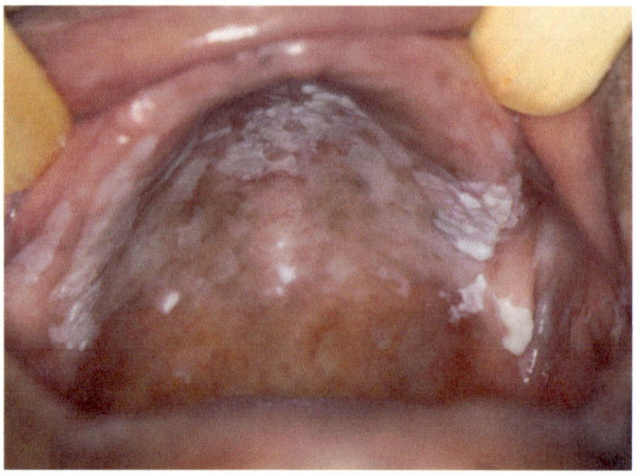

Figure 4.
Proliferative verrucous leukoplakia affecting the hard palate and alveolar ridge. Source: author's file.

plaque at the onset, which gradually becomes erythematous and exophytic with the progression of the disorder, affecting mainly the gingiva, alveolar mucosa, and palate (**Figure 4**) [4, 6, 11].

Regarding the histopathological characteristics of leukoplakia, a thick layer of keratin in the epithelium (hyperkeratosis) is present, with or without thickening of the thorny layer (acanthosis). It is still possible to observe in some leukoplakia the presence of hyperkeratosis with epithelial atrophy. Generally, leukoplastic lesions do not exhibit epithelial dysplasias, but the presence of them would be a worrying sign for a possible malignant transformation, a fact that is most observed among nonhomogeneous leukoplakias [4, 6].

The diagnosis of leukoplakia is basically by excluding other diseases or disorders that do not carry increased risk of malignant transformation. In order to perform an accurate diagnosis of leukoplakia, different levels of leukoplakia must be followed by certainties (factor C) that lead us from a primary clinical diagnosis to the definitive diagnosis based on the histopathological examination of the lesion [4, 6].

Thus, in the van der Waal factor, C1 evidence is obtained in a single visit, in the first contact between the dental surgeon and patient, applying only palpation and inspection as the primary means for diagnosis, in addition to anamnesis to collect data that may make up this provisional clinical diagnosis. In the certainty factor C2, evidence is obtained from negative results of elimination of etiological factors such as mechanical irritation, during a period of follow-up of 2–4 weeks or in the absence of any suspicious etiological factors (definitive clinical diagnosis). Factor C3 is similar to C2 but complemented by incisional biopsy (provisional histopathological diagnosis), and C4 is the evidence obtained from surgical excision of the lesion followed by histopathological examination of the resected specimen (definitive histopathological diagnosis) [11, 12]. Performing biopsy in the diagnosis of leukoplakia is important because only through this examination it is possible to determine whether to perform the histopathological diagnosis or not of epithelial dysplasias, thus guiding the treatment [12].

The treatment of leukoplastic lesions is dependent on the result found in the histopathological examination; in this way, the treatment plan is often individualized according to the histological findings, such as the degree of dysplasia found in the epithelium. The WHO in its latest manual for the classification of head and neck tumors (2017) defines dysplasias as architectural and cytological epithelial changes caused by an accumulation of genetic alterations associated with an increased risk of progression to squamous cell carcinoma. Therefore, in lesions that present mild dysplasia or do not present dysplasia, more conservative measures should be taken, such as clinical follow-up of the lesion every 6 months throughout life, evaluation of the need for new biopsies, and end of smoking [3, 10]. In leukoplakias that present moderate or severe dysplasia/carcinoma in situ, it is recommended that the lesion be removed completely, if possible, or by CO2 laser therapy. However, even with the surgical treatment, there appears to be no reduction in the risk of developing a carcinoma or even relapse of the leukoplakial lesion [6, 7, 10].

Regarding the prognosis of leukoplastic lesions, recurrence rates after any type of treatment can range from almost 0 to 30%, which means regular follow-up of patients every 6 months [10].

3. Erythroplakia

Erythroplakia is defined as "a red spot that can't be characterized clinically or pathologically like any other definable disease" [4]. When a mixture of red and white changes occurs, this lesion would be classified as a nonhomogeneous leukoplakia called erythroleukoplakia [10]. Erythroplakia is multifactorial, since no isolated etiological factor has been evident, but several intrinsic and extrinsic etiological factors have contributed to the origin of this disorder, such as smoking, alcohol consumption, candida infection, and even nutritional deficiencies such as iron and vitamin A deficiency [6].

Erythroplakia in comparison to leukoplastic lesions is rare and has a prevalence rate in South and Southeast Asia ranging from 0.02 to 0.83% but presents a high percentage of malignant transformation ranging from 14 to 50%, and about 90% of cases already present moderate or severe dysplasia/carcinoma in situ. Because of the high rates of malignant transformation and the presence of high-grade dysplasias, many specialists have already considered it a primordial clinical sign of squamous cell carcinoma. It is a prevalent disorder in middle-aged adults in the elderly, aged between 45 and 74 years, with no prevalence among the genders [6, 10, 13].

Clinically, erythroplakia presents as a well delimited, asymptomatic, reddish, smooth and shiny stain or plaque with a soft and velvety texture [3, 6]. If hardened areas are observed in the lesion, it is already indicative of the presence of a possible invasive carcinoma at the site. The preferred anatomical location is the floor of the mouth, but it can be observed anywhere in the oral cavity, such as the lip, hard palate, or oral mucosa [3]. The clinical presentation of a solitary lesion is consistently useful to clinically differentiate erythroplakia from erosive lichen planus, lupus erythematosus, and erythematous candidiasis, as these lesions always appear bilaterally and are more or less symmetrical (**Figure 5**) [10].

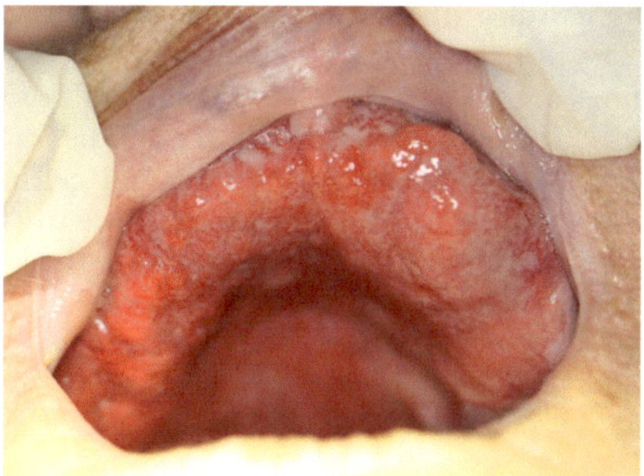

Figure 5.
Erythroplakia affecting palate and superior alveolar ridge. Source: author's file.

Histopathologically, 90% of erythroplakia present as severe epithelial dysplasias/carcinomas in situ or squamous cell carcinomas. The epithelium will show no production of keratin and is regularly atrophic. This absence of keratin associated with epithelial atrophy allows the underlying microvasculature to be exposed, thereby elucidating the reddish coloration of the lesion. In relation to connective tissue, it regularly exposes chronic inflammation [9].

The diagnosis of erythroplakia, as well as leukoplakias, is made by exclusion. This disorder presents clinically very similar to other lesions commonly found in the oral cavity, such as vascular lesions, candidiasis, mucosites, and even Kaposi's sarcoma. Because it has so many options for differential diagnosis, as in leukoplakia, one can use the steps or factors of analysis guided by Isaac van der Waal (factors C1, C2, C3, and C4) [10]. In addition, lesions on the floor of the mouth and belly regions and lateral border of tongue should be biopsied, since in some anatomical locations, the highest rates of malignant transformation occur and the presence of high degree dysplasia. With the accomplishment of the biopsy, for diagnostic purposes, it will be possible to verify the presence or absence of dysplasias. According to Neville et al. [6], 90% of the erythroplakia already present severe epithelial dysplasias/carcinomas in situ [9].

As in leukoplakias, the treatment plan for erythroplakia is guided by the definitive diagnosis obtained only after the histopathological examination. In the absence of dysplasia or presence of mild dysplasias, the lesion is monitored every 6 months, and if there is any change, perform a biopsy to check if any dysplastic modification has occurred. In lesions presenting moderate to severe dysplasia/carcinoma in situ, complete removal of the lesion should be done with safety margin. As with leukoplakia, total excision of the lesion does not guarantee that there is no recurrence of erythroplakia; in addition to the fact that this disorder already has high levels of malignant transformation, its removal does not exclude the likelihood of future cancerous lesions on the site or in other oral locations. Something that should be very clear regarding the treatment of erythroplakia and other PMOD is that the patient who has one of these disorders will never be medically released, as these must be followed for life to assess whether or not there was any dysplastic or even the appearance of cancerous lesions in other oral sites [3, 6, 10].

4. Oral lichen planus

Oral lichen planus is a chronic and systemic mucocutaneous disease often found in the oral cavity, but it can also affect other body parts such as the skin, nails, scalp, and vaginal mucosa. The British physician, Erasmus Wilson, in 1869, was the first to describe lichen planus, and he believed that the cause of this disorder would be fungal infections [6, 14]. Thus, the pathophysiology of OLP for years has been a mystery, but it is known that this disorder occurs due to T-cell-mediated autoimmune destruction of the basal cells of the epithelium. Recently it was considered a PMOD, after several discussions among scholars, due to the fact that the lesion shows a low degree of malignant transformation, around 0.5% [13, 14].

The etiological factors for this disorder are still unknown, but it is believed to be related to stress, anxiety, diabetes, autoimmune diseases, and genetic predisposition [15]. Stress and anxiety may not have total influence on the pathogenesis of lichen planus, but it has been observed that patients with this disorder are usually subjected to high levels of stress [6].

Oral lichen planus affects between 0.5 and 2% of the population, having a predilection for women between the ages of 30 and 60 years, being a rare disorder in children [6, 15]. The main intraoral sites of lichen planus are the jugal mucosa, tongue, and gingiva. An important feature of this lesion is bilaterality and symmetry [14].

Clinically, oral lichen planus is characterized by six distinct forms: reticular, erosive, bullous, plaque, papular, and atrophic, with reticular and erosive forms being the most prevalent. The reticular OLP is routinely present in the posterior jugal mucosa bilaterally. Other anatomical areas may be affected, such as the lateral border and back of the tongue, gingiva, palate, and vermilion lips [6, 15]. This type of OLP is much more common than erosive, but the latter is the most studied because it is symptomatic, which leads more patients to seek treatment specialists [6]. The reticular type is thus defined by its appearance of intertwined and asymptomatic white striations, the pathognomonic sign of the disorder being the Wickham striae (**Figure 6**). In the erosive type, erythematous and atrophic areas are observed, with varying degrees of central ulceration, and at the periphery of the atrophic regions, fine irradiated white streaks are usually observed (**Figure 7**) [6, 14, 15]. If the erosive state is aggravated, a separation between the epithelium and the underlying connective tissue may occur, resulting in a rare clinical presentation of oral bullous lichen planus [6].

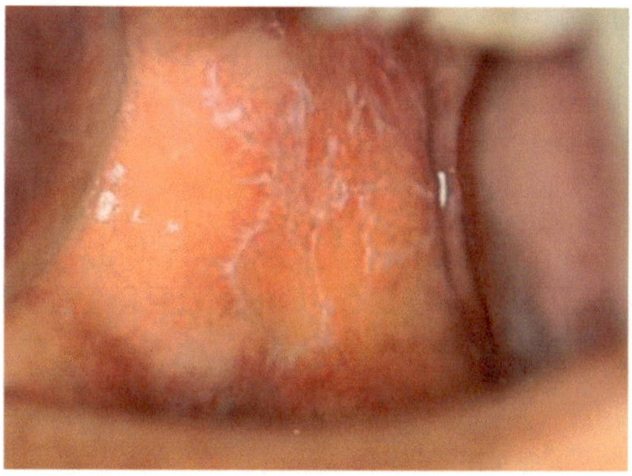

Figure 6.
Lichen planus on jugal mucosa, showing Wickham striations. Source: author's file.

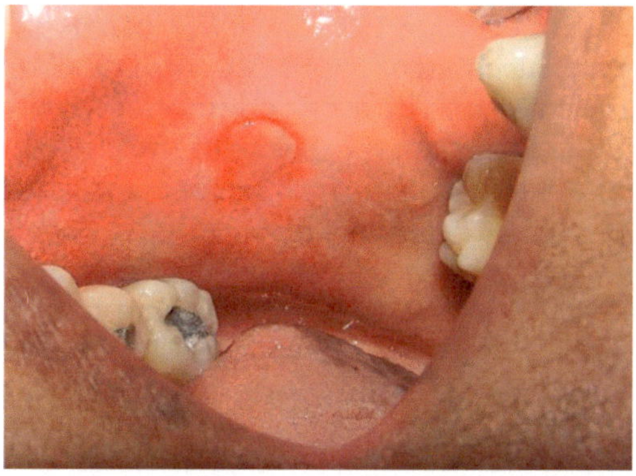

Figure 7.
Erosive lichen planus on jugal mucosa. Source: author's file.

Lichen planus has typical histopathological characteristics, but they are not specific for the lesion. Its epithelium has varying degrees of orthokeratosis and parakeratosis, and depending on whether the lesion is reticular or erosive, the thickness of the thorny layer may vary. Epithelial ridges may be absent, atrophic, or hyperplastic but usually exhibit sharp, serrate-like progressions. Another striking feature is the presence of hydropic degeneration, that is, the destruction of the basal cell layer of the epithelium and an intense infiltration of banded inflammatory cells predominantly composed of T lymphocytes. Some lesions of lichen planus may show some degree of dysplasia, being able to present aberrant mitoses and nuclear and cellular pleomorphisms, among other dysplastic alterations [6, 16].

The diagnosis of OLP is basically made by clinical findings, mainly in the reticular type, by the presence of the pathognomonic signal (Wickham striae). In addition to the clinical diagnosis, the histopathological examination may be requested for a definitive diagnosis. One thing that can make it difficult to diagnose OLP is the existence of candidiasis overlapping with lichen lesion, and for this, it is recommended that the treatment for candidiasis be carried out first and only subsequently the definitive diagnosis of OLP and the respective treatment plan of the same [6, 15].

As the reticular type does not present symptoms, there is no need for specific treatment, but as already mentioned, candidiasis can occur overlapping with lesions of lichen planus; in this way it is proposed that the antifungal treatment be performed based on topical nystatin, and mouthwash with nystatin or application of Miconazole gel is recommended. In erosive lichen planus, because it has painful symptomatology, treatment with topical corticosteroids initially, such as triamcinolone acetonide and beclomethasone, is suggested. The second line of treatment would be the use of retinoids, cyclosporine, and calcineurin inhibitors prescribed for about 2 weeks. In addition to drug treatment, photodynamic therapy is usually used to relieve symptoms [6, 13]. Lastly, patients with this disorder should be evaluated periodically for 3–6 months, especially in atypical cases with some degree of dysplasia [6].

5. Queilite actinic

Actinic cheilitis is a PMOD that frequently presents in vermilion of the lower lip, attributed to modifications in the keratinocytes of the labial mucosa. The expression cheilitis was first used in 1923, meaning inflammation on the lips, being multicausal, which include prolonged exposure to solar UV rays, allergic reactions, and systemic diseases. The term actinic refers to changes generated by radiant energy [6, 17, 18]. The etiopathogenesis of this disorder is multifactorial, but it is undeniable that the main etiological factor associated with actinic cheilitis lesions is prolonged exposure to the sun's rays, with UV radiation and with its wavelength of 200–400 nm acting as a carcinogenic factor, as it can cause cell damage, thereby generating mutations in the DNA and tumor suppressor genes, especially in the p53 gene. Lately, other risk factors have been associated with actinic cheilitis, such as smoking, immunosuppression, chronic lupus, and lichen planus [17, 18].

This disorder occurs in light-skinned individuals exposed for long periods to solar UV rays, which is more common in men and those performing outdoor work, such as rural and construction workers, or have a history of progressive exposure in the sun. The lesions mainly affect individuals in the age range between 50 and 70 years. As previously mentioned, the primary anatomical site is the lower lip, and this is due to the fact that its epithelium is thinner, has a discrete layer of keratin, has fewer melanocytes, and receives direct radiation. Actinic cheilitis has a malignant transformation rate of 17%, with squamous cell carcinoma growing gradually, and metastasis occurs only in the late stages of the lesion [3, 6, 16, 19].

This disorder develops slowly, and the first noticeable clinical changes are atrophy of the border of vermilion of the lower lip, exhibiting a smooth surface with spots of whitish staining. As the lesion progresses, the margin between the vermilion area and the cutaneous portion of the lip is erased. In more advanced states, rough areas with the presence of ulceration can be observed, in addition to the association with leukoplastic lesions. In these late states, in many cases, clinical signs may already be found that indicate malignant transformation, such as recurrent ulcers which do not heal (**Figure 8**) [3, 6, 17].

Actinic cheilitis can histologically be characterized by the presence of an atrophic stratified epithelium, hyperkeratinization, atrophy, or thickening of the thorny layer and varying degrees of epithelial dysplasia. In the underlying connective tissue, it is possible to observe an infiltration of chronic inflammatory cells and also collagenous bundles exhibiting basophilic changes resulting from the change from an eosinophilic collagen to a basophilic granular material, called solar elastosis [3, 6, 17].

The diagnosis of actinic cheilitis is basically clinical; because it is a very characteristic lesion, patients usually report a nonelastic sensation of the lips, followed by dryness and increase of volume; besides, the accomplishment of the incisional biopsy is mandatory mainly for its high rate of malignant transformation and also to propose a suitable treatment plan for the lesion. In the absence of dysplasias or presence of mild dysplasia, the use of 5-fluorouracil (Efudix®), which can be applied twice a day for 2–4 weeks, is recommended. Cryotherapy, which consists in freezing a tissue area to potentiate cell destruction without damaging the healthy tissues around the lesion, and the use of laser therapy are possible therapeutic alternatives. In the occurrence of moderate or severe dysplasia/carcinomas in situ, a vermilionectomy is indicated, the affected vermilion mucosa is removed, and the vermilion reconstruction of the lip occurs from the internal labial mucosa [3, 6, 17, 19]. In addition, all patients with actinic cheilitis should be directed to use sunscreens and other forms of protection against UV rays; thus, in the same way as with other PMODs, individuals who have actinic cheilitis should be monitored routinely throughout life.

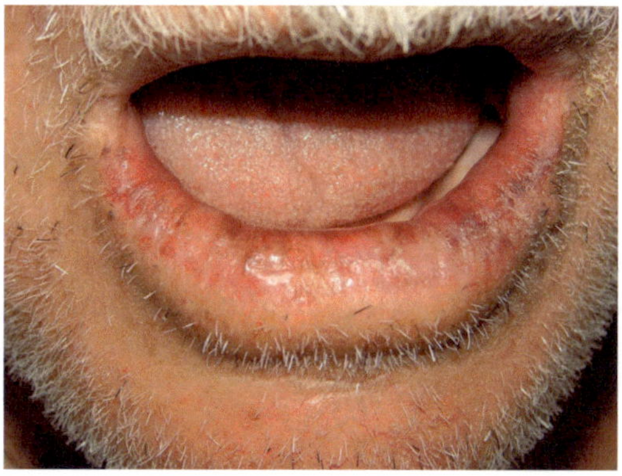

Figure 8.
Actinic cheilitis in the lower lip exhibiting epithelial atrophy and loss of sharpness of the demarcation line between the labial mucosa and the epidermis. Source: author's file.

6. Oral submucous fibrosis

Oral submucous fibrosis is a chronic disorder of the mucosa that lines the upper digestive tract that surrounds the oral cavity, oropharynx, and routinely the upper third of the esophagus, and is often found in individuals living in Southwest Asian countries [6, 13]. Before the etiology of this disorder was considered multifactorial and complex, it is now recognized that its appearance is due to the chewing of areca nut; this sachet is composed of areca palm nut and hydrated lime, sometimes with sweeteners and condiments, wrapped in a betel leaf [6, 20]. Because this custom is common in Southwest Asia, the highest frequency of this disorder is in the population of this region, mainly in India. Its frequency is about 0.5% in the population, and estimates suggest that about 2.5 million people are affected. The predominant age group is between 20 and 40 years, since the rural villagers begin the habit of chewing areca nuts very early and for long periods of time, around 16 hours. Oral submucous fibrosis has a malignant transformation rate between 2.3 and 7.6% [3, 11, 19].

Initially oral submucous fibrosis presents as vesicles and ulcers, often on the hard palate and buccal mucosa. With the progression of the disorder, the patient may present with xerostomia, difficulty in moving the tongue, and decreased elasticity of the oral mucosa, lips, and floor of the mouth, and some patients may report oral burning sensation. On palpation examination, dense fibrous bands may be felt, and a change in the color of the buccal mucosa with whitish and opaque tones. In the final stage, generalized fibrosis of the oral cavity and progressing trismus are observed [14].

Histologically, oral submucous fibrosis is described as a submucous deposition of dense collagenous connective tissue that shows little presence of blood vessels but with large numbers of chronic inflammatory cells. In lesions in soft states, the present epithelial alterations are subepithelial vesicles, whereas in lesions in more advanced states, it is possible to observe epithelial atrophy and hyperkeratosis. In addition, about 10–15% of FSO lesions present some level of dysplasia and even present carcinoma in situ [6].

The diagnosis is based on clinical findings and confirmed by biopsy and subsequent histopathological examination. There is no specific treatment for oral submucous fibrosis, but it is imperative that the diagnosed individual ceases the harmful habits. However, it is important to note that the lesion will not regress only with the removal of the habit, but it will prevent a possible malignant transformation. In patients who have mild or moderate cases of the disorder, treatment with corticosteroids applied to the lesion is recommended in order to reduce the symptoms. For later stages, surgical therapy is the most recommended, aiming to relieve trismus by releasing fibrous tissue through conventional techniques of tissue reconstruction, covering local/regional advancement flaps and microvascular flaps. Other treatment options include iron and multivitamin supplements and intralesional injections of lycopene alone or in combination with steroids, and some studies have shown the efficacy of interferon use for improved mouth opening [6, 11, 14, 19, 20]. Patients with oral submucous fibrosis are at least 19 times more likely to develop squamous cell carcinoma than individuals who do not have squamous cell carcinoma that even after the treatment for the symptomatology of the disease, the patients should be monitored routinely [6].

7. Conclusion

Potentially malignant oral disorders are the first indications of micro- and macroscopic alterations of possible malignant transformations, so knowledge about these lesions is of great importance for specific care and prevention against any type of carcinoma. The transformation of normal mucosa to dysplastic mucosa occurs through a complex set of interactions between the individual's organism and environmental factors. Risk factors involving PMOD such as sun exposure, smoking habits, alcohol ingestion, and infection by microorganisms are issues that need to be addressed in order to better treat, prevent, and reduce malignant transformation rates. Thus, it is suggested that clinicians design educational plans aimed at the prevention of PMOD, as well as possible malignant transformations, in this way, enabling their patients against exposure to the causal factors of the disorders. In summary, the diagnosis and treatment plan for potentially malignant oral disorders are fundamental, since lesions that have high degrees of dysplasia should be treated with surgical procedures and those with no or slight degrees of dysplasia should undergo conservative treatments, such as drug therapy or phototherapy.

Acknowledgments

Oral Cancer Nucleus of the State University of Feira de Santana, and Research Group on Head and Neck Cancer of Feira de Santana, Bahia, Brazil.

Conflict of interests

The authors declare that there is no conflict of interest.

Author details

Márcio Campos Oliveira*, Igor Ferreira Borba de Almeida, Almira Oliveira Pereira and Maria da Conceição Andrade
Universidade Estadual de Feira de Santana, Feira de Santana, Brazil

*Address all correspondence to: marciopatologiaoral@gmail.com

References

[1] World Health Organization (WHO), International Agency for Research on Cancer (IARC). A Digital Manual for the Early Diagnosis of Oral Neoplasia [Internet]. France: IARC; Available from: http://screening.iarc.fr/atlasoral.php?lang=1

[2] Ministério da Saúde, Instituto Nacional de Câncer, Brasil. Números Do Câncer: Incidência de Câncer no Brasil: Estimativa 2018. Rio de Janeiro: Inca; 2018

[3] Silva AT, Rezende SD. Lesões potencialmente malignas da cavidade oral: revisão de literatura. Revista Brasileira de Cirurgia da Cabeça e Pescoço. 2016;**45**(2):67-71

[4] Naggar Adel K et al. WHO Classification of Head and Neck Tumors. 4th ed. Lyon: International Agency for Research on Cancer (IARC); 2017. p. 343

[5] van Der WI. Oral leukoplakia, the ongoing discussion on definition and terminology. Medicina Oral, Patología Oral y Cirugía Bucal. 2014;**6**:685-692. DOI: 10.4317/medoral.21007

[6] Brad N et al. Patologia Oral e Maxilofacial. 3rd ed. Vol. 1. Rio de Janeiro: Elsevier; 2009. p. 989

[7] van Der WI. Oral potentially malignant disorders: Is malignant transformation predictable and preventable? Medicina Oral, Patología Oral y Cirugía Bucal. 2014:386-390. DOI: 10.4317/medoral.20205

[8] Susan M. Oral epithelial dysplasia, atypical verrucous lesions and oral potentially malignant disorders: Focus on histopathology. Oral Surgery, Oral Medicine, Oral Pathology, Oral Radiology. 2018;**125**(6):591-602. DOI: 10.1016/j.oooo.2018.02.012

[9] van Der WI. Knowledge about oral leukoplakia for use at different levels of expertise, including patients. Oral Diseases. 2018;**24**(1-2):174-178. DOI: 10.1111/odi.12695

[10] van Der WI. Potentially malignant disorders of the oral and oropharyngeal mucosa; present concepts of management. Oral Oncology. 2010;**46**(6):423-425. DOI: 10.1016/j.oraloncology.2010.02.016

[11] Lenzi CD et al. Proliferative verrucous leukoplakia: Diagnosis, management and current advances. Brazilian Journal of Otorhinolaryngology. 2017;**83**(5):585-593. DOI: 10.1016/j.bjorl.2016.12.005

[12] Dantas da SÉJ et al. Lesões orais com potencial de malignização: análise clínica e morfológica de 205 casos. Jornal Brasileiro de Patologia e Medicina Laboratorial. 2009;**45**(3):233-238. DOI: 10.1590/s1676-24442009000300008

[13] Michael A et al. Management update of potentially premalignant oral epithelial lesions. Oral Surgery, Oral Medicine, Oral Pathology, Oral Radiology. 2018;**125**(6):628-636. DOI: 10.1016/j.oooo.2018.03.010

[14] Aline T et al. Potencial de transformación maligna del liquen plano oral: Estudio retrospectivo. International Journal of Odontostomatology. 2015;**9**(3):511-517. DOI: 10.4067/s0718-381x2015000300025

[15] Vilmer C, Cavelier-Balloy B. Renaud-les lésions précancéreuses épithéliales buccales. Annales de Dermatologie et de Vénéréologie. 2017;**144**(2):100-108. DOI: 10.1016/j.annder.2016.07.017

[16] Neumann S et al. Paiva Oral lichen planus: Clinical profile and determination of oral

epithelial dysplasia. International Journal of Odontostomatology. 2016;**10**(1):99-106. DOI: 10.4067/s0718-381x2016000100016

[17] Hernández OC, Fuentes PB, Ricardo C-V. Queilitis actínica: Aspectos histológicos, clínicos y epidemiológicos. Revista Cubana de Estomatología. 2016;**53**(2):45-55. Disponible en: http://www.revestomatologia.sld.cu/index.php/est/article/view/824

[18] Yazdani A M-a et al. Photodynamic therapy for actinic cheilitis. Dermatologic Surgery. 2015;**41**(2):189-198. DOI: 10.1097/dss.0000000000000254

[19] Speight Paul M, Ali KS, Omar K. Oral potentially malignant disorders: Risk of progression to malignancy. Oral Surgery, Oral Medicine, Oral Pathology, Oral Radiology. 2018;**125**(6):612-627. DOI: 10.1016/j.oooo.2017.12.011.

[20] Fedorowicz Z et al. Interventions for the management of oral submucous fibrosis. Cochrane Database of Systematic Reviews. 2008;**1**:1-17. DOI: 10.1002/14651858.cd007156

Chapter 7

Oral Cancer: The State of the Art of Modern-Day Diagnosis and Treatment

Quang Van Le, Duy Quoc Ngo, Toan Duc Tran and Quy Xuan Ngo

Abstract

Diagnosing and treating lesions of the mouth and gums is challenging for most clinicians because of the wide variety of disease processes that can present with similar appearing lesions and the fact that most clinicians receive inadequate training in mouth diseases. Oral cancer, a common lesion in oral cavity, is not correctly diagnosing a clinical picture of an early squamous cell carcinoma. The prevalence of oral cancer continues to rise worldwide, related to the increase in consumption of tobacco, alcohol and other carcinogenic products. However, there has also been a significant reduction in mortality due to increasing awareness, early diagnosis and advances in treatments. This chapter is an attempt to provide a comprehensive update encompassing the spectrum of etiologic/risk factors, current clinical diagnostic tools, management philosophies, and molecular biomarkers and progression indicators of oral cancer.

Keywords: oral cancer, oral cavity cancer, head and neck cancer, squamous cell carcinoma, oral lesions

1. Introduction

Oral cancer is one of the most prevalent diseases worldwide, accounting for 30–40% of the head and neck cancer. There are an estimated 200,000 cases of oral cancer worldwide each year, which cause an estimated 100,000 deaths [1]. Particularly, these are malignant lesions of the oral structure including anterior two thirds of tongue, lips (upper lip, lower lip and edge), the upper and lower gingiva, retromolar trigone, buccal mucosa and floor of the mouth. The most common histopathology of oral cancer is squamous cell carcinoma, contributing to approximately 90% of cases. Multidisciplinary oncologic treatment, such as surgery, radiation therapy and chemotherapy, plays important roles in treatment for oral cavity cancer [2].

2. Oral cavity anatomy

The oral cavity is composed of the mucosa of the lips (not outer, dry lips), the buccal mucosa, the anterior tongue, the floor of the mouth, the hard palate and the

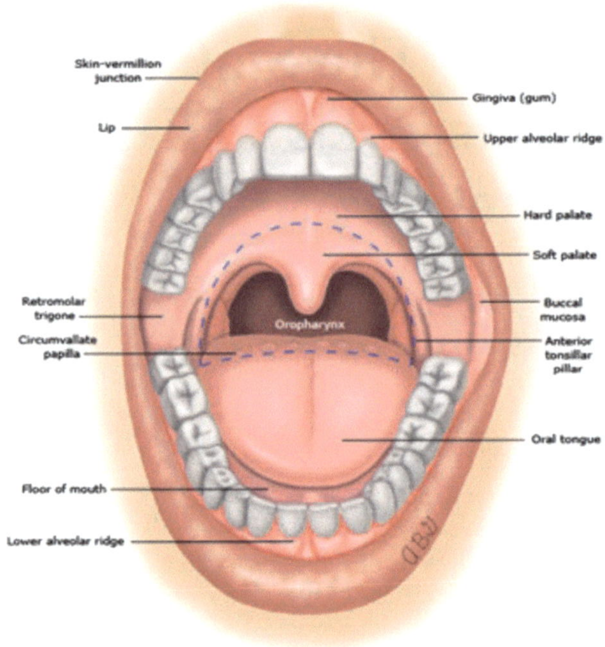

Figure 1.
Oral cavity anatomy.

upper and lower gingiva. The anterior boundary is determined by the portion of the upper lip connected to the lower lip (wet mucosa). While, the posterior side is bound by the V-groove of the tongue, the anterior tonsillar pillars (palatoglossus muscles) and the posterior margin of the hard palate. Inferiorly, the oral cavity is formed by mylohyoid muscles. Additionally, the lateral border of the oral cavity spans between the buccomasseteric area (buccal mucosa) and retromolar trigone (**Figure 1**).

3. Epidemiology and etiology of pathogenesis

An estimated 200,000 cases of oral cancer every year worldwide resulted in around 100,000 lethal cases [1]. Oral cavity tumors frequently occur with the local invasions, destructions of the surrounding tissue and lymph node metastases, but there is not often have distant metastasis at the time of diagnosis. Smoking and alcohol assumption are two major risks of the oral squamous cell carcinoma [3]. Likewise, in Asia, especially in India, chewing nut quid is also an important key factor [4]. Furthermore, oral tobacco use, periodontal disease, radiation and immunodeficiency have been considered as risks linked to oral cancer. By the same token, sun exposure (ultraviolet radiation) is also a causal factor. Both of tobacco assumption and chewing nut quid are predominant risks of buccal mucosa cancers [3, 4]. **Figure 2** illustrates Region-Specific Incidence Age-Standardized Rates by Sex for Cancers of the Lip and Oral Cavity in 2018 [1].

Interestingly, human papillomavirus (HPV) infection, especially HPV 16, is associated with the incidence rates of tonsilloma and tongue cancer. Yet, the ratio of HPV infection related to oral cancer is significantly lower and there was an unclear

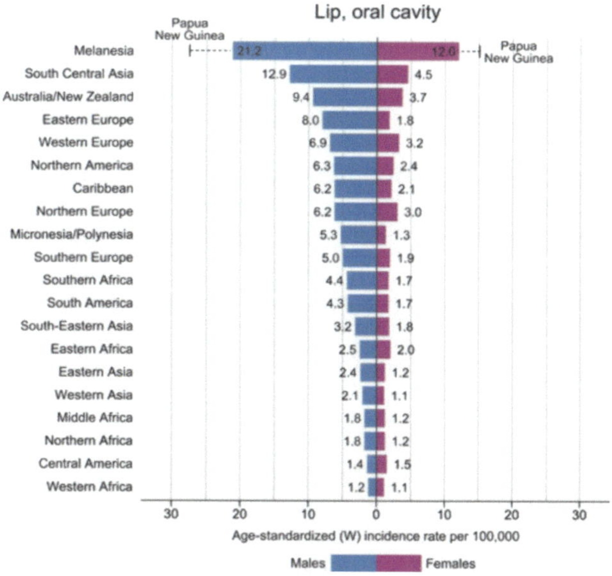

Figure 2.
Bar chart of region-specific incidence age-standardized rates by sex for cancers of the lip and Oral cavity in 2018. Source: GLOBOCAN 2018 [1].

relationship between clinical pathology and prognosis. Therefore, the HPV test has not been recommended for oral cancer [5].

4. Pathology

A total of 90 to 95% of all malignant lesions in the oral cavity are the squamous cell carcinoma. Moreover, it can be classified into three main groups: good differentiation (above 75% keratinization), moderate differentiation (25–75% keratinization) and poorly differentiated tumors (below 25% keratinization). Besides, less common types of histopathology could be mentioned such as verrucous carcinoma (a variant of squamous cell carcinoma), adenocarcinoma, adenoid cystic carcinoma and mucoepidermoid carcinomas.

On the other hand, the squamous cell carcinoma of the head and neck ordinarily undergo several developments of precancerous lesions due to exposure to carcinogenic factors.

- Oral leukoplakia is a precancerous lesion that presents as white patches in the oral mucosa. Notably, this damage is relatively common at a rate of 4% in the population [6]. Leukoplakia is divided into two types: homogenous lesions and heterogeneous lesions, in which cancer is highly induced by heterogeneous lesions. The diagnosis of leukoplakia usually relies on a biopsy to diagnose histopathology. Aside from that, biopsy is a standard criterion of the histopathological diagnosis in the clinical leukoplakia [7]. Surgery was indicated to any cases with small heterogeneous leukoplakia or lesions with severe dysplasia. Likewise, conservative treatments are regularly indicated for widespread leukoplakia or lesions with moderate or mild dysplasia [8]. Not to mention is oral proliferative verrucous leukoplakia (OPVL), a rare case found in patients. This is a malignant lesion of heterozygous leukoplakia with multifocal-type surface characteristics, slow progression and immense rate of malignant transformation. Some of the treatments such as surgery, laser, radiation or bleomycin-contained-chemotherapy facilitate to temporarily control the damage. Nonetheless, the relapse rate or malignant transformation is up to 70% of patients and the lethal rate contributes to higher than 30% for around a decade [9].

- Erythroplakia, a type of relatively uncommon lesions, has a relatively high rate of malignant transformation (above 80%) [10]. This lesion can be recognized with a red strip, relatively smooth, no symptoms in the floor of the mouth, the surface of the tongue and the soft palate in elder patients routinely using tobacco and alcohol. Thus, a complete removing surgery is a major recommendation in this case [11].

5. Clinical features and staging

5.1 Clinical presentation

The clinical manifestations of the oral cavity cancer are greatly contingent on the location of the primary tumor. Particularly, some of the symptoms could be found such as mouth sores or mouth ulcers, loose teeth, dysphagia, weight loss and bleeding. What's more, tumors of the mucosal surface, at the initial stage, recurrently appear as an unhealed ulcer with varying degrees of pain and occasionally bleed. These lesions regularly appear in the range of prior weeks to months that patients realized and go to the examination.

Above 66% of patients with tongue cancer have local lymph node metastases, depending on stage T and invasive depth, whereas the rate of lymph node metastasis is significantly lower than that of the hard palate cancer patients [12]. Similarly, the location and extent of the primary tumor attribute to the variants of clinical symptoms:

- Tongue cancer may develop as an ulcerative and/or infective lesion (**Figure 3**). Clinical signs are regular pain, with or without swallowing dysfunction. Markedly, the occurrence of those symptoms indicates that the tumor has deeper invaded into underlying other muscle layers of the tongue. In another way, it is seen that the disease is not at the early stage but reveals the history of leukoplakia or erythema in patients as well.

- Buccal mucosa cancer (**Figure 4**) can be presented with parotitis resulted from the pinched tumor-pinched-Stensen's duct sign.

- Oral cancer can induce one or both sides of the gland inflammation due to tumor compression and/or blockage of the Wharton duct leading to a palpable mass in the submandibular area, which may be the symptom.

- Upper gingival cancer at the early stage is easily bewildered with perianal infections which are inefficiency when being antibiotics-treated. Furthermore, sores, wounds and tooth loss could happen at the advanced stage.

- Lip cancer is generally presented with an exophytic or an ulcerative lesion, occasionally associated with bleeding or pain. Some cases indicate the nerve-associated-chin numbness because of invasion of the mental nerve [12].

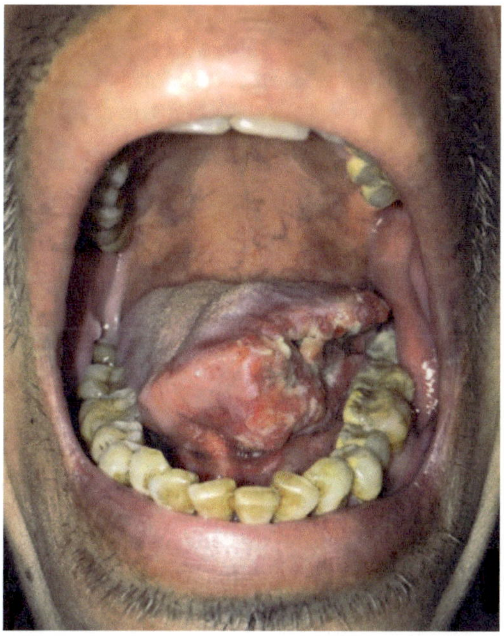

Figure 3.
Cancer of anterior two thirds of tongue.

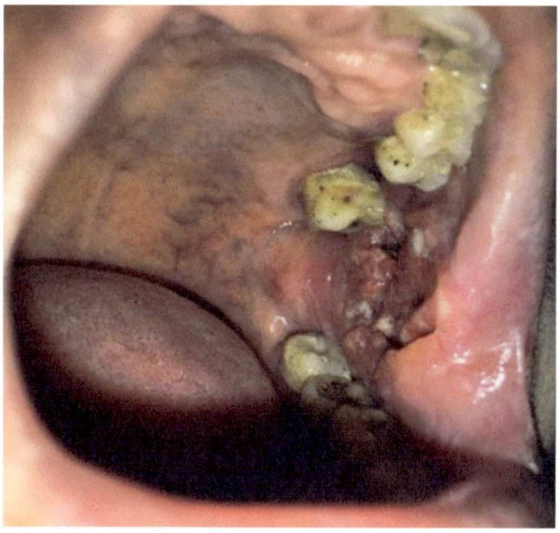

Figure 4.
Buccal mucosa cancer.

5.2 Physical examination

All patients with the oral tumor should have a completely general examination for both head and neck areas which includes finding and evaluating secondary tumors in the upper gastrointestinal tract as well as regional lymph nodes.

5.2.1 Intraoral examination

The process of the oral examination requires to systematically observe and touch the buccal mucosa, the anterior tongue, the floor of the mouth, the hard palate, and the upper, lower gingiva and the retromolar trigone. It is advisable to use a tongue depressor with good light (headlight) to fully observe all positions of the oral cavity. Then again, the size and characteristics of the lesion are evaluated, including the extent of invasion (endophytic or exophytic) and the relationship of lesion with surrounding structures.

5.2.2 Extraoral examination

With patients suffering from oral tumors, it is strongly advised that the facial skin and scalp are strongly advised to carefully observe and palpate. Besides, the major salivary glands and metastatic lymph nodes of the neck are evaluated. For instance, the sensation of the forehead, cheeks, upper lip, chin and lower lip should be assessed to find the clinical evidence of tumor-invaded-nerve.

The lymph nodes of the head and neck should be thoroughly and systematically such as preauricular, periparotid, submental, prevascular facial, submandibular, deep jugular and posterior triangle lymph nodes. Having said that, neck lymph nodes I, II and III are concerned as the most metastatic lymph-node groups of oral cancer. Whenever abnormal lymph nodes are detected, a conscientious assessment of the location, size, amount and clinical signs of the invasive lymph nodes is conducted.

5.3 Tissue diagnosis

In the oral tumor case, the histopathological diagnosis is preferentially carried out by a "bite" or excisional biopsy with few pieces from the boundary of benign and malignant lesions. This procedure should be performed in a specialized clinic with anesthetics. Similarly important is that the biopsy piece must be resected at the margin of positive and negative lesions. Additionally, the biopsy piece is necessary to take a sufficient depth to ensure the quality and necrotic area should be averted. If the anatomy is negative but clinically suspected to be cancerous, a biopsy is advisory performed until the procedure is positive. Notably, the fine needle aspiration biopsy applied into the metastasis-suspected lymph nodes in the neck also facilitates to identify and diagnose the disease stage. Nevertheless, this technique should be conducted under ultrasound guidance to enhance accuracy.

5.4 TNM staging system

The tumor, node, metastases (TNM) staging system of the American Joint Committee on Cancer (AJCC) and the Union for International Cancer Control (UICC) is used to classify cancers of the head and neck (**Table 1**) [13]. The T classifications indicate the extent of the primary tumor and are site specific; there is considerable overlap in the cervical N classifications.

5.5 Staging evaluation

Diagnostic imaging tools coupled with clinical examination help to accurately assess the stage of the disease, especially the extent of tumor invasion, lymph node metastasis, distant metastasis and the occurrence of second primary cancer. The most common metastatic areas are the lungs, liver and bone. Meanwhile, the second primary cancer is often found in the head and neck area, following the lung and esophagus.

Primary tumor (T)

T category	T criteria
TX	Primary tumor cannot be assessed
Tis	Carcinoma *in situ*
T1	Tumor ≤2 cm with depth of invasion (DOI)* ≤5 mm
T2	Tumor ≤2 cm, with DOI* >5 mm and ≤10 mm; **or** Tumor >2 cm and ≤4 cm, with DOI* ≤10 mm
T3	Tumor >2 cm and ≤4 cm with DOI* >10 mm; **or** Tumor >4 cm with DOI* ≤10 mm
T4	Moderately advanced or very advanced local disease
T4a	Moderately advanced local disease. Tumor >4 cm with DOI* >10 mm; **or** Tumor invades adjacent structures only (eg, through cortical bone of the mandible or maxilla, or involves the maxillary sinus or skin of the face). *NOTE:* Superficial erosion of bone/tooth socket (alone) by a gingival primary is not sufficient to classify a tumor as T4.
T4b	Very advanced local disease. Tumor invades masticator space, pterygoid plates, or skull base and/or encases the internal carotid artery.

* DOI is depth of invasion and **not** tumor thickness.

Regional lymph nodes (N)

Clinical N (cN)

N category	N criteria
NX	Regional lymph nodes cannot be assessed
N0	No regional lymph node metastasis
N1	Metastasis in a single ipsilateral lymph node, 3 cm or smaller in greatest dimension ENE(−)
N2	Metastasis in a single ipsilateral node larger than 3 cm but not larger than 6 cm in greatest dimension and ENE(−); **or** Metastases in multiple ipsilateral lymph nodes, none larger than 6 cm in greatest dimension and ENE(−); **or** In bilateral or contralateral lymph nodes, none larger than 6 cm in greatest dimension, and ENE(−)
N2a	Metastasis in a single ipsilateral node larger than 3 cm but not larger than 6 cm in greatest dimension, and ENE(−)
N2b	Metastases in multiple ipsilateral nodes, none larger than 6 cm in greatest dimension, and ENE(−)
N2c	Metastases in bilateral or contralateral lymph nodes, none larger than 6 cm in greatest dimension, and ENE(−)
N3	Metastasis in a lymph node larger than 6 cm in greatest dimension and ENE(−); **or** Metastasis in any node(s) and clinically overt ENE(+)
N3a	Metastasis in a lymph node larger than 6 cm in greatest dimension and ENE(−)
N3b	Metastasis in any node(s) and clinically overt ENE(+)

NOTE: A designation of "U" or "L" may be used for any N category to indicate metastasis above the lower border of the cricoid (U) or below the lower border of the cricoid (L). Similarly, clinical and pathological ENE should be recorded as ENE(−) or ENE(+).

Pathological N (pN)

N category	N criteria
NX	Regional lymph nodes cannot be assessed
N0	No regional lymph node metastasis
N1	Metastasis in a single ipsilateral lymph node, 3 cm or smaller in greatest dimension and ENE(−)
N2	Metastasis in a single ipsilateral lymph node, 3 cm or smaller in greatest dimension and ENE(+); **or** Larger than 3 cm but not larger than 6 cm in greatest dimension and ENE(−); **or** Metastases in multiple ipsilateral lymph nodes, none larger than 6 cm in greatest dimension and ENE(−); **or** In bilateral or contralateral lymph node(s), none larger than 6 cm in greatest dimension, ENE(−)
N2a	Metastasis in single ipsilateral node 3 cm or smaller in greatest dimension and ENE(+); **or** A single ipsilateral node larger than 3 cm but not larger than 6 cm in greatest dimension and ENE(−)
N2b	Metastases in multiple ipsilateral nodes, none larger than 6 cm in greatest dimension and ENE(−)
N2c	Metastases in bilateral or contralateral lymph node(s), none larger than 6 cm in greatest dimension and ENE(−)
N3	Metastasis in a lymph node larger than 6 cm in greatest dimension and ENE(−); **or** Metastasis in a single ipsilateral node larger than 3 cm in greatest dimension and ENE(+); **or** Multiple ipsilateral, contralateral, or bilateral nodes any with ENE(+); **or** A single contralateral node of any size and ENE(+)
N3a	Metastasis in a lymph node larger than 6 cm in greatest dimension and ENE(−)
N3b	Metastasis in a single ipsilateral node larger than 3 cm in greatest dimension and ENE(+); **or** Multiple ipsilateral, contralateral, or bilateral nodes any with ENE(+); **or** A single contralateral node of any size and ENE(+)

NOTE: A designation of "U" or "L" may be used for any N category to indicate metastasis above the lower border of the cricoid (U) or below the lower border of the cricoid (L). Similarly, clinical and pathological ENE should be recorded as ENE(−) or ENE(+).

Distant metastasis (M)

M category	M criteria
M0	No distant metastasis
M1	Distant metastasis

Prognostic stage groups

When T is...	And N is...	And M is...	Then the stage group is...
Tis	N0	M0	0
T1	N0	M0	I
T2	N0	M0	II
T3	N0	M0	III
T1, T2, T3	N1	M0	III
T4a	N0, N1	M0	IVA
T1, T2, T3, T4a	N2	M0	IVA
Any T	N3	M0	IVB
T4b	Any N	M0	IVB
Any T	Any N	M1	IVC

Table 1.
The tumor, node, metastases (TNM) staging system of the American Joint Committee on Cancer (AJCC) and the Union for International Cancer Control (UICC) is used to classify cancers of the head and neck [13].

5.5.1 Fine needle aspiration (FNA) biopsy

Fine needle aspiration biopsy was used in the case with a patient with metastatic cervical lymph nodes. This technique has high sensitivity and specificity, markedly, diagnostic accuracy is in the range of 89–98% [14, 15]. Yet, if a metastatic neck lymph node was suspected contrary to the negative FNA result, FNA needed to be re-conducted before an open biopsy being performed.

5.5.2 Diagnostic methods

5.5.2.1 Primary tumor

Both of CTs with intravenous contrast and magnetic resonance imaging can diagnose the tumor's invasion to surrounding organs. Indeed, axial and sagittal MRI scan can accurately assess tumor depth. However, CT scan with contrast allows an accurate approach to measure how deep bone could be invasive such as tumors in the hard palate, gums or floor of the mouth [16]. While, magnetic resonance is superior to CT that could evaluate the degree of soft tissue invasion, nerve invasion [17].

5.5.2.2 Nodal metastases

CT with intravenous contrast and MRI can facilitate the diagnosis of metastatic lymph node and extranodal spread circumstances. In other words, the lymph nodes with an increase in size enhancement, round, rim enhancement and central necrosis are suspected as malignant ones [18, 19].

5.5.2.3 Distant metastasis

Diagnosis of the presence of distant metastasis is highly important to determine the treatment and prognosis of the patients. Chest X-rays may be indicated to the early-staged cases or patients with low-risk lesions and non-smokers. However, in the advance-staged patients, the risk of lymph nodes N2,3 and bilateral lymph nodes are under a higher possibility of a distant invasion. Hence, chest CT or PET/CT are recommended to this group [20]. No differences have been found in the diagnosis of metastatic lung lesions between chest CT and PET/CT [21].

6. Treatment

The comprehensive management of oral cancer requires a disciplinary specialty including head and neck surgery, radiotherapy, medical oncology, imaging, pathology, microsurgery, nutrition, social workers and nurses. Generally, surgery is the primary treatment for oral squamous cell carcinoma. Surgery allows an accurate assessment of the anatomical stage, margins, invasive status and histopathological characteristics, based on the pros and cons that can determine the strategy. Adjuvant radiotherapy $\pm$ chemotherapy is used on locoregionally advanced tumors if being indicated. Multidisciplinary coordination is also extraordinarily important to ensure treatment outcomes. To individualize treatment, several factors need to be carefully considered, in which the risk of treatment-related complications should be assessed based on age, comorbidities (e.g., cardiovascular condition, respiration ...), lifestyle (smoking, alcohol assumption ...), surgical resectability and expectation of patients.

6.1 Surgery

Generally, surgery is the primary treatment for oral cancer. Remarkably, the general principles of surgical treatment will be discussed in this article such as the surgical approach to oral cancer, management of the mandible, management of neck lymph nodes and reconstruction of defects after oral surgery.

6.1.1 Management of primary tumor

The surgical purpose is to completely remove the primary tumor with negative margins as well as evaluate the stage and treatment of regional lymph nodes [22]. Every attempt should be made to ensure negative resection margins since positive margins are associated with a worse prognosis. The rate of local control significantly increased when the resection distance to the tumor was greater than 0.5 cm compared to less than 0.5 cm (36 and 18%, respectively) [23]. Moreover, the surgical approach is determined by the location and size of the tumor (**Figure 5**). The possibility of complete resection with a negative margin in the three dimensions is the most important factor in determining the approach. Lesions located in the anterior or lateral oral tongue, superficial tumors of the anterior floor of mouth are resected transorally. However, in the case, the invasion intensively toward posterior and/or on patients with trismus and/or obstructive dentition may require a more invasive approach such as the lip-splitting paramedian mandibulotomy approach [24]. The upper cheek flap and midfacial degloving approaches are indicated for gaining access to the maxilla.

6.1.2 Management of the mandible

Management of the mandible is an important consideration in oral cancer surgery since the proximity of the primary tumor to the mandible or invasion of the mandible by primary tumor requires resection of some part of the mandible. The mandibular invasion can occur at an early stage of tumors of the floor of the mouth, lower gingiva. Thus, assessment of the mandible is essential for appropriate surgical planning and treatment. In some circumstances, the floor of the mouth tumors can be removed via transoral approach, regularly combined with marginal or segmental mandibulectomy. The local control rate is declined to own to the mandibular invasion. That said, this resection is based on an assessment of the invasive cortex and bone marrow before surgery. The current indications for marginal mandibulectomy are: (1) for obtaining satisfactory three-dimensional margins around the primary tumor, (2) when the primary tumor approximates the mandible and (3) for minimal erosion of the alveolar process of the mandible (**Figure 6**).

The current indications for segmental mandibulectomy include: (1) gross invasion by oral cancer; (2) proximity of oral cancer to the mandible in a previously irradiated patient; (3) invasion of the inferior alveolar nerve or canal by tumor [12, 25, 26].

6.1.3 Management of neck lymph nodes

Management of the neck is a key component of oral cavity cancer treatment. Sixty percentage of patients with metastatic cervical lymph nodes (cN0) in the early stage of oral cancer cannot be clinically detected. Additionally, approximately 20–30% has evidence of microscopic lymph node metastasis on pathology after the selective neck dissection (SND). The risk of neck lymph node metastasis is associated with several factors such as tumor size, histologic grade, depth of invasion,

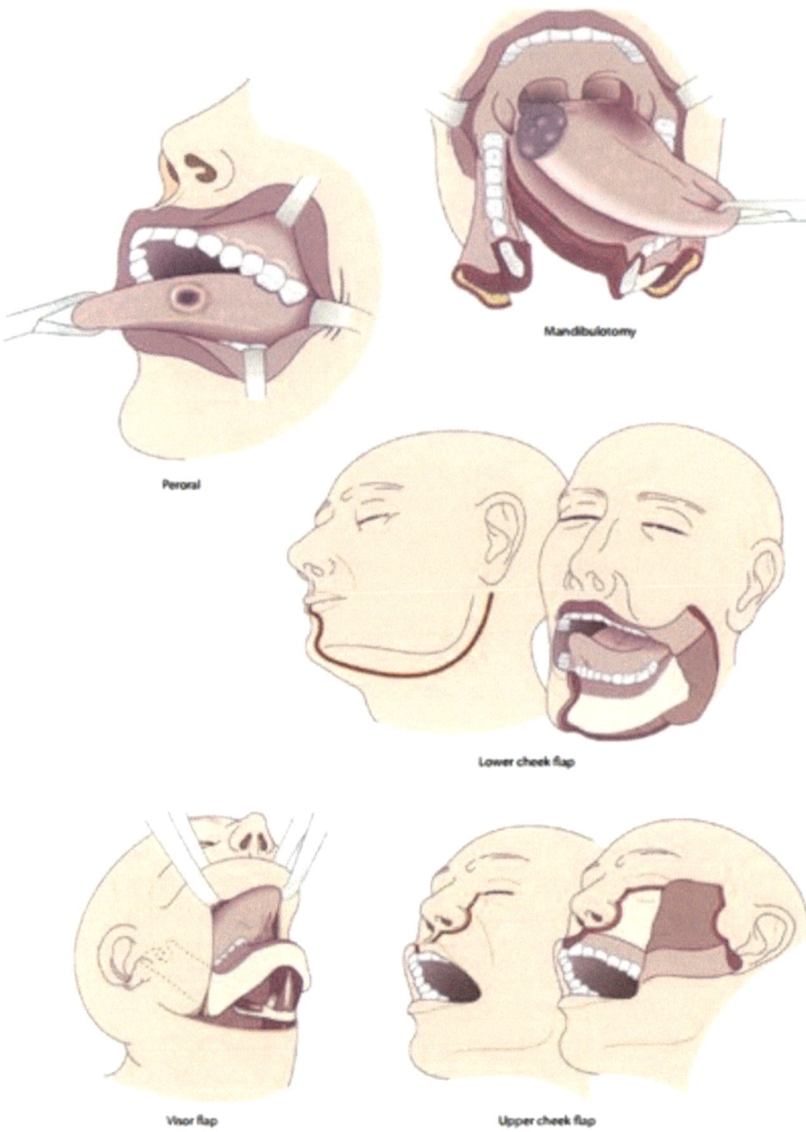

Figure 5.
Surgical approaches to oral cavity [12].

perineural invasion and vascular invasion [27, 28]. Cervical lymph node metastasis is the most essentially prognostic aspect of oral cancer. To give an illustration, comparing to a similar primary tumor without lymph node metastases, the chance of survival is declined by 50% [29]. Squamous cell carcinoma of the mobile tongue and the floor of the mouth are likely to metastases of the cervical lymph nodes, so these patients should have a selective neck removal surgery even with early-stage tumors, especially, the tumor thickness > 4 mm [30]. The SND is not indicated in the circumstances of the hard palate and maxillary gland tumors owing to their less possibility to have lymph node metastasis. Sentinel node biopsy may be an alternative to SND in patients with early stage (cT1,2 N0) squamous cell carcinoma. Notably, this technique was initially published in 2001 by Shoaib and colleagues, then analyzed in several single-center studies and two multi-center clinical trial

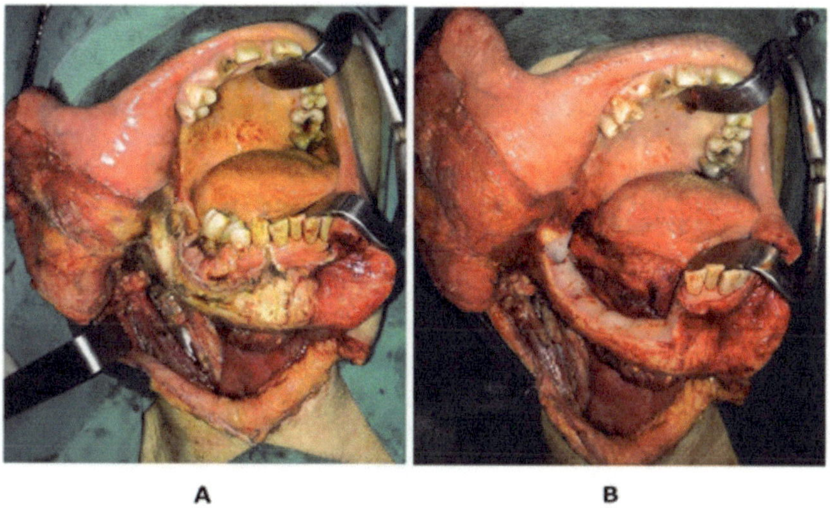

Figure 6.
(A) Cancer of lower gingiva. (B) Marginal mandibulectomy for cancer of lower gingiva.

studies, one in the US and one in Europe [31]. On the other hand, the procedure is still a big technical challenge and unsustainable success in identifying lymph nodes and metastases which highly dependent on the experience and competence of surgeons. That is to say, this technique could only be performed in some of the intensive centers with proficient skills. In some patients with lymph node metastasis on clinical examination or diagnostic imaging, therapeutic comprehensive neck dissection is indicated, including cervical lymph node group I to V group. The conservation or destruction of other structures such as the spinal accessory nerve, sternocleidomastoid muscle, or internal jugular is vein reliant on the location as well as the metastatic characteristics. The most common type of comprehensive neck dissection is the modified radical neck dissection, MRND Type 1. Radical neck dissection is rarely performed unless there is a direct extranodal spread of the lymph nodes to evade into the corresponding organs. Likewise, in patients without clinical lymph node metastases, the underlying risk of lymph node metastasis is mainly in the group I-III, rarely in the groups IV and V. Thus, supraomohyoid neck resection (SOHND) is commonly sufficient for stage cN0. Similarly, the rate of neck recurrence is 10–24% was found in patients who have positive lymph nodes under SND treatment [32]. Then again, patients are appropriately chosen to optimize postoperative radiation therapy. Particularly, the failure control rate is reported less than 10% in patients with cN0 demonstrated no lymph node metastasis on pathology [33].

6.1.4 Reconstructive surgery

Reconstructive surgery plays an important role in treatment for oral cavity cancer. The defects after surgery can cause significant issues in airway management, mastication, speech and cosmesis. The aim of reconstructive surgery is to restore presurgical function and cosmesis. Primary reconstruction, rather than a secondary surgery, has become the first choice of treatment for most cases with oral cancer. Primary closure or the use of skin graft can indicate for defects after oral surgery of early stage tumors. Contrarily, with large and complex defects after the oral tumor resection, plastic surgery needs the participation of an expert reconstructive surgeon. Microvascular free flap surgery is the prevailingly preferential technique. For instance, application of the free radial forearm flap into patients with soft tissue defects of tongue, the floor of mouth or retromolar trigone apparently performs an excellent result. In addition to the purpose of covering the soft tissue, the free flap is also a reliable method for recovering the bone defects, such as the fibula free flap used as post-surgical reconstruction after segmental mandibulectomy. Other combined microvascular flanges could be considered as radial forearm osteocutaneous flap, iliac crest and scapula free flaps. What's more, a few studies have demonstrated the effectiveness and safety of microsurgery [34]. The potency to recover major defects after surgery has contributed to improving the oncologic outcomes in patients with locally advanced stage due to increased ability to complete resection [35]. Pedicled myocutaneous flaps such as the pectoralis major, latissimus dorsi or trapezius flaps may also be a promising alternative when there is no reconstructive surgeon or the patient's condition is inappropriate for microvascular surgery.

6.2 Adjuvant treatment

Postoperative adjuvant therapy is indicated to patients with high risks of the local, regional recurrence, including pT3,4 primary tumors, pN2,3 lymph node metastases, level IV or V lymph node metastases, positive margins, lymphovascular invasion, perineural invasion and extracapsular spread. Indeed, external beam radiation is the traditional adjuvant treatment, with doses of 60–70 Gy often providing positive control. Two clinical trials have shown that adjuvant radiotherapy with cisplatin significantly improves the control rates along with survival time compared to the single adjuvant radiation therapy in those who have invasive head and neck cancer with extracapsular spread [36, 37]. But for all that concomitant radiotherapy has more severe side effects, so it should be carried out in the large centers with an expert team and appropriate infrastructure.

7. Prognosis

The clinical stage is the key predictor of survival. The Surveillance, Epidemiology and End Results (SEER) Cancer Statistics reveal that a 5-year survival for locally advanced oral cavity cancer of 54.7%, in contrast to 82.5% for early-stage cancer patients treated from 1975 to 2007 [38]. Lymph node metastasis is the single most important prognostic factor for oncologic outcome in oral cancer [39]. Besides, the number and size of positive lymph nodes, the presence of extranodal extension higher histologic grade, the presence of perineural invasion and increasing size have been correlated with worse outcomes [40–42].

8. Following

Oral cancer has a high risk of local, regional recurrence and development of a secondary primary cancer, but the recurrent rate due to distant metastases is relatively low. The contingency of the second cancer is about 4–7% annually [43]. A comprehensive clinical examination and high vigilance are the cornerstones of the early diagnosis. That's said, lifestyle modifications, such as smoking and drinking management should be a priority since these factors increase the risk of treatment failure and the appearance of second cancer. Unfortunately, preventive chemicals are ineffective and follow-up is the second crucial step. Basic imaging is usually indicated every 3–6 months after the end of treatment or clinical signs are suspected. Chest radiographs are not routinely used but may be useful in some patients with a history of tobacco addiction. Additional assessments could be included oral and swallowing rehabilitation if being indicated, thyroid hormone test if neck-area radiation and periodic dental examinations are performed.

9. Conclusions

The treatment outcome of oral cancer in recent decades has compellingly improved with the advancement in reconstructive surgery and adjuvant treatment. Further improvement in prolonging survival is hampered by an increase in the second-cancer incidence in long-term patients. With this in mind, oral cancer prevention is the first step, following that a requirement of enhancing awareness, promoting education, improving lifestyle and developing early diagnosis tools should have high consideration.

Conflict of interest

The authors declare no conflict of interest.

Author details

Quang Van Le[1,2], Duy Quoc Ngo[1*], Toan Duc Tran[1] and Quy Xuan Ngo[1]

1 Department of Head and Neck Surgery, Vietnam National Cancer Hospital, Hanoi, Vietnam

2 Hanoi Medical University, Hanoi, Vietnam

*Address all correspondence to: duyyhn@gmail.com

References

[1] http://globocan.iarc.fr/Pages/fact_sheets_population.aspx [Accessed: 20 February 2018]

[2] Harrison LB, Sessions RB, Hong WK. Head and Neck Cancer: A Multidisciplinary Approach. 3rd ed. Philadelphia, PA: Lippincott, William & Wilkins; 2009

[3] Warnakulasuriya S. Global epidemiology of oral and oropharyngeal cancer. Oral Oncology. 2009;**45**:309

[4] Guha N, Warnakulasuriya S, Vlaanderen J, Straif K. Betel quid chewing and the risk of oral and oropharyngeal cancers: A meta-analysis with implications for cancer control. International Journal of Cancer. 2014;**135**:1433

[5] Castellsagué X, Alemany L, Quer M, et al. HPV involvement in head and neck cancers: Comprehensive assessment of biomarkers in 3680 patients. Journal of the National Cancer Institute. 2016;**108**:djv403

[6] Mello FW, Miguel AFP, Dutra KL, et al. Prevalence of oral potentially malignant disorders: A systematic review and meta-analysis. Journal of Oral Pathology & Medicine. 2018;**47**:633

[7] van der Waal I. Oral leukoplakia, the ongoing discussion on definition and terminology. Medicina Oral, Patología Oral y Cirugía Bucal. 2015;**20**:e685

[8] Holmstrup P, Dabelsteen E. Oral leukoplakia-to treat or not to treat. Oral Diseases. 2016;**22**:494

[9] Pentenero M, Meleti M, Vescovi P, Gandolfo S. Oral proliferative verrucous leucoplakia: Are there particular features for such an ambiguous entity? A systematic review. British Journal of Dermatology. 2014;**170**:1039

[10] Kalavrezos N, Scully C. Mouth cancer for clinicians part 6: Potentially malignant disorders. Dental Update. 2015;**42**:866

[11] Yang SW, Lee YS, Chang LC, et al. Outcome of excision of oral erythroplakia. The British Journal of Oral & Maxillofacial Surgery. 2015;**53**:142

[12] Shah JP, Patel SG, Singh B. Jatin Shah's Head and Neck Surgery and Oncology. 5th ed. Philadelphia, PA: Elsevier Mosby; 2019

[13] Part II Head and Neck. In: Amid MB, editor. AJCC Cancer Staging Manual. 8th ed. New York: Springer; 2017, 2018. p. 53. Corrected at 4th printing

[14] Tandon S, Shahab R, Benton JI, et al. Fine-needle aspiration cytology in a regional head and neck cancer center: Comparison with a systematic review and meta-analysis. Head & Neck. 2008;**30**:1246

[15] Pisharodi LR. False-negative diagnosis in fine-needle aspirations of squamous-cell carcinoma of head and neck. Diagnostic Cytopathology. 1997;**17**:70

[16] Arya S, Rane P, Deshmukh A. Oral cavity squamous cell carcinoma: Role of pretreatment imaging and its influence on management. Clinical Radiology. 2014;**69**:916-930

[17] Ong C, Chong V. Imaging of perineural spread in head and neck tumours. Cancer Imaging. 2010;**10**(1A):S92-S98

[18] King A, Tse G, Ahuja A, et al. Necrosis in metastatic neck nodes: Diagnostic accuracy of CT, MR imaging, and US. Radiology. 2004;**230**(3):720-726

[19] King A, Tse G, Yuen E, et al. Comparison of CT and MR imaging for the detection of extranodal neoplastic spread in metastatic neck nodes. European Journal of Radiology. 2004; **52**(3):264-270

[20] Coca-Pelaz A, Rodrigo JP, Suarez C. Clinicopathologic analysis and predictive factors for distant metastases in patients with head and neck squamous cell carcinomas. Head & Neck. 2012;**34**:771-775

[21] Krabbe CA, Pruim J, van der Laan BF, et al. FDG-PET and detection of distant metastases and simultaneous tumors in head and neck squamous cell carcinoma: A comparison with chest radiography and chest CT. Oral Oncology. 2009;**45**:234-240

[22] National Comprehensive Cancer Network: NCCN Practice Guidelines in Oncology: Head and Neck Cancers. 2019. Available from: http://www.nccn.org/professionals/physician_gls/f_guidelines.asp

[23] Loree TR, Strong EW. Significance of positive margins in oral cavity squamous carcinoma. American Journal of Surgery. 1990;**160**:410-414

[24] Cilento BW, Izzard M, Weymuller EA, et al. Comparison of approaches for oral cavity cancer resection: Lip-split versus visor flap. Otolaryngology and Head and Neck Surgery. 2007;**137**:428-432

[25] Wax MK, Bascom DA, Myers LL. Marginal mandibulectomy vs segmental mandibulectomy: Indications and controversies. Archives of Otolaryngology – Head & Neck Surgery. 2002;**128**:600-603

[26] Wang CC, Cheng MH, Hao SP, et al. Osteoradionecrosis with combined mandibulotomy and marginal mandibulectomy. Laryngoscope. 2005; **115**:1963-1967

[27] Woolgar JA, Scott J. Prediction of cervical lymph node metastasis in squamous cell carcinoma of the tongue/ floor of mouth. Head & Neck. 1995; **17**(6):463-472

[28] Spiro RH, Huvos AG, Wong GY, et al. Predictive value of tumor thickness in squamous carcinoma confined to the tongue and floor of the mouth. American Journal of Surgery. 1986;**152**(4):345-350

[29] Robbins KT, Ferlito A, Shah JP, et al. The evolving role of selective neck dissection for head and neck squamous cell carcinoma. The European Archives of Oto-Rhino-Laryngology. 2013; **270**(4):1195-1202

[30] Huang SH, Hwang D, Lockwood G, et al. Predictive value of tumor thickness for cervical lymphnode involvement in squamous cell carcinoma of the oral cavity: A meta-analysis of reported studies. Cancer. 2009;**115**(7):1489-1497

[31] Shoaib T, Soutar DS, MacDonald DG, et al. The accuracy of head and neck carcinoma sentinel lymph node biopsy in the clinically N0 neck. Cancer. 2001;**91**(11): 2077-2083

[32] Tupchong L, Scott CB, Blitzer PH, et al. Randomized study of preoperative versus postoperative radiation therapy in advanced head and neck carcinoma: Long-term follow-up of RTOG study 73–03. International Journal of Radiation Oncology, Biology, Physics. 1991;**20**(1): 21-28

[33] Andersen PE, Shah JP, Cambronero E, et al. The role of comprehensive neck dissection with preservation of the spinal accessory nerve in the clinically positive neck. American Journal of Surgery. 1994; **168**(5):499-502

[34] Hanasono MM, Friel MT, Klem C, et al. Impact of reconstructive microsurgery in patients with advanced oral cavity cancers. Head & Neck. 2009; **31**:1289-1296

[35] Hanasono MM, Friel MT, Klem C, et al. Impact of reconstructive microsurgery in patients with advanced oral cavity cancers. Head & Neck. 2009; **31**(10):1289-1296

[36] Cooper JS, Pajak TF, Forastiere AA, et al. Postoperative concurrent radiotherapy and chemotherapy for high-risk squamous-cell carcinoma of the head and neck. The New England Journal of Medicine. 2004;**350**(19): 1937-1944

[37] Bernier J, Domenge C, Ozsahin M, et al. Postoperative irradiation with or without concomitant chemotherapy for locally advanced head and neck cancer. The New England Journal of Medicine. 2004;**350**(19):1945-1952

[38] Available from: http://seer.cancer.gov/csr/1975_2007/ [Accessed: 14 March 2011]

[39] Shah JP, Cendon RA, Farr HW, Strong EW. Carcinoma of the oral cavity. Factors affecting treatment failure at the primary site and neck. American Journal of Surgery. 1976;**132**: 504

[40] Gil Z, Carlson DL, Boyle JO, et al. Lymph node density is a significant predictor of outcome in patients with oral cancer. Cancer. 2009;**115**:5700

[41] Myers JN, Greenberg JS, Mo V, Roberts D. Extracapsular spread. A significant predictor of treatment failure in patients with squamous cell carcinoma of the tongue. Cancer. 2001; **92**:3030

[42] Arduino PG, Carrozzo M, Chiecchio A, et al. Clinical and histopathologic independent prognostic factors in oral squamous cell carcinoma: A retrospective study of 334 cases. Journal of Oral and Maxillofacial Surgery. 2008;**66**:1570

[43] Leon X, Martinez V, Lopez M, et al. Second, third, and fourth head and neck tumors. A progressive decrease in survival. Head & Neck. 2012;**34**(12): 1716-1719

Chapter 8

Non-Invasive Methods for Early Diagnosis of Oral Cancer

Manoela Garcia Dias da Conceição, Ana Cláudia Figueiró and Vera Lucia Luiza

Abstract

Oral cancer is a public health problem because of its high morbidity and mortality, and when not treated in a timely manner, it is significantly mutilating, causing damage to the physical and psychological aspects of patients and directly interfering with their quality of life. Several factors influence the early diagnosis of this pathology, including lack of self-care related to oral health, especially among people with prolonged use of dental prosthesis; delayed perception of the lesion; delayed search for professional assistance since the lesion is noticed by the patient; lack of information about oral cancer, its risk and protective factors, and oral lesions that may be suggestive of cancer; lack of health promotion and prevention activities aimed at oral cancer; and lack of training in oral cancer among oral health professionals. These factors must be tackled to promote the timely diagnosis of this pathology. The use of reliable noninvasive diagnosis methods is also important because they can be easily made available in low resource settings, increasing the coverage of people who are under risk of developing oral cancer.

Keywords: oral health, prevention, primary health care, secondary health care, oral cancer

1. Introduction

Oral health is part of general health and is essential to people's well-being. Good oral health implies being free from chronic orofacial pain, oral and pharyngeal cancer, soft tissue changes in the mouth, congenital disabilities, and other issues affecting the craniofacial complex [1].

Oral cancer (OC) is considered a public health problem because of its high mortality and morbidity rates. This problem also affects most people with low sociocultural level and who are alcoholics and smokers. However, there are other associated risk factors: chewing tobacco, use of a dental prosthesis, infection with human papilloma virus (HPV) type 16, nutritional deficiency, age, gender, poor oral hygiene, excess body fat, and chewing betel nut, among others [2, 3].

Data published by the International Agency for Research on Cancer (IARC) regarding cancer cases in general reported in 2012 about 14.1 million new cases, 8.2 million deaths within 5 years of diagnosis, and 32.6 million people living with cancer in the world. Of these, approximately 57% of new cases, 65% of deaths, and 48% of cases diagnosed in the last 5 years are in developing countries [4].

In 2018, new data were released, indicating an increase in new cases of cancer, with 18.1 million new cases and 9.6 million deaths [5]. The significant increase of this disease is clear, indicating the need for new plans for prevention and early diagnosis.

Regarding oral cancer, the highest rates have been observed in populations of Melanesia, Central-South Asia, Eastern and Western Europe, Africa, and Central America. Oral cancer is the sixth most common in the world, and most cases occur in India and Southeast Asia, according to the estimates for 2012 [6]. A change was seen in 2018 when oral cancer ranked in the 11th position among the most common cancers in the world. This type of cancer is quite common in Brazil, which has the third highest incidence in the world, behind only India and former Czechoslovakia [5].

Oral cancer is a condition that negatively interferes with the general and oral health of the individual. These oral problems cause pain and infection, leading to psychological and physical distress. It is important to note that such dental conditions express social exclusion. In general, they are associated with poor education, low income, unemployment, and difficulty in accessing care services [7]. Thus oral cancer patients represent a group of people that should receive differentiated attention because, besides cancer itself, they are highly susceptible to other ills [2]. When this disease affects individuals, they may have to face consequences such as facial mutilation. Also, they may render them unable to work, with severe damage to their quality of life. The disease may sometimes be lethal, mainly because of late diagnosis.

This pathology causes essential changes in the daily lives of the affected people, interfering with their body image, body functioning, and psychological, social, and family structure. The disease mostly affects the population in their working phase of life, causes indirect damage to the country. Late diagnosis is directly associated with shorter survival. However, if diagnosed early, it has a good prognosis and an average 5-year survival rate of 77.3% in stages I and II, but of 32.2% in stages III and IV [2].

Morbidity and mortality rates are high, with diagnosis in advanced phases in 65–85% of the cases, reducing the likelihood of cure [2, 8–11]. For most of these patients, palliative care is the only option available to achieve a better quality of life and control symptoms.

Protective factors against this condition include general and specific measures. The adoption of healthy lifestyle habits, including adequate nutrition, physical exercise, and self-care, is part of the prevailing standards. In turn, specific practices include oral health care, routine inspection of the oral cavity, periodic dental evaluation, and cessation of smoking and alcoholism, and recent studies have shown the consumption green tea as a protective measure [12, 13].

Although oral cancer is easily detected, its diagnosis is late in most cases. It is possible to improve diagnosis through the use of health promotion and prevention measures and improved access to health services, to promote early diagnosis [7, 14, 15]. Diagnosis is followed by curative treatment, preventing mutilating and disabling sequelae.

The relevance of this disease and its early diagnosis should be considered for the possibility of curative treatment and promotion of the quality of life of patients. It is essential to know and recommend methods that act in favor of the early diagnosis of this pathology. It may mean identifying early malignant and even premalignant lesions, leading to the cure of these patients and rehabilitation to their social routine. It is equally important to act on factors that influence to late diagnosis of this pathology, through the planning of actions.

2. Factors related to late diagnosis of oral cancer

The problem of delayed diagnosis of OC is known worldwide, and each country or region has different strategies to address it. These factors are described in several studies [16, 17], showing that this is a global problem. Factors related to late diagnosis of OC concern the social determinants, health literacy, and characteristics of the health system:

1. Profile of the affected people concerning lifestyle habits: most people who develop OC were smokers and alcoholics and are in situations associated with other unhealthy lifestyles, such as poor diet and physical inactivity [2].

2. Lack of self-care in oral health: the most vulnerable populations, which are those with a low socioeconomic level, frequently have poor self-care due to their living conditions, especially in terms of oral health, besides other health problems. This problem directly interferes with their quality of life and interaction with peers. They also present a low search for health care, leading to the worsening of health problems and, in this case, late diagnosis of oral cancer [18].

3. Delayed perception of the lesion: due to poor self-care, most do not identify the presence of initial lesions in the oral cavity. Thus, injuries are only perceived when they cause discomfort, pain, bleeding, or other symptoms, and at that point, in most cases, the disease is already in an advanced stage [18].

4. Lack of information about oral cancer and its protective and risk factors: many campaigns for the dissemination of information on disease have been promoted, but specifically on oral cancer is still incipient. People asked to appear to not know about oral cancer, suspected lesions or risk, and protective factors, even patients who are undergoing treatment for this type of cancer [14, 19].

5. Lack of health promotion and prevention activities aimed at oral cancer: a few specific actions to promote and prevent this type of cancer are carried out. These actions are usually linked to other campaigns such as those focused on vaccination, smoking, and oral health in general [14].

6. Lack of training in oral cancer among oral health professionals and deficits in addressing this content in the curricula of undergraduate courses: oral health professionals are not routinely updated and trained on this content. Still, the approach during undergraduate training is deficient, producing professionals with little experience to approach patients with suspected lesions [14, 16].

7. Delayed search for professional assistance when the patient perceives the lesion: people usually notice the presence of the injury but do not seek a professional for confirmation. Often they refer to fear of confirming the diagnosis of the disease. This delay in seeking the diagnosis causes the lesion to continue growing, leading to late diagnosis [14].

8. Difficulties in accessing dental treatment: many people are unable to get adequate dental care due to the difficulty in accessing health services. In general, it is due to their vulnerable conditions or even because they do not seek health services [14].

Regarding oral cancer prevention and health promotion activities, it is essential to highlight the urgency of designing public policies for long-term health education actions. If education is not changed, concepts and habits will not change after short campaigns. That points out to the need for permanent education programs, since the best way to combat oral cancer is prevention, early diagnosis, and the attempt to eliminate risk factors. Health education through programs aimed at valuing periodic evaluations and the importance of examining the oral cavity are the significant weapons available to reduce the high incidence of oral cancer in the community [14].

The biopsy is undoubtedly the gold standard for the diagnosis of OC. However, there are several questions related to this method used in screening. It is an aggressive procedure, not readily accepted by people, especially when the lesion is asymptomatic and, even more so if it is proposed in oral health campaigns. The biopsy is limited by morbidity, once the procedure provokes another injury that may cause pain, bleeding, or other symptoms. Still, due to the resources required and the possibility of underdiagnosis, this method demands trained professionals to perform the procedure, trained pathologist, and facilities for the necessary reading of the exam. These characteristics mean a long time to receive the diagnosis, and patients experience discomfort caused by all the process [20].

Although the factors related to early detection of OC have different natures, it is noteworthy that, after all, the primary responsibility lies with the health system. For that, health service and program must organize its strategies according to the characteristics of the users.

Studies have been conducted to support measures aimed at solving the problem of late diagnosis, and the various approaches used to solve this problem are related to the factors abovementioned. In this text, we will address in particular the issue of noninvasive methods.

3. Prevention of oral cancer

Considering factors that interfere with the pathology diagnosis in question, the actions should be directed to them, to improve the care to the population.

Prevention and early diagnosis of oral cancer are critical. Equally important is the need for a differentiated look in this issue, given the characteristics of the affected population, the role of the dentist, the continuing training of oral health professionals, and the implementation of new strategies for early detection of this pathology [16, 21].

Actions related to the prevention of oral cancer and early diagnosis are foreseen within concepts widely worked in public health, which are health promotion and disease prevention. Health prevention requires firstly action based on knowledge of the natural history of the disease to prevent its progress [22]. Primary prevention is defined as a set of interventions to minimize the risk of specific ailments, reducing incidence and prevalence rates in the population and focusing on keeping individuals free from diseases.

Health promotion, on the other hand, is broader, as it refers to measures that act in the health disease process. Here, the intention is to modify the lifestyle and living conditions of the population, thus not working on a specific disease. Health promotion depends on the individuals, the community, and the sectors of society, health professionals, and oral health professionals [23].

Preventive measures may have a collective or individual approach. The collective approach includes interventions focused on health promotion. It means educational actions, periodic examinations of the most vulnerable people to the development of oral cancer, integration of the oral health team into smoking control programs, and other actions related to control of oral cancer. Besides that is a systematic provision of information on reference sites to the population about the diagnostic examination of oral cancer. In turn, the individual approach includes early diagnosis, treatment, and rehabilitation [17, 18].

Some primary intervention and prevention measures would be ideal for reducing cancer, such as combating lifestyle, environmental, and occupational factors and investigating the genetic factors associated with some specific types of cancer [14]. Population screening is indicated as an important preventive measure. This process can favor the diagnosis of suspicious lesions, which are to be referred for differential diagnosis, making it possible to implement early intervention and increase the chance of cure [14, 24]. Studies indicate the relevance of the screening of this pathology in risk populations, such as smokers and alcoholics. And it is even more relevant given the delay in diagnosis. Although evidence from the use of the visual examination of the mouth on mortality rates is weak by OC, some authors

Risk factors for oral cancer	Primary and secondary prevention methods
Unhealthy lifestyle habits: tobacco and alcohol use, physical inactivity, nutritional deficiency, tobacco chewing, betel nut chewing, poor oral hygiene	Active performance of the dentist in care and prevention actions
Population characteristics: low sociocultural level, age, and gender	Training of the oral health team on oral cancer
HPV infection	Implementation of new early detection strategies, according to the population served
Prolonged use of dental prosthesis, especially in the absence of routine monitoring and evaluation by a professional	Individual and collective educational actions on healthy living habits
Lack of information about the disease, its risk factors and protection	Routine screening for early detection of cancer, especially among the most vulnerable to oral cancer
Lack of information to the population about health services and their flow when a suspected injury is diagnosed	Integration of the oral health team with smoking control programs and other actions related to oral cancer control
Lack of training of professionals working in care	Systematic information to the population on reference sites for oral cancer diagnostic examination
Lack of specific campaigns and information about oral cancer, its risk factors and protection	Fight against lifestyle, environmental, and occupational factors that may be related to oral cancer
	Investigation of genetic factors associated with some specific types of cancer for the risk group
	Tracking of this pathology in at-risk populations by the health team
	Offering opportunities for evaluation of oral lesions (active search—through home visits or specific campaigns)
	Follow-up of suspected cases, creating a reference service if necessary and establishing partnerships between universities and other organizations for prevention, diagnosis, treatment, and recovery
	Training of professionals working in the front line of health care

Table 1.
Summary of risk factors related to oral cancer and primary and secondary prevention methods.

suggest proceeding to the screening on individuals who are exposed to risk factors. For these people, it may result in an increased positive predictive factor [7].

The approach to OC should involve prevention and control measures, including routine screening for early detection; offer of opportunities for evaluation of oral lesions (active search—through home visits or specific campaigns); follow-up of suspected cases, creating a referral service if necessary; and establishing partnerships between universities and other organizations for prevention, diagnosis, treatment, and recovery [18].

Actions with this objective can be organized as primary prevention. They include activities geared at disseminating information to the population, intending to change unhealthy lifestyle habits to healthy ones and to reduce the prevalence and incidence rates. At this level, the emphasis is placed on drinking, smoking, diet, and exposure to sun and human papillomavirus (HPV) infection.

Secondary prevention, in turn, occurs through the identification of precancerous lesions. For correct identification, it is essential to train health-care professionals with an emphasis on assessing potentially malignant cell lesions/disorders (PMD) (DPM) [17].

Below in **Table 1** is a summary of the risk factors and prevention methods.

4. Noninvasive methods for diagnosis of OC

Easy-to-handle, noninvasive diagnostic methods are useful for identifying precancerous lesions. The following noninvasive methods are cited: toluidine blue testing, exfoliative cytology, autofluorescence, contact endoscopy, and in vivo microscopy. However, there is no scientific evidence that these methods are more effective than oral inspection and palpation. Thus, more extensive studies are needed to justify the widespread use of these methods in the population. However, studies have shown that these methods can be useful if used in people with risk factors and non-healing lesions, favoring a faster diagnosis [20, 25, 26].

The following noninvasive diagnostic methods should be used according to the possibilities and conditions of the context.

4.1 Toluidine blue test

Toluidine blue is a basic thiazine metachromatic dye that selectively marks acidic groups of tissue components (carboxylic radicals, sulfates, and phosphates), showing an affinity for nuclear DNA and cytoplasmic RNA, which fix the dye, becoming richly stained. The intensity of toluidine blue staining depends on the degree of involvement of the epithelial surface. In benign lesions, there is a faint coloration; in dysplasia and epithelial lesions and carcinomas, the coloration is more intense.

The application maneuver consists of drying and isolating the region to be examined from salivary contamination by grasping the site with the fingers and using gauze. Employing a flexible cotton swab, 1% acetic acid (acid solution) is applied to clean the lesion surface, remove the glycoprotein barrier of cells, and promote slight dehydration of the mucosa. After 1 minute, the AT dye is applied with the other side of the cotton swab, and after 1 minute, the excess is cleaned with 1% acetic acid again and washed with plenty of water.

The result is intended to highlight intensely stained areas compatible with areas of tissue degeneration. Indications: detection of epithelial dysplasias, in situ or early invasive carcinomas, delimitation of neoplastic epithelium margins, assessment of tumor recurrence after surgical or radiotherapy treatment, delimitation of areas of cancer action, screening of oral lesions in population groups exposed to risk factors for oral cancer, and in intraoperative actions for marginal control of carcinomas.

It has the advantages of being painless, low-cost, and easy to apply, giving fast results, and having high sensitivity. As for disadvantages, it may generate false-positive or false-negative results and be of low and little specificity [10, 27].

4.2 Exfoliative cytology

It can be defined as the morphological and morphometric study of desquamated cells of the mucosa, mainly suprabasal cells, through optical microscopy. It consists in the examination of cells from various parts of the body to determine the cause or nature of the disease that affects them.

There are reports of numerous methods for collection of these cells in the literature. Conventional exfoliative cytology and liquid-based exfoliative cytology are two of the most disseminated among them.

Collecting the material in exfoliative cytology involves scraping the surface of the lesion with a spatula or brush, which is then smeared over the glass slide, and the material is fixed to the slide using 95% alcohol or 1:1 alcohol/ether solution.

Exfoliation cytology in liquid media has been developed in recent years as a method that could replace the conventional exfoliative cytology proposed by Papanicolaou. Collection by this method is done using a brushing device with soft bristles arranged in a conical shape, which is then dipped in a methanol-based preservative liquid contained in a hermetically sealed tube. Such liquid has the function of preserving the cellular structure, the proteins, and principally the genetic material. The liquid undergoes a centrifugation or homogenization process, which helps to shrink some artifacts, and it is then filtered. The residual material in the filters is put in blades by contact imprinting. Debris, red blood cells, and mucus pass through the filter pores, which retain the epithelial cells to be analyzed.

It has the advantages of being painless, harmless, noninvasive, and low-cost. As for disadvantages, it does not have the same efficacy as biopsy concerning identifying the type of lesion, but it is beneficial when the biopsy is not possible [20, 28, 29].

4.3 Fluorescence/autofluorescence

Optical fluorescence can be used as an aid to oral clinical examination. It allows, by autofluorescence, the detection of numerous changes in the oral cavity that could go unnoticed by the dentist or even be difficult to perceive with the visual method alone.

The oral fluorescence system allows the observation of changes in dental hard tissues such as stains, dental plaque and calculus, incipient lesions, and marginal infiltrations and facilitates the differentiation between restorative materials such as composite resin and ceramic.

In soft tissues, it is possible to detect potentially malignant lesions and tumoral lesions. Therefore, the optical fluorescence system allows the simple, noninvasive, and real-time diagnosis and identification of structures and alterations in the oral cavity, revealing lesions that would not be easily detected with conventional illumination.

As advantages, this method is highly sensitive to cancer and dysplasia, allows the evaluation of large areas of the oral mucosa during a consultation, and is noninvasive and painless. However, it has the disadvantage of false-positive results [20].

4.4 Contact endoscopy

It is also known as contact microstomatoscopy. It consists of the contact of the endoscope lens with the mucosa, the vermilion, and or the lesion.

It has the advantages of being painless and providing a fast diagnosis. However, a study by showed that the difficulties encountered about the device and the anatomical structures examined (lip and oral cavity) were related to the contact of the lens surface, fine tremors, and the sliding of the device; these difficulties varied according to topography. The quality depended on the site of the lesion, the extent of the ulceration, the volume of crusts, prior cleaning of the site, patient collaboration, the presence of more or less saliva, the mobility of the examined structure, and the support for the device [28, 30].

4.5 In vivo microscopy

High-resolution microendoscopy, optical coherence tomography, confocal reflectance microscopy, and multiphoton imaging are considered in this classification. These methods allow practitioners to see many of the same microscopic features used for histopathological evaluation at the consultation.

Each technology measures different optical properties of the tissue and offers various features in parameters such as image depth, resolution, visual field, and acquisition time. Their development is at an early stage. We cite Raman spectroscopy as a promising technique for cancer diagnosis. This device is an analytical noninvasive technique that provides information about the molecular structure of the investigated sample, considering that the molecular structures of proteins and lipids differ between normal and neoplastic tissues.

The advantage of these technologies is their accuracy, but the high cost of acquisition is a significant disadvantage [20, 31].

4.6 Tumor biomarkers

Tumor biomarkers are substances found in blood, urine, or other body fluids and tissues that may be in increased amounts when a particular type of cancer is present. These biomarkers are used for diagnostic elucidation through serology and histological methods. They are cellular, structural, and biochemical components that can be quantitatively measured by biochemical, immunological, and molecular methods in body fluids and tissues associated with neoplasms and possibly the organs where cancer originates.

At present, no marker is used for cancer detection in the general population, only for people who are in the risk group for certain types of cancer. In this case, biomarkers can help to diagnose the disease in early stages.

Research on the diagnosis of saliva using nanotechnology and molecular technologies to detect oral squamous cell carcinoma (OSCC) is currently being expanded. Collecting saliva for this assessment is a secure, noninvasive method, which is considered advantageous.

Diagnosing saliva using nanotechnology and molecular technologies to detect OSCC has become an attractive field of study. New cancer-related proteins have been reported, as well as potent biomarkers for early diagnosis, further facilitating the application of quantification in proteomics for carcinogenesis research. Identifying transcripts and pathways that change at early stages of carcinogenesis provides potentially useful information for early diagnosis and prevention strategies.

At the beginning of the research on this method, the hope was that all cancers could be detected at an early stage, preventing the death of millions of people. But only a few markers can detect cancer at an early stage. The disadvantages of this method are most people have a small amount of these markers that prevents detection, the levels of these markers tend to increase when the disease progresses, some cancer patients may never have high levels of markers, and even in the presence of elevated levels, they do not always indicate cancer, as they may be related to other disorders [6, 32–36].

4.7 Oral inspection and palpation

The main areas examined for oral cancer are the face, neck, lips, nostrils, and oral cavity. Before the screening, the patient should remove all removable dental appliances and devices to leave the entire area exposed. The patient must be seated or lying down, and the dentist must look for signs of asymmetry, edema, swelling, staining, ulceration, or other abnormalities.

To examine the inside of the mouth, the practitioner will use good lighting and a mirror to see clearly; he will also use a tongue depressor to immobilize the organ and look at the back of the mouth. After or during the visual examination, the dentist will palpate the head, face, around the jaw, under the chin, and the oral cavity. The aim is to detect unusual lumps or masses. Another sign of a potential problem is immobility in some regularly moving tissue.

The advantages are the fast, painless, low-cost characteristics of the method, and the disadvantage is that it relies heavily on the examiner's skills and knowledge. Conventional oral examination (COE) alone is insufficient for risk stratification. COE is generally useful for identifying lesions but not for subsequent clinical follow-up for treatment planning [20].

Despite the importance of the methods described above as adjuvants in the process of diagnosis of suspected lesions, the biopsy is considered the gold standard for definitive diagnosis [20].

All of these methods have their advantages and disadvantages and can be used in care to facilitate diagnosis. These noninvasive alternatives are not much disseminated in health services, and visual inspection under white light and palpation by a physician or dentist remain as the gold standard for screening of oral cancer. This procedure, however, has the limitation of being dependent on the examiner's experience; this limitation underlies the development of more objective diagnostic techniques.

Despite the scarcity of evidence about the abovementioned noninvasive methods as the diagnosis of a lesion front line, they can be useful in several situations. For instance, in cases where the biopsy is not a reasonable procedure, either for cost or complexity, most of these methods can make a difference.

They used to be inexpensive, can be performed by less specialized professionals, are generally handled with lighter technology, and are more easily implemented in less resourceful regions and within primary health care [25, 26]. In these situations, the aim is to replace noninvasive techniques where a biopsy cannot be performed promptly. More, it can facilitate the screening of lesions in apparently healthy people, with or without risk factors for cancer, since it is a recommended noninvasive method that makes it possible to differentiate malignant to benign lesions. Despite the several possibilities of diagnostic methods, the rates still indicate that patients are diagnosed in advanced stages of cancer [25, 26, 37].

These adjuvant diagnostic methods may help dentists better evaluate lesions suggestive of oral cancer before a definitive biopsy. The existing adjuvants such as

Method	Indication	Advantage	Disadvantage
Toluidine blue test	Diagnosis and surgical approach to various mucosal tumors	Painless, low-cost, easy application, fast result, and high sensitivity	It can generate false-positive or false-negative results, being of low specificity
Exfoliative cytology	Initial assessment of incipient lesions and follow-up of areas that underwent previous surgical resection	Painless, harmless, noninvasive, inexpensive	It does not have the same efficacy as biopsy in the identification of the type of lesion; however it is very useful when biopsy is not possible. It can generate false-positive or false-negative results
Fluorescence/autofluorescence	Adjuvant method in oral clinical examination for detection of cellular disorders	High sensitivity for cancer and dysplasia, ability to evaluate large areas of the oral mucosa at the moment of consultation, noninvasive, painless	It can generate false-positive results
Contact endoscopy	A colposcope with optical magnification of up to 40 times is applied to help diagnose oral cavity lesions	Painless, fast diagnosis	Difficulties in relation to the device and the anatomical structures examined (lip and oral cavity) related to the contact of the lens surface, fine tremors, and slippage of the device
In vivo microscopy	Histopathological evaluation of suspected lesions at the moment of consultation	High precision	High cost
Tumor biomarkers	Diagnostic elucidation, tumor recurrence evaluation, or follow-up of treatment progress	Early detection, noninvasive	It can generate false-positive or false-negative results

Method	Indication	Advantage	Disadvantage
Oral inspection and palpation	Identification of lesions, monitoring of oral health of the individual, screening of suspicious lesions for oral cancer	Fast, painless, and low-cost	It depends on the examiner's skill and knowledge

Table 2.
Noninvasive methods for diagnosis of oral cancer.

toluidine blue, acetowhitening, and autofluorescence imaging are not much specific and, therefore, generally not recommended. Recently, new in vivo microscopy technologies such as high-resolution microendoscopy, optical coherence tomography, reflectance confocal microscopy, and multiphoton imaging have shown to offer promising improvements and more accurate diagnosis of these lesions and are not invasive procedures. The advantages of these technologies are that they allow the visualization of the microscopic characteristics used for histopathological evaluation at the moment of consultation, making the diagnosis faster, besides being painful or uncomfortable to patients [20].

Other measures discussed are those related to the reorganization of health services, screening of risk groups, and awareness campaigns. These measures are used in many countries around the world, but the problem of late diagnosis is still a worldwide reality [38, 39].

New strategies to approach the population and to identify suspicious lesions are paramount in the dissemination of information and for the increase of early diagnosed cases. The cooperation of primary health-care teams and not only of oral health professionals is essential for the fight against late diagnosis. Because other sectors of the health area often assist the population and can identify the risk, and even suspicious lesions, they also should be able to refer patients to the oral health sector. Thus, with all professionals working together in primary health care, identifying risk factors and suspicious lesions, and referring to the responsible sector, this collaborative work may bring a great positive gain for the population [14, 38].

Below in a **Table 2** is a summary of the methods discussed above.

4.8 Considerations

Considering the real problem of oral cancer worldwide, actions aimed at reducing the negative impact on society should be carried out with planning to achieve excellence of care to the population.

Some factors lead to late diagnosis of oral cancer. Thus, such elements must be identified in each population so that health professionals can act to interfere with these factors, leading to better care for the community. Knowing population profile to be assisted is required, as much to identify factors that interfere with the diagnosis of the pathology as in the action planning.

Although the biopsy is considered as the gold standard for definitive diagnosis, there are some constraints for your full application. This method is invasive and expensive, the results may take some days to be disclosed, and it requires specialized training, thus limiting its use for screening. Therefore, noninvasive methods are valuable, becoming more suitable in specific contexts.

Nomenclature

OC	oral cancer
HPV	human papilloma virus
IARC	International Agency for Research on Cancer
MPD	malignant cell lesions/disorders
COE	conventional oral examination

Author details

Manoela Garcia Dias da Conceição[1,2]*, Ana Cláudia Figueiró[3] and Vera Lucia Luiza[4]

1 Sergio Arouca National School of Public Health, ENSP, Oswaldo Cruz Foundation, FIOCRUZ, Rio de Janeiro, RJ, Brazil

2 National Cancer Institute, Brazil

3 Endemic Department Samuel Pessoa, Sergio Arouca National School of Public Health, ENSP, Oswaldo Cruz Foundation, FIOCRUZ, Rio de Janeiro, RJ, Brazil

4 Department of Drug Policy and Pharmaceutical Care, Sergio Arouca National School of Public Health, ENSP, Oswaldo Cruz Foundation, FIOCRUZ, Rio de Janeiro, RJ, Brazil

*Address all correspondence to: manu_dias1984@yahoo.com.br

References

[1] World Health Organization. The World Oral Health Report 2003. Continuous improvement of oral health in the 21st century-the approach of the WHO Global Oral Health Programme. 2003

[2] Toscano de Brito R, França Perazzo M, Santos PeixotoT, Weege-NonakaCF, deMeloBrito Costa EM, Granville-Garcia AF. Profile of patients and factors related to the clinical staging of oral squamous cell carcinoma. Revista de Salud Pública Bogota. dezembro de. 2018;**20**(2):221-225

[3] Chaturvedi P, Singh A, Chien C-Y, Warnakulasuriya S. Tobacco related oral cancer. BMJ. junho de. 2019;**365**:l2142

[4] Ferlay J. Globocan 2012: Cancer Incidence and Mortality Worldwide. IARC; 2013

[5] Ferlay J. Globocan 2018: Cancer Incidence and Mortality Worldwide. IARC; 2019

[6] Mishra R. Biomarkers of oral premalignant epithelial lesions for clinical application. Oral Oncology. 06PY - 2012 de. 2012;**48**(7):578-584

[7] Bhatt S, Isaac R, Finkel M, Evans J, Grant L, Paul B, et al. Mobile technology and cancer screening: Lessons from rural India. Journal of Global Health. 2018;**8**(2):020421-020421

[8] Carvalho AL, Singh B, Spiro RH, Kowalski LP, Shah JP. Cancer of the oral cavity: A comparison between institutions in a developing and a developed nation. janeiro de. 2004;**26**(1):31-38

[9] Kowalski LP, Brentani MM, Coelho FRG. Bases da oncologia. São Paulo: Lemar; 2003

[10] Ramos GHA, de Oliveira BV, Biasi LJ, Sampaio Júnior LA. Avaliação da citologia e do teste do azul de toluidina no diagnóstico dos tumores malignos da mucosa oral. Revista Brasileira de Cirurgia da Cabeça e Pescoço. 03PY - 2007 de. 2007;**36**(1):27-29

[11] da Silva MC, Marques EB, de Melo LC, de Bernardo JMP, Leite ICG. Fatores relacionados ao atraso no diagnóstico de câncer de boca e orofaringe em Juiz de Fora/MG. Revista Brasileira de Cancerologia. 2009;**55**(4):329-335

[12] Rafieian N, Azimi S, Manifar S, Julideh H, ShirKhoda M. Is there any association between green tea consumption and the risk of head and neck squamous cell carcinoma: Finding from a case-control study. Archives of Oral Biology. 2019;**98**:280-284

[13] Zhou H, Wu W, Wang F, Qi H, Cheng Z. Tea consumption is associated with decreased risk of oral cancer: A comprehensive and dose-response meta-analysis based on 14 case-control studies (MOOSE compliant). Med Baltimore. dezembro de. 2018;**97**(51):e13611

[14] Amorim NGC, Sousa AS, Alves SM. Prevenção e diagnóstico precoce do câncer bucal: Uma revisão de literatura. Revista Uningá. junho de. 2019;**56**(2):70-84

[15] Narvai PC, Frazão P. Saúde Bucal no Brasil muito além do céu da boca. Rio de Janeiro: Fiocruz; 2008. 148 p

[16] Rangel EB, Lucietto DA, Stefenon L. Autopercepção de cirurgiões-dentistas sobre conhecimentos e práticas em relação ao câncer de boca. Revista Rede de Cuidados em Saúde. dezembro de. 2018;**12**(2):28-40

[17] Torres-Pereira CC, Angelim-Dias A, Melo NS, Lemos CA Jr, de Oliveira EMF.

Abordagem do câncer da boca: Uma estratégia para os níveis primário e secundário de atenção em saúde Strategies for management of oral cancer in primary and secondary healthcare services. Cadernos de Saúde Pública. 2012;**28**(supl):s30-s39

[18] Dias MG. Avaliação da Atenção em Saúde Bucal: contribuições para o controle do câncer de boca no município do Rio de Janeiro. Rio de Janeiro: Escola Nacional de Saúde Pública; 2018

[19] Al-Kaabi R, Gamboa ABO, Williams D, Marcenes W. Social inequalities in oral cancer literacy in an adult population in a multicultural deprived area of the UK. Journal of Public Health—Oxford Academic. 2016;**38**(3):474-482

[20] Yang EC, Tan MT, Schwarz RA, Richards-Kortum RR, Gillenwater AM, Vigneswaran N. Noninvasive diagnostic adjuncts for the evaluation of potentially premalignant oral epithelial lesions: Current limitations and future directions. Oral Surgery, Oral Medicine, Oral Pathology, and Oral Radiology. abril de. 2018;**125**(6):670-681

[21] Alvarenga ML, Couto MG, de Ribeiro AO, Milagres RCM, Messora MR, Kawata LT. Avaliação do conhecimento dos cirurgiões-dentistas quanto ao câncer bucal. RFO UPF [Internet]. 04PY - 2012 de 2012;17(1). Disponível em: http://files.bvs.br/upload/S/1413-4012/2012/v17n1/a2980.pdf

[22] Leavell H, Clark EG. Preventive Medicine for the Doctor in His Community. MacGraw Hill: Nova York; 1965

[23] Silva, da AN, Senna, de MAA, Jorge RC, da Albuquerque DMS, de Queiroz TF. Promoção da Saúde. In: Fundamentos em Saúde Bucal Coletiva. Rio de Janeiro: Medbook; 2013. pp. 1-14

[24] Brasil Instituto Nacional de Câncer—INCA. A Situação do câncer no Brasil. INCA; 2006

[25] Walsh T, Liu JL, Brocklehurst P, Glenny AM, Lingen M, Kerr AR, et al. Clinical assessment to screen for the detection of oral cavity cancer and potentially malignant disorders in apparently healthy adults. Cochrane Database of Systematic Reviews. 12PY - 2013 de. 2013;**11**:CD010173-CD010173

[26] Sweeny L, Dean NR, Magnuson JS, Carroll WR, Clemons L, Rosenthal EL. Assessment of tissue autofluorescence and reflectance for oral cavity cancer screening. Otolaryngology–Head and Neck Surgery. 12PY - 2011 de. 2011;**145**(6):956-960

[27] Sharbatdaran M, Abbaszadeh H, Siadati S, Ranaee M, Hajian-Tilaki K, Rajabi-Moghaddam M. Assessment of oral cytological features in smokers and nonsmokers after application of toluidine blue. Diagnostic Cytopathology. março de. 2017;**45**(6):513-519

[28] Dias MG, Figueiró AC, Luiza VL. Prevention and early diagnosis of oral cancer—A literature review. Revista Odonto Ciência. 25 de julho de. 2018;**32**(4):204

[29] Lucena EE de S, Miranda AM, Araújo FA da C, Galvão CAB, de Medeiros AMC. Método de coleta e a qualidade do esfregaço de mucosa oral. Revista de Cirurgia e Traumatologia Buco Maxilo Facial. junho de. 2011;**11**(2):55-62

[30] Ramos GHA, Tavares MR, Dedivitis RA, França CM, Oliveira BV, Pedruzzi PA. Endoscopia de contato (microestomatoscopia) nas lesões da boca e do lábio: Avaliação do método. Revista do Colégio Brasileiro de Cirurgiões. 2008;**35**(6):355-360

[31] Pelc R, Masek V, Llopis-Torregrosa V, Bour P, Wu T. Spectral counterstaining in luminescence-enhanced biological Raman microscopy. Chemical Communications. julho de. 2019;**55**(57):8329-8332

[32] Jiang W-P, Wang Z, Xu L-X, Peng X, Chen F. Diagnostic model of saliva peptide finger print analysis of oral squamous cell carcinoma patients using weak cation exchange magnetic beads. Julho de. 2015;**35**(3). Disponível em: http://www.ncbi.nlm.nih.gov/pmc/articles/PMC4613719/?tool=pubmed

[33] Guerrero-Preston R, Soudry E, Acero J, Orera M, Moreno-López L, Macía-Colón G, et al. NID2 and HOXA9 promoter hypermethylation as biomarkers for prevention and early detection in oral cavity squamous cell carcinoma tissues and saliva. Cancer Prevention Research (Phila). 07PY - 2011 de. 2011;**4**(7):1061-1072

[34] Mankapure PK, Barpande SR, Bhavthankar JD, Mandale M. Serum big endothelin-1 as a biomarker in oral squamous cell carcinoma patients: An analytical study. Journal of Applied Oral Science. novembro de. 2015;**23**(5):491-496

[35] Lingen MW. Screening for oral premalignancy and cancer: What platform and which biomarkers? Cancer Prevention Research (Phila). 09PY - 2010 de. 2010;**3**(9):1056-1059

[36] Brinkmann O, Kastratovic DA, Dimitrijevic MV, Konstantinovic VS, Jelovac DB, Antic J, et al. Oral squamous cell carcinoma detection by salivary biomarkers in a Serbian population. Oral Oncology. 02PY - 2011 de. 2011;**47**(1):51-55

[37] Mehrotra R, Gupta DK. Exciting new advances in oral cancer diagnosis: Avenues to early detection. Head and Neck Oncology. 2011;**3**

[38] Bulgareli JV, Diniz OCCF, de Faria ET, de Vazquez FL, Cortellazzi KL, Pereira AC. Prevenção e detecção do câncer bucal: planejamento participativo como estratégia para ampliação da cobertura populacional em idosos. Ciênc Saúde Coletiva. 12PY - 2013 de. 2013;**18**(12):3461-3473

[39] de Scheufen RC, Almeida FCS, da Silva DP, de Araujo ME, Palmiere M, Pegoretti T, et al. Prevenção e detecção precoce do câncer de boca: Screening em populações de risco. Pesquisa Brasileira em Odontopediatria e Clínica Integrada. 02PY - 2012 de. 2012;**11**(02). Disponível em: http://revista.uepb.edu.br/index.php/pboci/article/viewFile/1442/683

Chapter 9

Vascular Endothelial Growth Factor Expression in the Pathological Angiogenesis in Oral Squamous Cell Carcinoma

Biagio Rapone and Elisabetta Ferrara

Abstract

Tumor angiogenesis and tumor progression to late oral squamous cell carcinoma are closely related. Vascular endothelial growth factor (VEGF), a heparin-binding growth factor with mitogenic activity specific for vascular endothelial cells, regulates key events of the pathological angiogenesis involved in the metabolic functions of malignant tissues. The level of high-affinity tyrosine kinase receptor for VEGF, *flt*, in tumor endothelial cells *in vivo* is seen upregulated, supporting the role of VEGF as a potential signaling tumor angiogenesis axis *in vivo* and sustaining the notion that paracrine mechanisms are responsible for the regulation of tumor angiogenesis. The expression of VEGFs is increased in the processes of oral squamous cell carcinoma (OSCC) progression and proliferation. Vascular endothelial growth factor C (VEGF-C)/VEGF3 expression induced by chemokine CCL4 is connected to lymph node metastasis in OSCC. This chapter was aimed to summarize and analyze the findings on the role of vascular endothelial growth factor in oral squamous cell carcinoma and briefly discuss the potential of vascular endothelial growth factor that targets this pathway as treatment for OSCC.

Keywords: angiogenesis, vascular endothelial growth factor, oral cancer, overexpression, VEGF polymorphism

1. Introduction

The angiogenesis process involves approximately twenty factors, such as basic fibroblast growth factor, placenta growth factor (PIGF-1), epidermal growth factor (EP), as platelet-derived GF (PDGF), and the most important angiogenic factor: vascular endothelial growth factor (VEGF). Studies of restricted expression patterns and functional roles have implicated VEGFs in the generation of new blood vessels from pre-existing vasculature complex genetic pathways. VEGF has since been documented as being a potent stimulator of endothelial cells proliferation and migration and to induce the expression of interstitial collagenases. Specifically, VEGFs regulate physiological angiogenesis, including the vessel and the organ development, the lymphogenesis, and the differentiation during embryogenesis, as well the pathogenesis of a multiplicity of disorders. The hypothesis that VEGF action is required for tumor angiogenesis has been first provided by the findings of the vascular development of tumor xenografts in mice. These results were confirmed through in situ hybridization studies, showing a correlation between the degree of defective angiogenesis and VEGF mRNA upregulation. These studies uniformly concur that VEGF expression enhances tumor growth. In this chapter, we provide a brief historical overview of the discovery of VEGF, structural characterization of the other members of VEGF family and their receptor, and to summarize the main features of the role of vascular endothelial growth factor in angiogenesis of oral cancer development.

2. Discovery of VEGF

VEGF was first described in 1983 as a factor secreted by hepatocarcinoma cell lines [1] that increased microvascular permeability to plasma proteins in the skin of guinea-pigs. It was highly purified to homogeneity from pituitary folliculostellate cells and characterized in 1989 [2]. Other authors supported evidence that this protein potently stimulated endothelial cell migration [3–5]. It was named "vascular permeability factor" or VPF, potent inducers of vascular hyperpermeability (especially venular endothelium) to fibrinogen and other plasma proteins [6], which upon secretion by tumor cells, promotes vascular leakage [7]. More years later, it was demonstrated that VPF has potent mitogenic activity in a diversity of cell types, and also versus endothelial cells [8]. Vascular endothelial growth factors (VEGFs) are predominantly produced by endothelial, hematopoietic, and stromal cells in response to hypoxia and upon stimulation by growth factors such as transforming growth factor β (TGFβ), interleukins, or platelet-derived growth factors (PDGFs). VEGFs specifically interact with one or several receptor tyrosine kinases (RTKs), VEGF receptor −1, −2, and −3 (VEGFR-1, −2, −3), and with distinct coreceptors such as neuropilins or heparan sulfate glycosaminoglycans. VEGF receptors are classified as type V RTKs whose extracellular domains consist of seven immunoglobulin-like (Ig-like) domains [9, 10]. The intracellular domain consists of seven immunoglobulin-like domains (I–VII), a single transmembrane (TM) region, and a tyrosine kinase consensus sequence (TK) interrupted by a cytoplasmatic kinase domain [11, 12].

3. The VEGF gene and isoforms

The VEGFs term identifies a large and heterogeneous family of secreted polypeptides, named VEGF-A, VEGF-B, VEGF-C, VEGF-D, VEGF-E and placenta growth factor (PGF), characterized by a highly conserved receptor-binding cystine-knot structure similar to that of the platelet-derived growth factors [13, 14]. Of those six members, VEGF-A plays a key role in vasculogenesis and angiogenesis [15]. PGF is mainly expressed in placenta, heart and lungs; it is a ligand for VEGFR-2 and it is involved in angiogenesis regulation. VEGF-B binds VEGFR-1 and neuropilin-1, mostly expressed in the extracellular matrix and abundantly expressed in brown fat, in the myocardium and skeletal muscle; it is implicated in high cellular energy metabolism. VEGF-C is produced as a precursor protein [16, 17]. VEGF-C promotes mitogenesis, migration and survival of ECs [18], and regulates the lymphatic vessel growth by binding to VEGF-receptor-3 (VEGFR-3, Flt-4) [19, 20]. VEGF-D, binds and activates VEGFR-2 and VEGFR-3, because is mitogenic for EC, angiogenic, and lymphangiogenic. Its expression was demonstrated mainly in the lung and skin during embryogenesis. VEGF-E expression, binding the VEGFR-2, promotes the release of tissue factors, proliferation, chemotaxis and sprouting of cultured vascular ECs in vitro and angiogenesis in vivo [6, 21]. The major function of VEGF-C consist in regulation VEGF exerts its effect on tissues at several levels; mechanisms range from a plethora of physiological processes which regulate blood vessel growth, such as during pregnancy and in tissue repair to pathological conditions, including chronic inflammation, would healing process, and cancer [6, 22]. It has been proven that VEGF causes a pronounced angiogenic response in a variety of in vivo models, including the chick chorioallantoic membrane [23, 24]. Native VEGF is a basic, heparin-binding, homodimeric glycoprotein of 45,000 daltons. Interestingly, the VEGF gene has been mapped to chromosome 6 at position p21.3 [25] and consists of eight exons and seven introns in the coding sequence, which covers a region of 14 kilobases. Among these, there is evidence that the −634G/C, −1154G/A, and −2578C/A *VEGF* polymorphisms have been shown to be associated with increased VEGF production. Alternative splicing of the mRNA from the gene of VEGF, VEGF-B, and PIGF results in the expression of five known human isoforms with differential diffusibility and heparin-binding properties containing 121, 145, 165, 183, 189 and 206 amino acids with different biological properties: $VEGF_{121}$, $VEGF_{165}$, $VEGF_{189}$, and $VEGF_{206}$ [26]. The $VEGF_{121}$ is a weakly acidic polypeptide with a 44 *amino-acid insertion* encoded by exon 7a, that fails to bind to heparin [27]; *$VEGF_{189}$ has* a further *insertion* of 24 *amino acids, highly enriched in basic residues* encoded by exon 6a. $VEGF_{121}$ and $VEGF_{165}$ have been detected predominantly in normal tissue, but VEGF121 isoform is both more angiogenic and tumorigenic than being the 165 and 189 isoforms [27, 28]. In particular, the isoform 121 has been shown to predominate in primary human breast carcinomas (Relf M) $VEGF_{189}$ expression has been shown to be dominant in normal lung [29] and the 183 isoform predominates in heart [30, 31]. Several studies have reported that the expression of $VEGF_{206}$ occurs mainly in fetal liver.

3.1 Biological effects of VEGF expression

The VEGF and the "fibroblastic growth factor" (bFGF) demonstrate a powerful synergism in the promotion of angiogenesis in vitro, as shown by models using microvascular endothelial cells invading the *three-dimensional collagen* gel system [32, 33]. Also, VEGF exerts its effect by coordinating of angiopoietins, another class of angiogenic factors. Specifically, VEGF is involved in the early sequences of events leading to the vessel development, whereas angiopoietin 1 (Ang1), an agonist ligand for the endothelial-specific Tie2 receptor, binds and activates Tie2 to promote vessel maturation, vascular stability and leakiness [34]; Ang2 acts as a Tie2 agonist in lymphatic endothelial cells generating an important vascular signaling pathway involved in angiogenesis, vascular stability and quiescence. VEGF achieves its functions of endothelial cell differentiation and proliferation by binding a family of tyrosine kinases receptors (VEGFRs), known as Flt-1 receptor (VEGF receptor-1) and VEGF receptor-2 (VEGF-2 or KDR/Flk-1). VEGFR-1 binds VEGF, VEGF-B and PlGF with high affinity and induces weak mitogenic signals in ECs. [23, 35] VEGFR-1 expression is up-regulated by hypoxia via (transcription hypoxia inducible factor) HIF-dependent mechanism [36, 37]. In the lung, VEGFR-1 provokes secretion of Matrix Metalloproteinase 9 (MMP9) at the vascular bed, thus empowering metastasis. Also, it has been discovered the role of VEGFR-1 in releasing tissue specific factors in a perivascular specific pattern at the level of vascular endothelium [38]. VEGFR-2, the major mediator of endothelial cell mitogenesis, proliferation and survival [39, 40] binds VEGF, VEGF-C, VEGF-D, VEGF-E and PlGF [22, 39]. VEGFR-2 expression is down-regulated in the adult blood vascular ECs, and is again up-regulated in the endothelium of angiogenic process. VEGF, VEGF-C and VEGF-D are bound VEGFR-3 and are involved in regulation of lymphangiogenesis, the growth of new lymphatic vessels [41–45]. The expression of VEGFR-3 (or Flt-4) is relevant in lymphatic vessels [44] and in hematopoietic cells of monocytic lineage [6, 42], and is also expressed in a subset of capillary endothelia [19]. Studies on animal models showed that VEGF-C/VEGFR-3 axis plays a crucial role in cancer metastasis by inducing lymphangiogenesis [46–48], but further investigations would be necessary. Furthermore, it has been documented the link between mutations in VEGFR-3 with hereditary lymphedema, an autosomal dominant disorder of the lymphatic system that can lead to lymphangiosarcomas [13, 49]. Neuropilins-1 and -2 are more important in immunology and neuronal development, but they are also involved in angiogenesis [19, 44]. Neuropilins, bind especially class 3 semaphorins but the Neuropilin-1 also binds VEGF, VEGF-B and PlGF, while Neuropilin-2 binds VEGF, VEGF-C and PlGF [50]. When is coexpressed in cells together with VEGFR-2, Neuropilin-1 enhances the binding of VEGF165 to VEGFR-2 and augments tumor angiogenesis in vivo [51, 52]. Nrp-2 is expressed also on lymphatic ECs, and mutated Nrp-2 forms induce abnormalities in the formation of small lymphatic vessels and lymphatic capillaries in mice [53]. In addition, some isoforms bind to known as non-tyrosine kinase receptors, known as neuropilins (NRPs) (neuropilin-1 and neuropilin-2 (22–44)). Neuropilins-1 and -2 are also involved in immunology and neuronal development [50, 54]. Neuropilins bind, especially class 3 semaphorins but the Neuropilin-1 also binds VEGF, VEGF-B and PlGF, while Neuropilin-2 binds VEGF, VEGF-C and PlGF [50]. Neuropilin-1 is capable to improve the binding of VEGF165 to VEGFR-2 and increase tumor angiogenesis in vivo [51, 53]. Nrp-2 is expressed also on lymphatic ECs, and it has been shown in vivo that mutated Nrp-2 form alters the formation of small lymphatic vessels and lymphatic capillaries in mice [54]. The binding results in stimulation of cell-signaling pathways that act to increase cell nucleus division, and contributing to angiogenesis through extracellular matrix dissolution, and endothelial cell movement.

4. Role of VEGF in oral squamous cell carcinoma

4.1 The role of VEGF in invasion

Angiogenesis, the formation of new blood vessels, is not only a normal physiological process, but it is closely linked to both tumor growth and metastasis, providing the principal pathway through tumor cells exit the primary tumor site and enter the circulation. A multiplicity of molecular determinants is involved in these different mechanisms of vascular growth, and VEGFs play a significant role in pathological angiogenesis. In particular, the role of VEGF-A in tumor angiogenesis are clarified by several studies [23, 55], but the results concerning VEGF-expression in normal and dysplastic oral epithelium, as well as about the potential role of VEGF in oral squamous cell carcinoma progression shown contradictions. VEGF-A overexpression has been reported in most types of cancer, including oral squamous cell carcinoma, and it is thought to be a prognostic factor for survival. Some studies revealed no altered VEGF expression in the normal and mildly dysplastic oral epithelium, or the expression was significantly lower than neoplastic epithelium [16–18]. A considerable upregulation of VEGF expression during the transition from normal oral epithelium through dysplasia to OSCC, but no correlation was found between VEGF expression and the grade of dysplasia. Many researchers demonstrated an upregulation of VEGF expression in cancerous tissues in comparison to the normal oral mucosa. These results suggest that VEGF could be implicated in tumor progression by expanding the vascularity during the process of transition from the normal oral mucosa to invasive carcinoma [18, 51–56].

Immunohistochemical study of VEGF expression in oral squamous cell carcinomas clarify the relationship between vascular endothelial growth factor (VEGF) expression and clinicopathological factors in oral squamous cell carcinoma (OSCC), showing that serum VEGF levels were significantly higher in oral cancer patients as compared to normal controls that further showed an increasing trend with clinical stage and lymph node involvement, suggesting that VEGF level may be a reliable biomarker and may be a potential target for development of chemotherapeutic strategies for patients with oral carcinoma.

4.2 The role of VEGF in metastasis

Lymphangiogenesis plays a vital role in tumor growth and systemic dissemination of different carcinomas [2]. Although vascular endothelial growth factor C (VEGF-C) is well known to be associated with lymph node metastasis in patients with OSCC, inducing the production of urokinase by cancer and playing a crucial role in the extracellular matrix remodeling and tumor cell invasion, the specific mechanisms of lymphangiogenesis in OSCC are largely unknown. Further, it has been implicated in inducing the growth of both blood and lymphatic vessels and in regulation of proliferation, differentiation and migration of lymphatic endothelial cells in many physiological and pathological conditions [19, 20]. Overexpression of VEGF-C has been detected in various malignancies and is frequently associated with lymphatic invasion, nodal and distant metastasis and consequently poor survival [23, 33]. VEGF-C signaling is involved in the progression of several malignancies that put forward VEGF-C as a potential target for the development of new anticancer therapies to prevent local invasion and metastatic spread of disease. The progression of several malignancies involves VEGF-C signaling. The immunohistochemical analysis and real-time quantitative RT-PCR studies showed a significant correlation between the levels of VEGF-C mRNA expression in a human OSCC cell line, through the phosphoinositide 3-kinase-Akt pathway. The angiogenic action of this growth factor is achievable by binding to two receptor tyrosine kinases (RTK), VEGFR-1 (Flt-1) and VEGFR-2 (KDR, Flk-1) [17, 22]. VEGFR-2 is the major mediator of the mitogenic, angiogenic and permeability-enhancing effects of VEGF-A, while the role of VEGFR-1 in the regulation of angiogenesis is controversial. It is implicated in a paracrine release of growth factors, but the central role of this receptor is to prevent the interaction of VEGF with VEGFR-2. Also, it may promote angiogenesis by recruitment in tumor vasculature of monocytes and other bone marrow-derived cells [48, 52, 57]. Moreover, VEGFR-1 is involved in the induction of matrix metalloproteinases [49] that retrovirus-mediated expression of a dominant negative VEGFR-2, because of inhibition of signal transduction through wild-type VEGFR-2, suppression of the growth of glioblastoma multiforme and other tumor cell lines in vivo. Correlation of VEGF expression with clinical stage of OSCC is controversial. Clinicopathologic findings suggest that evaluation of VEGF expression is of prognostic value in patients with OSCC. VEGF expression was found to increase significantly with advancing stage of the tumor. Elevated expression of VEGF was associated with aggressive phenotype and advanced stage of the tumor [58], as well as demonstrated by Yu Hong Li et al. which found a higher VEGF expression in stage 3 and 4 tumors as compared to stage 1 and 2 [59]. An explanation could be attributed to the correlation with the intensity of VEGF expression and the degree of differentiation or invasiveness of carcinoma. The results support the findings of previous *results* on the average density of immunohistochemistry (IHC), indicating that in normal oral squamous cells, VEGF expression was detected only in the vascular endothelial cells in the mesenchymal tissues [60, 61]. According to these results, to Kim's study on the up-regulation of vascular endothelial growth factor (VEGF) expression in oral squamous cell carcinoma, immunohistochemical staining with VEGF, found a very little expression of VEGF in normal oral squamous cell tissues and a significant positive relationship between VEGF expression and the degree of differentiation or invasiveness of carcinoma [62]. In addition, histopathological findings showed that the VEGF had *higher expression* levels in less-differentiated invasive oral squamous cell carcinoma, while it was expressed at slightly higher levels in well-differentiated and less-invasive intraepithelial carcinoma tissues or highly differentiated oral squamous cell carcinoma than in normal cells [62]. In contrast, Shang and Li found that VEGF expression was significantly higher in patients in patients with stage 1 and 2 tumors as compared to when there were a stage 3 and 4 tumors [63].

4.3 The role of VEGF in prognosis

Interestingly, some studies have focused on the potential prognostic importance of *VEGF* polymorphisms in head and neck cancers [14, 20, 21]. Results showed the association between −1154GG *VEGF* genotype, located in the promoter region of the gene, and higher VEGF production [12]. A study conducted by Ku et al., reported an association of −460C/T polymorphism and VEGF overexpression in oral cancer, showing a higher risk for oral cancer in the patients with a high −460TC ratio [66, 67]. Further investigations showed an association between +960C/T *VEGF* polymorphism and oral cancer [23], indicating that the low production of VEGF by the T allele is correlated with increased risk of oral cancer, and vascular invasion in oral squamous cell carcinoma. In contrast, Vairaktaris et al. [56], did not demonstrate an influence of gene polymorphism on the oral cancer in the logistic regression models. However, the genotype *VEGF* −460CT was associated with early stage tumors. Nasr et al. analyzed the polymorphism *VEGF* −2578C/A and suggested that carriers of *VEGF* −2578C allele may play a role in susceptibility to nasopharyngeal carcinoma [64, 65]. The risk for laryngeal squamous cell carcinoma seems to be linked with the increase of the −1154G/G genotype of the *VEGF* gene, in the −1154G/A polymorphism of the *VEGF* [27]. Moreover, the polymorphism −1154G/A *VEGF* has been shown to be associated with differential expression of VEGF *in vitro*. However, some of the data are contradictory.

4.4 Vascular endothelial growth factor and advances in developing novel therapeutic strategies for oral squamous cell carcinoma

There is a great need for therapies to prevent and/or slow the progression of OSCC. Recent studies focused on potential of drugs that target VEGF or its receptors-signaling system because their angiogenesis-promoting activity at the level of endothelial cells. Therefore, modulation of these factors to inhibit tumor angiogenesis, currently, is a major focus in developing OSCC therapies. The development of angiogenesis inhibitors as anticancer agents have been developed with data showing promising efficacy at reducing OSCC in in vitro models [13, 14]. Recent studies found that administration of angiogenesis inhibitors agents in association with chemotherapy and radiotherapy can improve the efficacy of these treatments. For example, Teicher et al. observed that coadministration of the TNR-470, angiogenesis inhibitor agent, induces a substantial cyclophosphamide-induced tumor cell-killing. Jain's study confirmed these findings suggesting that it was a consequent normalization of the tumor vasculature, as a result of endothelial cell death. Different therapeutic strategies to induce the inhibition of VEGF or its receptor signaling system are being emerging for treatment of OSCC, as VEGFR-1 ribozymes, VEGF toxin conjugates, and soluble VEGF receptors.

5. Conclusions

Angiogenesis is *essential* for the growth and metastasis of solid *tumors*, including oral squamous cell *carcinoma*. The main factor responsible for angiogenesis is *VEGF* and its receptors. Specifically, *VEGF*-A is known to be a *key* angiogenic factor, and its overexpression has been reported in most types of *cancer*, including *oral squamous cell carcinoma*, and it is thought to be a prognostic factor for survival. It was pointed out that VEGF as an attractive candidate for therapeutic intervention, but more studies are needed to clarify the real potential of angiogenesis inhibitors agents in OSCC, to determine optimal timing for VEGF, and to search for drug candidates.

Conflict of interest

The authors declare no conflict of interest.

Author details

Biagio Rapone[1]* and Elisabetta Ferrara[2]

1 Department of Basic Medical Sciences, Neurosciences and Sense Organs, "Aldo Moro" University of Bari, Bari, Italy

2 Complex Operative Unit of Odontostomatology, Hospital S.S. Annunziata, Chieti, Italy

*Address all correspondence to: biagiorapone79@gmail.com

References

[1] Senger DR, Galli SJ, Dvorak AM, Perruzzi CA, Harvey VS, Dvorak HF. Tumor cells secrete a vascular permeability factor that promotes accumulation of ascites fluid. Science. 1983;**219**(4587):983-985

[2] Hamilton WJ, Boyd JD, Mossman HW. Human Embryology. Baltimore: William & Wilkins; 1962

[3] Gilbert SF. Developmental Biology. Sunderland, MA: Sinauer; 1988

[4] Folkman J, Klagsbrun M. Angiogenic factors. Science. 1987;**235**:442-447

[5] Ferrara N, Henzel WJ. Pituitary follicular cells secrete a novel heparin-binding growth factor specific for vascular endothelial cells. Biochemical and Biophysical Research Communications. 1989;**161**(2):851-858

[6] Davis S, Aldrich TH, Jones PF, Acheson A, Compton DL, Jain V, et al. Isolation of angiopoietin-1, a ligand for the TIE2 receptor, by secretion-trap expression cloning. Cell. 1996;**87**:1161-1169

[7] Thurston G, Daly C. The complex role of angiopoietin-2 in the angiopoietin-tie signaling pathway. Cold Spring Harbor Perspectives in Medicine. 2012;**2**:a006550

[8] Favard C, Moukadiri H, Dorey C, Praloran V, Plouët J. Purification and biological properties of vasculotropin, a new angiogenic cytokine. Biology of the Cell. 1991;**73**(1):1-6

[9] Criscuolo GR, Merrill MJ, Oldfield EH. Further characterization of malignant glioma-derived vascular permeability factor. Journal of Neurosurgery. 1988;**69**(2):254-262

[10] Keck PJ, Hauser SD, Krivi G, Sanzo K, Warren T, Feder J, et al. Vascular permeability factor, an endothelial cell mitogen related to PDGF. Science. 1989;**246**(4935):1309-1312

[11] Robinson CJ, Stringer SE. The splice variants of vascular endothelial growth factor (VEGF) and their receptors. Journal of Cell Science. 2001;**114**(Pt 5): 853-865

[12] Bates DO, Cui TG, Doughty JM, Winkler M, Sugiono M, Shields JD, et al. VEGF165b, an inhibitory splice variant of vascular endothelial growth factor, is down-regulated in renal cell carcinoma. Cancer Research. 2002;**62**:4123-4131. The discovery of a novel inhibitory VEGF-A_{165} variant resulting from analternative exon 8

[13] Robinson CJ, Stringer SE. The splice variants of vascular endothelial growth factor (VEGF) and their receptors. Journal of Cell Science. 2001;**114**:853-865. A review of the splice variants of VEGF-A and their functions

[14] Gluzman-Poltorak Z, Cohen T, Herzog Y, Neufeld G. Neuropilin-2 and neuropilin-1 are receptors for the 165-amino acid form of vascular endothelial growth factor (VEGF) and of placenta growth factor-2, but only neuropilin-2 functions as a receptor for the 145-amino acid form of VEGF. The Journal of Biological Chemistry. 2000;**275**:18040-18045. This study shows that the VEGF-A_{145} isoform selectively recognizes NRP2. DOI: 10.1074/jbc.M909259199

[15] Ferrara N, Gerber HP, Lecouter J. The biology of VEGF and its receptors. Nature Medicine. 2003;**9**(6):669-676

[16] Fong GH, Zhang L, Bryce DM, Peng J. Increased hemangioblast commitment, not vascular disorganization, is the primary defect in flt-1 knock-out mice. Development. 1999;**126**(13):3015-3025

[17] Leung DW, Cachianes G, Kuang W-J, Goeddel DV, Ferrara N. Vascular endothelial growth factor is a secreted angiogenic mitogen. Science. 1989;**246**:1306-1309

[18] Keck PJ, Hauser SD, Krivi G, Sanzo K, Warren T, Feder J, et al. Vascular permeability factor, an endothelial cell mitogen related to platelet derived growth factor. Science. 1989;**246**:1309-1312

[19] Tischer E, Mitchell R, Hartman T, Silva M, Gospodarwicz D, Fiddes JC, et al. The human gene for vascular endothelial growth factor. Multiple protein forms are encoded through alternative exon splicing. The Journal of Biological Chemistry. 1991;**266**:11947-11954

[20] Turley H, Scott PAE, Watts VM, Bicknell B, Harris AL, Gatter KG. Expression of VEGF in routinely fixed material using a new monoclonal antibody VG1. The Journal of Pathology. 1998;**186**:313-318

[21] Zhang H, Craft P, Scott PAE, Ziche M, Weich HA, Harris AL, et al. Enhancement of tumor growth and vascular density by transfection of vascular endothelial cell growth factor into MCF-7 human breast carcinoma cells. Journal of the National Cancer Institute. 1995;**87**:213-219

[22] Park JE, Keller GA, Ferrara N. The vascular endothelial growth factor (VEGF) isoforms: Differential deposition into the subepithelial extracellular matrix and bioactivity of extracellular matrix-bound VEGF. Molecular Biology of the Cell. 1993;**4**:1317-1326

[23] Meyer M, Clauss M, Lepple-Wienhues A, Waltenberger J, Augustin HG, Ziche M, et al. A novel vascular endothelial growth factor encoded by Orf virus, VEGF-E, mediates angiogenesis via signalling through VEGFR-2 (KDR) but not VEGFR-1 (Flt-1) receptor tyrosine kinases. The EMBO Journal. 1999;**18**(2):363-374

[24] Gille H, Kowalky J, LI B, Lecouter J, Moffat B, Zioncheck TF, et al. Analysis of biological effects and signaling properties of Flt-1 (VEGFR-1) and KDR (VEGFR-2). A reassessment using novel receptor-specific vascular endothelial growth factor mutants. The Journal of Biological Chemistry. 2001;**276**(5):3222-3230

[25] Wise LM, Veikkola T, Mercer AA, Savory LJ, Fleming SB, Caesar C, et al. Vascular endothelial growth factor (VEGF)-like protein from orf virus NZ2 binds to VEGFR2 and neuropilin-1. Proceedings of the National Academy of Sciences of the United States of America. 1999;**96**(6):3071-3076

[26] Partanet TA, Alitalo K, Miettinen M. Lack of lymphatic vascular specificity of vascular endothelial growth factor receptor 3 in 185 vascular tumors. Cancer. 1999;**86**(11):2406-2412

[27] Cross MJ, Claesson-Welsh L. FGF and VEGF function in angiogenesis: Signalling pathways, biological responses and therapeutic inhibition. Trends in Pharmacological Sciences. 2001;**22**(4):201-207

[28] Matsumoto T, Claesson-Welsh L. VEGF receptor signal transduction. Science's STKE. 2001;**2001**(112):re21

[29] Alitalo K, Carmeliet P. Molecular mechanisms of lymphangiogenesis in health and disease. Cancer Cell. 2002;**1**(3):219-227

[30] Yuan F, Chen Y, Dellian M, Safabakhsh N, Ferrara N, Jain RK. Time-dependent vascular regression and permeability changes in established human tumor xenografts induced by an anti-vascular endothelial growth factor/ vascular permeability factor antibody.

Proceedings of the National Academy of Sciences of the United States of America. USA. 1996;**93**:14765-14770

[31] Carmeliet P, Ng Y-S, Nuyens D, Theilmeier G, Brusselmans K, Cornelissen I, et al. Impaired myocardial angiogenesis and ischemic cardiomyopathy in mice lacking the vascular endothelial growth factor isoforms VEGF164 and VEGF188. Nature Medicine. 1999;**5**:495-502

[32] Cheung N, Wong MP, Yuen ST, Leung SY, Chung LP. Tissue-specific expression pattern of vascular endothelial growth factor isoforms in the malignant transformation of lung and colon. Human Pathology. 1998;**29**:911-914

[33] Coltrini D, Gualandris A, Nelli EE. Growth advantage and vascularisation induced by basic fibrolblast growth factor overexpression in endometrial HEC-1-B cells: An export -dependent mechanism of action. Cancer Research. 1995;**55**:4729-4738

[34] Gitay-Goren H, Cohen T, Tessler S, Soker S, Gengrinovitch S, Rockwell P, et al. Selective binding of VEGF121 to one of the three vascular endothelial growth factor receptors of vascular endothelial cells. The Journal of Biological Chemistry. 1996;**271**:5519-5523

[35] Relf M, LeJeune S, Scott PAE, Fox S, Smith K, Leek R, et al. Expression of the angiogenic factors vascular endothelial cell growth factor, acidic and basic fibroblast growth factor, transforming growth factor β-1, platelet-derived endothelial cell growth factor, placenta growth factor and pleiotrophin in human primary breast cancer and its relation to angiogenesis. Cancer Research. 1997;**57**:963-969

[36] Plate K. From angiogenesis to lymphangiogenesis. Nature Medicine. 2001;**7**(2):151-152

[37] Shibuya M, Claesson-Welsh L. Signal transduction by VEGF receptors in regulation of angiogenesis and lymphangiogenesis. Experimental Cell Research. 2006;**312**(5):549-560

[38] Skobe M, Hawighorst T, Jackson DG, Prevo R, Janes L, Velasco P, et al. Induction of tumor lymphangiogenesis by VEGF-C promotes breast cancer metastasis. Nature Medicine. 2001;**7**(2):192-198

[39] Taipale J, Makinen T, Arighi E, Kukk E, Karkkainen M, Alitalo K. Vascular endothelial growth factor receptor-3. Current Topics in Microbiology and Immunology. 1999;**237**:85-96

[40] Partanen TA, Arola J, Saaristo A, Jussila L, Ora A, Miettinen M, et al. VEGF-C and VEGF-D expression in neuroendocrine cells and their receptor, VEGFR-3, in fenestrated blood vessels in human tissues. The FASEB Journal. 2000;**14**(13):2087-2096

[41] Klagsbrun M, Folkman J. Angiogenesis. In: Sporn MB, Roberts AB, editors. Peptide Growth Factors and their Receptors. New York: Springer-Verlag; 1991. pp. 549-586

[42] Soker S, Takashima S, Miao HQ, Neufeld G, Klagsbrun M. Neuropilin-1 is expressed by endothelial and tumor cells as an isoform-specific receptor for vascular endothelial growth factor. Cell. 1998;**92**(6):735-745

[43] Yuan L, Moyon D, Pardanaud L, Bréant C, Karkkainen MJ, Alitalo K, et al. Abnormal lymphatic vessel development in neuropilin 2 mutant mice. Development. 2002;**129**(20):4797-4806

[44] Safran M, Kaelin WG. HIF hydroxylation and the mammalian oxygen-sensing pathway. The Journal of Clinical Investigation. 2003;**111**(6):779-783

[45] Rak J, Mitsuhashi Y, Bayko L, Filmus J, Shirasawa S, Sasazuki T, et al. Mutant ras oncogenes upregulate VEGF/VPF expression: Implications for induction and inhibition of tumor angiogenesis. Cancer Research. 1995;**55**(20):4575-4580

[46] Coultas L, Chawengsaksophak K, Rossant J. Endothelial cells and VEGF in vascular development. Nature. 2005;**438**(7070):937-945

[47] Chen JC, Chang YW, Hong CC, Yu YH, Su JL. The role of the VEGF-C/VEGFRs axis in tumor progression and therapy. International Journal of Molecular Sciences. 2013;**14**(1):88-107

[48] Abdul-Aziz MA, Amin AK, El-Rouby DH, Shaker OG. Lymphangiogenesis in oral squamous cell carcinoma: Correlation with VEGF-C expression and lymph node metastasis. International Journal of Dentistry. 2017:10. Article ID: 7285656

[49] Bryne M. Is the invasive front of an oral carcinoma the most important area for prognostication? Oral Diseases. 1998;**4**(2):70-77

[50] Abdo MM, Gaballah ET, Fikry HE, Mosbah MM. Expression of VEGF-C in oral precancerous lesions and oral squamous cell carcinoma. Mansoura Journal of Dentistry. 2014;**1**(3):105-108

[51] Wang Z, Chen Y, Li X, Li X, Ma W, et al. Expression of VEGF-C/VEGFR-3 in human laryngeal squamous cell carcinomas and its significance for lymphatic metastasis. Asian Pacific Journal of Cancer Prevention. 2012;**13**(1):27-31

[52] Khaleel ME, Raza A, Ehsan A, Masood R, Javed M. Clinicopathological spectrum of oral squamous cell carcinoma at a public sector health facility. Biomédica. 2015;**31**(1):21-26

[53] Krishna A, Singh RK, Singh S, Verma P, Pal US, et al. Demographic risk factors, affected anatomical sites and Clinicopathological profile for oral squamous cell carcinoma in a north Indian population. Asian Pacific Journal of Cancer Prevention. 2014;**15**(16):6755-6760

[54] Benke EM, Ji Y, Patel V, Wang H, Miyazaki H, et al. VEGF-C contributes to head and neck squamous cell carcinoma growth and motility. Oral Oncology. 2010;**46**(4):e19-e24

[55] Ding MX, Lin XQ, Fu XY, Zhang N, Li JC. Expression of vascular endothelial growth factor-C and angiogenesis in esophageal squamous cell carcinoma. World Journal of Gastroenterology. 2006;**12**(28):4582-4585

[56] Vairaktaris E, Serefoglou Z, Avgoustidis D, Yapijakis C, Critselis E, Vylliotis A, et al. Gene polymorphisms related to angiogenesis, inflammation and thrombosis that influence risk for oral cancer. Oral Oncology. 2009;**45**:247-253

[57] Cheng CY, Chang CS, Liu CJ, Kao SY. Vascular endothelial growth factor 936 C/T polymorphism is associated with vascular invasion in oral squamous cell carcinoma. Oral Surgery, Oral Medicine, Oral Pathology, Oral Radiology, and Endodontics. 2008;**106**:79-84

[58] Faratzis G, Tsiambas E, Rapdis AD, et al. VEGF and KI 67 expression in squamous cell carcinoma of tongue–An immunohistochemical and computerized image analysis study. Oral Oncology. 2009;**45**(7):584-588

[59] Li YH, Hu CF, Shao Q, et al. Elevated expression of survival and VEGF protein are strong independent predictors of survival in advanced nasopharyngeal carcinoma. Journal of Translational Medicine. 2008;**6**:1

[60] Ferrara N, Davis-Smyth T. The biology of vascular endothelial growth factor. Endocrine Reviews. 1997;**18**:4-25

[61] Ferrara N. Vascular endothelial growth factor as a target for anticancer therapy. The Oncologist. 2004;**9**(Suppl 1): 2-10

[62] Kim SK, Park SG, Kim KW. Expression of vascular endothelial growth factor in oral squamous cell carcinoma. Journal of the Korean Association of Oral and Maxillofacial Surgeons. 2015;**41**(1):11-18. DOI: 10.5125/jkaoms.2015.41.1.11

[63] Shang ZJ, Li JR. Expression of endothelial nitric oxide synthase and vascular endothelial growth factor in oral squamous cell carcinoma its correlation with angiogenesis and disease progression. Journal of Oral Pathology & Medicine. 2005;**34**(3):134-139

[64] Nasr HB, Chahed K, Bouaouina N, Chouchane L. Functional vascular endothelial growth factor −2578 C/A polymorphism in relation to nasopharyngeal carcinoma risk and tumor progression. Clinica Chimica Acta. 2008;**395**:124-129

[65] Unal ZN, Unal M, Bagdatoglu OT, Polat G, Atik U. Genetic polymorphism of VEGF-1154 (A/G) in laryngeal squamous cell carcinoma. Archives of Medical Research. 2008;**39**:209-211

[66] Ku KT, Wan L, Peng HC, Tsai MH, Tsai CH, Tsai FJ. Vascular endothelial growth factor gene-460 C/T polymorphism. Acta Haematol. 2010;**123**:91-95

[67] Shintani S, Li C, Ishikawa T, et al. Expression of vascular endothelial growth factor A, B, C and D in oral squamous cell carcinoma. Oral Oncology. 2004;**40**(1):13-20

Chapter 10

The Role of Neck Dissection in Oral Cavity Carcinoma

Alfredo Quintin Y. Pontejos Jr. and Daryl Anne A. del Mundo

Abstract

Nodal status at the time of presentation for oral cavity carcinoma is the most important prognostic factor. Neck dissection is warranted for T3/T4 oral cavity carcinoma but there has been an ongoing controversy in the treatment of clinically negative neck in T1/T2. The risk of occult metastases in N0 squamous cell carcinoma of the oral cavity is 20–30%, and was found highest for tongue carcinoma. Elective neck dissection is recommended for T2N0 tongue carcinoma, and Stage I clinically N0 oral cavity carcinoma with tumor thickness >3 mm. CT scan has the highest sensitivity in detecting occult cervical lymph node metastases. Sentinel lymph node biopsy, as well as identification of biomarkers, continue to show increased utility. This chapter aims to discuss the methods of detecting nodal metastasis, the need for elective neck dissection for clinically neck node negative T1/T2 oral cavity carcinoma, the role of watchful waiting in N0 necks, the impact of tumor thickness in the risk for cervical lymph node metastasis, the role of sentinel lymph node biopsy in the detection of occult lymph node metastasis, and the role of biomarkers as predictors of occult lymph node metastasis.

Keywords: oral cavity carcinoma, neck dissection, elective neck dissection, occult cervical metastases

1. Introduction

Nodal status at the time of presentation for oral cavity carcinoma is the most important prognostic factor [1]. If the nodes are affected, the chance for cure is reduced by half [1, 2]. Historically, Shah et al., as early as 1990, demonstrated that levels I, II, and III were at greatest risk for nodal metastases from primary squamous cell carcinoma of the oral cavity [3]. Yuen et al. showed that the rate of cervical metastases is greatest for carcinoma of the oral tongue and floor of mouth, with the rate increasing with increasing T stage [4]. Curative surgery involves wide excision of the primary and neck dissection [1]. For T3/T4 oral cavity carcinoma, neck dissection is warranted even for clinically negative necks [1]. There has long been an ongoing controversy in the treatment of clinically negative neck in early stage oral cavity carcinoma (T1/T2) [1, 4, 5].

This chapter will discuss the methods of detecting nodal metastasis, the need for elective neck dissection for clinically neck node negative T1/T2 oral cavity carcinoma, the role of watchful waiting in N0 necks, the impact of tumor thickness in the risk of cervical lymph node metastasis, the role of sentinel lymph node biopsy in the detection of occult lymph node metastasis, and the role of biomarkers as predictors of occult lymph node metastasis.

2. Detection of nodal metastasis

It has been shown that the sensitivity, specificity, and accuracy of detection of neck metastases by clinical examination are 70, 65, and 68%, respectively; with an overall error of 20–30% [6].

Various imaging modalities are being utilized to detect nodal metastasis and are found to be more reliable than clinical palpation. These include computerized tomography (CT) scan, magnetic resonance imaging (MRI), ultrasound, and positron emission tomography (PET) scan. These modern imaging modalities offer similar diagnostic accuracy to diagnose clinically N0 neck [7]. Sensitivity is comparable across all modalities but CT Scan has been shown to offer the highest specificity [8, 9]. A most recent study by Bae et al. in 2019 showed a higher sensitivity for detection of occult metastasis with PET CT than that for CT/MRI for 42 patients [10].

Despite the quality of current imaging modalities, the risk of occult metastases in necks categorized as N0 in patients with oral cavity squamous cell carcinoma (SCC) has been reported to be between 20 and 30% [8].

3. Elective neck dissection for clinically neck node negative T1/T2 Oral cavity carcinoma

The rate of occult lymph node metastasis in T1 to T2 oral cavity carcinoma reaches as high as 34% [11–13]. Personal data from the experience of the authors showed an occult regional neck nodal metastasis rate of 25% (n = 4) for Stage I and 27.8% (n = 18) for Stage II oral cavity carcinoma.

The decision to observe or treat the N0 neck is left to the choice of the patient and the head and neck oncologist [6]. In oral cavity carcinoma, the only clinically N0 necks for which observation is appropriate are those associated with T1/T2 lip carcinomas, T1/T2 oral tongue carcinomas that are less than 4 mm thick, and T1/T2 floor of mouth cancers less than or equal to 1.5 mm thick [6]. A most recent systematic review by Cao et al. showed that elective neck dissection could significantly decrease neck recurrence and improve disease-free survival and overall survival compared to watchful waiting for patients with cT1-T2N0 oral cavity carcinoma [14].

Particularly for early stage (Stage I and Stage II) oral cavity carcinoma, previous studies have shown a lower risk of regional recurrence rate with elective neck dissection compared to watchful waiting [11, 15–18]. Five-year survival rate is higher for elective neck dissection versus watchful waiting; and specific death rate from regional recurrence is less for elective neck dissection than watchful waiting [11, 17, 18]. Regional recurrence rate for 154 Stage I and II N0 patients was found to be higher for patients who did not receive elective neck dissection [11].

4. Neck dissection general recommendations for Oral cavity carcinoma

The standard treatment for N0 neck (and even N1) is neck dissection of levels I, IIA, and III [19]. However, when level IIA is involved, there is a 22% risk of level IIB involvement, therefore, level IIB has to be included in the dissection [19]. Controversy about level IV involvement has come into play which may justify its dissection because of a reported 15% risk of involvement [20, 21]. Level V is rarely involved in oral cavity that is why it is hardly resected.

For N2/N3, neck dissection of levels I to V are indicated with or without resection of IJV, SCM, or SAN [1].

5. The impact of tumor thickness in the risk of cervical lymph node metastasis and the role of sentinel lymph node biopsy

The National Comprehensive Cancer Network Guidelines (2019) recommends that elective neck dissection be based on the risk of occult metastasis in the appropriated nodal basin [1]. Selective neck dissection of at least levels I–III is recommended for N0 oral cavity carcinoma.

Particularly, for oral cavity squamous cell carcinoma, sentinel lymph node biopsy or the primary tumor depth of invasion should guide decision making and these are currently the best predictors of occult metastatic disease [1, 22]. Earlier versions of NCCN state that for Stage I clinically N0 oral cavity cancer, elective neck dissection is recommended for tumor thickness >4 mm but recent evidence supports the effectiveness of elective neck dissection in patients with oral cavity cancers >3 mm depth of invasion [1, 22].

It is worthy of mention that the recently proposed 8th edition of the American Joint Committee on Cancer (AJCC) staging system for oral cavity squamous cell carcinoma is the addition of depth of invasion (DOI) as a modifier for the T category in the TNM staging [23]. It remains a controversy whether it is reasonable to substitute tumor thickness for DOI, since tumors with a larger DOI or thickness are associated with an increased risk of nodal metastasis and worse survival outcomes [24]. It has been concluded in a 2017 study by Dervin et al. that the T category and TNM stage prognostic performance of the eighth edition AJCC staging of oral cancer is similar regardless of whether DOI or thickness is used as the T-category modifier; hence, in centers or institutions without complete DOI data, it is reasonable to use tumor thickness [24].

Accuracy of sentinel lymph node biopsy for nodal staging of early oral cavity carcinoma has been tested extensively against the reference standard of immediately performed neck dissection or subsequent extended follow-up, with a pooled estimate of sensitivity of 0.93 and negative predictive values ranging from 0.88 to 1, with comparable survival outcomes [1, 22, 25–29]. A more recent systematic review revealed that sentinel lymph node biopsy is advantageous because it improves the accuracy of tumor staging, is a minimally-invasive procedure, avoids unnecessary nodal dissection, and results in limited morbidity and mortality with negative predictive value of 90–95% [6]. The disadvantages include posing difficulty for peri-tumoral injection for bulky invasive primary tumors that invade adjacent anatomic subsites, difficulty in floor of mouth tumors and those with proximity to the draining lymphatic basin, clinically positive nodes that are difficult to be identified by sentinel node mapping because of poor uptake of tracer, and the need for additional second stage surgery in case of positive neck node [6].

In addition, sentinel lymph node biopsy is a technically demanding procedure, with its success rates for sentinel node and occult lymphatic metastasis identification much dependent on technical expertise and experience [1]. Thus, sufficient caution must be exercised when offering it as an alternative to elective neck dissection [1].

6. Biomarkers as predictors of occult lymph node metastasis

Table 1 shows the various biomarkers which have been studied to detect occult lymph node metastasis.

Harada et al. showed that in normal squamous epithelium, cyclin B1 was localized in the nucleus and was expressed only in several cells of the basal and parabasal layers. In tumor tissues, however, cyclin B1 was expressed mainly in the cytoplasm. Cyclin B1 overexpression was positively correlated with occult cervical lymph node metastases and the number of mitotic cells [30].

Predictor	Non-predictor
Cyclin B-1	Vascular endothelial growth factor-C (VEGF-C)
Secreted protein acidic and rich in cysteine (SPARC)	High mobility group box 1 (HMGB1)
E-cadherin (ECAD)	
Podoplanin	
Matrix metalloproteinase-7 (MMP-7)	
Activin A	
partial epithelial-to-mesenchymal transition	

Table 1.
Predictors and non-predictors of occult lymph node metastases in oral cavity carcinoma.

Zhang et al. showed that the secreted protein acidic and rich in cysteine (SPARC) has a positive rate in 49.1% of tongue cancer tissues and 0% in normal tissues. The expression of SPARC was positively correlated with occult lymph node metastasis and recurrence [31].

Huber et al. showed that the differentiation grade and down-regulation of E-cadherin expression significantly correlate with positive lymph node status in univariate and multivariate analyses. Thus, E-cadherin immunohistochemistry may be used as a predictor for lymph node metastasis in squamous cell carcinoma of the oral cavity and oropharynx [32].

Huber et al. showed that podoplanin expression correlated significantly with sentinel lymph node metastasis and remained a significant predictor for lymph node status even after controlling for tumor stage [33]. In relation to this, a more recent study revealed the association of podoplanin and SOX2 in the progression of oral squamous cell carcinoma [34]. OX2 is a transcription factor related to the maintenance of stem cells in a pluripotent state. Podoplanin is a type of transmembrane sialoglycoprotein, which plays an important role in tumor progression and metastasis [34]. There was a significant inverse correlation between the expression of SOX2 and podoplanin with the tumor grade, survival analysis showed that a high expression of SOX2 correlated positively with the disease-free survival, and a significant positive association between the pattern of SOX2 and podoplanin expression [34].

Mäkinen et al. showed that matrix metalloproteinase-7 (MMP-7) expression was associated with presence of occult metastases (OR 3.67; $p = 0.013$); increased invasion depth (OR 4.60; $p = 0.005$); high tumor grade (OR 3.30; $p = 0.007$). MMP-7 was predictive of poor outcome ($p = 0.021$) [35].

In a study by Kelner et al. in 2015, it was found that high immunohistochemical expression of activin A was significantly associated with presence of occult lymph node metastasis in oral tongue squamous cell carcinoma [36].

Non-predictors of occult lymph node metastases as shown in **Table 1** include vascular endothelial growth factor-C (VEGF-C) and High mobility group box 1 (HMGB1). No statistically significant difference was found between OSCC with and without occult lymph node metastasis in regard to VEGF-C immunoexpression by malignant cells [37]. Isolated VEGF-C expression by malignant cells is not of predictive value for occult lymph node metastasis in early stages of oral squamous cell carcinoma [37]. Likewise, Prediction of occurrence of late neck metastasis in early tongue squamous cell carcinoma by evaluating HMGB1 (high mobility group box 1) expression in the primary lesion showed that immunohistochemistry study of HMGB1 in early tongue squamous cell carcinoma did not appear to be very useful for predicting occult neck metastasis [38].

Most recently, immunohistochemistry quantification of partial epithelial-to-mesenchymal transition (p-EMT) in oral cavity squamous cell carcinoma primary tumors has been reliably shown to be associated with nodal metastases, perineural invasion, and high grade [39]. EMT is thought to be a potential driver of invasiveness and metastasis in a variety of epithelial cancers [39]. It has been said that with prospective validation, p-EMT biomarkers may aid in decision making over whether to perform a neck dissection in the N0 neck and/or for adjuvant therapy planning [39].

7. Post-operative follow-up

Based on the algorithm proposed by Paler et al., follow-up CT scan may be done for N1 disease and PET CT for N2/N3 disease 12 weeks after treatment [40]. CT scan may also be done for N0 neck [1].

The NCCN guidelines follow-up recommendations for oral cavity carcinoma include a complete head and neck examination every 1–3 months for the first post-operative year, every 2–6 months for the second post-operative year, every 4–8 months for years 3–5, and every 12 months beyond 5 years post-operatively. Speech/hearing and swallowing evaluation, nutritional evaluation and rehabilitation, smoking cessation and alcohol counseling, and surveillance for depression are included in the post-operative supportive care recommendations [1].

8. Conclusions

Despite advances in imaging studies in detecting occult metastasis, the risk of occult metastases in necks categorized as N0 in patients with oral cavity squamous cell carcinoma (SCC) remains and the need for neck dissection should carefully be examined. Elective neck dissection, specifically, selective neck dissection, is recommended for Stage II oral cavity carcinoma given the high risk of occult metastasis. For Stage I clinically N0 oral cavity carcinoma, elective neck dissection has been historically recommended for tumor thickness >4 mm but recent evidence supports the effectiveness of elective neck dissection in patients with oral cavity carcinoma >3 mm depth of invasion. The role of sentinel lymph node biopsy in detection of occult cervical lymph node metastasis is promising but requires technical expertise and experience. Identification of biomarkers in predicting the presence of cervical lymph node metastasis may prove to have increasing utility.

Author details

Alfredo Quintin Y. Pontejos Jr. * and Daryl Anne A. del Mundo
Department of Otorhinolaryngology, University of the Philippines
Manila-Philippine General Hospital, Manila, Philippines

*Address all correspondence to: docpontejosjr@yahoo.com

References

[1] National Comprehensive Cancer Network (NCCN). Clinical Practice Guidelines in Oncology. NCCN Guidelines. Version 1. 2019

[2] Bree R, Takes R, Shah J, Hamoir M, Kowalski L, Robbins KT, et al. Elective neck dissection in oral squamous cell carcinoma: Past, present, and future. Oral Oncology. 2019;**90**:87-93

[3] Shah JP, Candela FC, Poddar AK. The patterns of cervical lymph node metastases from squamous carcinoma of the oral cavity. Cancer. 1990;**66**:109-113

[4] Yuen AP, Wei WI, Won YM, Tang KC. Elective neck dissection versus observation in the treatment of early oral tongue carcinoma. Head & Neck. 1997;**19**:583-588

[5] Akhtar S, Ikram M, Ghaffar S. Neck involvement in early CA of tongue. Is neck dissection warranted? Journal of Pakistan Medical Association. 2007;**57**(6):305-307

[6] Hegab A, Elmasry M, Khallaf M. Management of the clinically negative neck in oral squamous cell carcinoma: A systematic review. Journal of Cancer Research and Therapeutic Oncology. 2013;**2**:1-12

[7] Liao LJ, Lo WC, Hsu WL, Wang CT, Lai MS. Detection of cervical lymph node metastasis in head and neck cancer patients with clinically N0 neck: A meta-analysis comparing different imaging modalities. BMC Cancer. 2010;**12**:236

[8] Saafan ME, Elguindy AS, Abdel-Aziz MF, Younes A, Albirmawy OA, Mandour M, et al. Assessment of cervical lymph nodes in squamous cell carcinoma of the head and neck. Surgery: Current Research. 2013;**3**:4

[9] Psychogios G, Mantsopoulos K, Bohr C, Koch M, Zenk J, Iro H. Incidence of occult cervical metastasis in head and neck carcinomas: Development over time. Journal of Surgical Oncology. 2012;**107**(4):384-387

[10] Bae MR, Roh J, Kim J, Lee J, Cho K, Choi S, et al. ^{18}F-FDG PET/CT versus CT/MR imaging for detection of neck lymph node metastasis in palpably node-negative oral cavity cancer. Journal of Cancer Research and Clinical Oncology. Germany: Springer-Verlag GmbH; 2019. DOI: 10.1007/s00432-019-03054-3

[11] Capote A, Escorial V, Muñoz-Guerra MF, Rodríguez-Campo FJ, Gamallo C, Naval L. Elective neck dissection in early-stage oral squamous cell carcinoma—Does it influence recurrence and survival? Head & Neck. 2006;**29**(1):3-11

[12] Akhtar S, Ikram M, Ghaffar S. Neck involvement in early carcinoma of tongue. Is elective neck dissection warranted? The Journal of the Pakistan Medical Association. 2007;**57**(6):305-307

[13] El-Naaj LY, Shveis M, Sabo E, Peled M. Incidence of oral cancer occult metastasis and survival of T1-T2N0 oral cancer patients. Journal of Oral and Maxillofacial Surgery. 2011;**69**(10):2674-2679

[14] Cao Y, Wang T, Yu C, Guo X, Li C, Li L. Elective neck dissection versus wait-and-watch policy for oral cavity squamous cell carcinoma in early stage: A systematic review and meta-analysis based on survival data. Journal of Oral and Maxillofacial Surgery. 2019;**77**(10):2154-2167

[15] Peng KA, Chu AC, Lai C, Grogan T, Elashoff D, Abemayor E, et al. Is there a role for neck dissection in T1 oral tongue squamous cell carcinoma? The UCLA experience. American Journal of Otolaryngology. 2014;**35**(6):741-746

[16] Mirea D, Grigore R, Safta D, Mirea L, Popescu C, Popescu B, et al. Elective neck dissection in patients with stage T1-T2N0 carcinoma of the anterior tongue. Hippokratia. 2014;**18**(2):120-124

[17] D'Cruz AK, Vaish R, Kapre N, Dandekar M, Gupta S, Hawaldar R, et al. Elective versus therapeutic neck dissection in node-negative oral cancer. The New England Journal of Medicine. 2015;**373**(6):521-529

[18] Abu-Ghanem S, Yehuda M, Carmel N-N, Leshno M, Abergel A, Gutfeld O, et al. Elective neck dissection vs observation in early-stage squamous cell carcinoma of the oral tongue with no clinically apparent lymph node metastasis in the neck. JAMA Otolaryngology – Head & Neck Surgery. 2016;**142**(9):857

[19] Coskun HH, Medina J, Robbins T, Siver C, Strojan P, Teymoortash A, et al. Current philosophy in the surgical management of neck metastases for head and neck squamous cell carcinoma. Head & Neck. 2015;**37**(6):915-926

[20] De Zinis LO, Bolzoni A, Piazza C, Nicolai P. Prevalence and localization of nodal metastases in squamous cell carcinoma of the oral cavity: Role and extension of neck dissection. European Archives of Oto-Rhino-Laryngology. 2006;**263**:1131-1640

[21] Byers RM, Weber RS, Andrews T, McGill D, Kare R, Wolf P. Frequency and therapeutic implications of "skip metastases" in the neck from squamous cell carcinoma of the oral tongue. Head & Neck. 1997;**19**:14-19

[22] Civantos FJ, Zitsch RP, Schuller DE, Agrawal A, Smith RB, Nason R, et al. Sentinel lymph node biopsy accurately stages the regional lymph nodes for T1-T2 oral squamous cell carcinomas: Results of a prospective multi-institutional trial. Journal of Clinical Oncology. 2010;**28**(8):1395-1400

[23] Amin MB et al. AJCC Cancer Staging Manual. 8th ed. American College of Surgeons. 2018

[24] Dirven R, Ebrahimi A, Moeckelmann N, Palme CE, Gupta R, Clark J. Tumor thickness versus depth of invasion—Analysis of the 8th edition American Joint Committee on Cancer Staging for Oral Cancer. Oral Oncology. 2017;**74**:30-33

[25] Alkureishi LWT, Ross GL, Shoaib T, Soutar DS, Robertson AG, Thompson R, et al. Sentinel node biopsy in head and neck squamous cell cancer: 5-year follow-up of a European Multicenter Trial. Annals of Surgical Oncology. 2010;**17**(9):2459-2464

[26] Govers TM, Hannink G, Merkx MAW, Takes RP, Rovers MM. Sentinel node biopsy for squamous cell carcinoma of the oral cavity and oropharynx: A diagnostic meta-analysis. Oral Oncology. 2013;**49**(8):726-732

[27] Pezier T, Nixon IJ, Gurney B, Schilling C, Hussain K, Lyons AJ, et al. Sentinel lymph node biopsy for T1/T2 oral cavity squamous cell carcinoma—A prospective case series. Annals of Surgical Oncology. 2012;**19**(11):3528-3533

[28] Broglie MA, Haerle SK, Huber GF, Haile SR, Stoeckli SJ. Occult metastases detected by sentinel node biopsy in patients with early oral and oropharyngeal squamous cell carcinomas: Impact on survival. Head & Neck. 2012;**35**(5):660-666

[29] Samant S. Sentinel node biopsy as an alternative to elective neck dissection for staging of early oral carcinoma. Head & Neck. 2013;**36**(2):241-246

[30] Harada H, Omura K, Nakajima Y, Hasegawa S, Mogi S. Cyclin B1 is useful to predict occult cervical lymph node metastases in tongue carcinoma. Journal of Experimental & Clinical Cancer Research. 2006;**25**:3

[31] Zhang J, Zhang Q, Zhang Q, Liu XK, Li CQ, Guo ZM. Expression and clinical significance of SPARC in clinical stage II tongue squamous cell carcinoma. Ai Zheng. 2009;**28**(1):68-71

[32] Huber GF, Züllig L, Soltermann A, Roessle M, Graf N, Haerle SK, et al. Down regulation of E-cadherin (ECAD)—A predictor for occult metastatic disease in sentinel node biopsy of early squamous cell carcinomas of the oral cavity and oropharynx. BMC Cancer. 2011;**11**:1-8. DOI: 10.1186/1471-2407-11-217

[33] Huber GF, Fritzsche FR, Züllig L, Storz M, Graf N, Haerle SK, et al. Podoplanin expression correlates with sentinel lymph node metastasis in early squamous cell carcinomas of the oral cavity and oropharynx. International Journal of Cancer. 2011;**129**(6):1404-1409

[34] Sonali P, Vasudeva G, Charlotte SM. Association of the co-expression of SOX2 and Podoplanin in the progression of oral squamous cell carcinomas—An immunohistochemical study. Journal of Applied Oral Science [Internet]. 2019;**27**:e20180348. [Cited: 17 November 2019]

[35] Mäkinen LK, Häyry V, Hagström J, Sorsa T, Passador-Santos F, Keski-Säntti H, et al. Matrix metalloproteinase-7 and matrix metalloproteinase-25 in oral tongue squamous cell carcinoma. Head & Neck. 2014;**36**(12):1783-1788

[36] Kelner N, Rodrigues PC, Bufalino A, Fonseca FP, dos Santos-Silva AR, Miguel MCC, et al. Activin A immunoexpression as predictor of occult lymph node metastasis and overall survival in oral tongue squamous cell carcinoma. Head & Neck. 2014;**37**(4):479-486

[37] Faustino SES, Oliveira DT, Nonogaki S, Landman G, Carvalho AL, Kowalski LP. Expression of vascular endothelial growth factor-C does not predict occult lymph-node metastasis in early oral squamous cell carcinoma. International Journal of Oral and Maxillofacial Surgery. 2008;**37**(4):372-378

[38] Hanakawa H, Orita Y, Sato Y, Takeuchi M, Takao S, Ohno K, et al. Does HMGB1 predict occult neck lymph node metastasis in early tongue carcinoma? A case–control study of 26 patients. The Journal of Laryngology and Otology. 2014;**128**(10):926-931

[39] Parikh AS, Puram SV, Faquin WC, Richmon JD, Emerick KS, Deschler DG, et al. Immunohistochemical quantification of partial-EMT in oral cavity squamous cell carcinoma primary tumors is associated with nodal metastasis. Oral Oncology. 2019;**99**:104458

[40] Paleri V, Urbano TG, Mehanna H, Repanos C, Lancaster J, Patel M, et al. Management of neck metastases in head and neck cancer: United Kingdom National Multidisciplinary Guidelines. The Journal of Laryngology & Otology. 2016;**130**(S2):S161-S169

Chapter 11

Modalities and State of Art in Oral Cancer Reconstruction

Andres Chala

Abstract

The treatment of the oral cancer is complex in terms of resection and reconstruction. Adequate multidisciplinary approach is needed to plan the oncological resection and functional reconstruction to obtain optimal results and adequate rehabilitation of the patient. Many factors should be considered in order to reconstruct the surgical defects, including patient factors, the expertise of the team, and other tumor and defect factors. Early cancer and its subsequent defects can be reconstructed merely with a primary closure or a skin graft, but as soon as the cancer stage worsens, the devastation of primary tumor is bigger needing a more complex surgery and skilled reconstructive techniques to implant a new safe tissue, starting from a local flap, a pediculate flap, and up to a free composite flap. Nowadays there is a trend to perform microvascular free flaps in most of the reconstructions, but if a rational approach is planned, even in the most advanced cases, it can be solved with locoregional flaps, limiting the need of a microvascular surgery and its subsequent overcost in care and special skills in reconstruction. This chapter pretends to give a rational approach to get that goal.

Keywords: oral cancer, head and neck reconstruction, local flaps, pediculate flaps, free flaps

1. Introduction

One of the most common cancers of the head and neck region is the oral cavity cancer. Globally, over 300,000 people are diagnosed with oral cancer each year, being the eight most common cause of malignancy [1]. In early stages, a cure is possible with minimum morbidity; unfortunately, such disease is not usually diagnosed until it has set to an advanced stage impacting survival, including in that stage morbidity due to tumor invasion or tissue devastation, and its consequent treatment negatively impacts the quality of life [2]. With that in mind, every effort must be done to reconstruct the defect of the primary resective procedure in order to restore swallowing, speech, esthetics, and color match, among others. A complete evaluation must be done to define the optimal reconstruction without compromising the oncological resection and first of all evaluating each patient in terms of age, functional capacity, adjuvant therapies, airway protection, survival, etc. There are many options to reconstruct the defect, so a comprehensive approach should be planned, principally considering its location in the oral cavity, the size of the anatomical structure resected, as well as the consequence of the defect that may affect a complex functional unit that could include the mucosa, muscle, bone, skin, or a combination of them, which additionally may develop a continuity solution that creates a communication between the oral cavity with the neck and its subsequent salivary fistula, infection, risk of a major vessel blood bleeding or carotid blowout, and death. The reconstruction might be done just with a primary closure and skin graft or may be left to heal by second intention with no closure; some cases will need a pediculate, local, or regional flap, and in complex and huge defects, a microvascular free flap might be needed. Currently there is a trend to perform a microvascular reconstruction for most of the defects, but even in a two-team approach, the microvascular reconstruction increases the cost and duration time of the surgery; furthermore some health centers lack surgeons with the necessary skills to perform a microvascular surgery. The purpose of this chapter is to review the state of art in oral cavity reconstruction after an oncological resection and especially provide a rational approach to reconstruct each defect in order to restore it as similar as normal tissue before resection, discussing pros and cons of reconstruction.

2. Anatomic landmark

The oral cavity begins at the lips and ends at the anterior surface of the faucial arch. It is lined by squamous epithelium with interspersed minor salivary glands. It contains the lips, buccal mucosa, mandibular and maxillary alveolar ridge, retromolar trigone, hard palate, floor of the mouth, and anterior oral tongue. Motor innervation of intrinsic musculature is supplied by the hypoglossal nerve and sensation is provided by trigeminal nerve V2 and V3 branches. The sensation of the anterior two-thirds of the tongue is provided by the lingual nerve (CN V3), and its taste comes via the chorda tympani (CN VII) [3]. For the purposes of this chapter, only the proper oral cavity is considered, so lip reconstruction is excluded.

3. Defect characteristics

Assessing the characteristics of the defect is the first step to decide which is the best option to reconstruct. The size and specific subsite of the primary resection including its function will determine the need for subsequent reconstruction. Small or medium defects may not disturb function, so minimal intervention to reconstruct is necessary; on the other hand, composite defects that include several units and structures like the muscle, mucosa, bone, or even skin can affect the function in many ways, so in order to restore it, a specific composite tissue is needed, which is also a technique to avoid scars, nonfunctional tissue, or retractions with its subsequent unit dysfunction. Previous treatment like chemotherapy and especially radiation will also entail special needs in terms of reconstruction since providing a new normal tissue is essential to prevent local complications like fistula, dehiscence, infection, or a permanent scar.

4. Specific subsites

With the aim to choose correctly from a range of different technics, although it is frequent to face a combination of subsites and structures after surgical resection, each subsite must be considered independently to assist the decision.

4.1 Floor of mouth

The subsite floor of mouth (FOM) is limited anteriorly by the inferior alveolar ridge, posteriorly by the ventral surface of the lingual tongue, and laterally by the anterior tonsil pillar. The FOM avoids the spillage of saliva to the neck and is also necessary to support the tongue in speech and deglutition as well as to maintain the humidity of the mouth due to the big amount of minor salivary glands and to the outlet of the submandibular gland duct. The resection may result in a small or big defect that could or could not include the mucosa, bone and skin. The main goal of reconstruction is to restore the anatomic limits of the sulcus to avoid communication with the neck with the corresponding spillage of saliva and food, and to avoid retraction or fixation of the tongue then maintaining the adequate tongue mobility to support articulation and speech as well as allowing the tongue to move freely to push the food bolus back.

4.1.1 Small defects

A very small deformity could be let alone without closure and permit healing by second intention with a granulation tissue. A facial artery myomucosal flap (FAMM), which blood supply is provided by the facial artery, could similarly be used for a defect limited up to a width of 2 cm and permit the primary closure of the donor site [4]. A split-thickness skin graft (STSG) or a full-thickness skin graft (FTSG) could be used for a defect smaller than 3–4 cm that does not spare the suprahyoid musculature or expose the bone (**Figure 1a** and **b**). The graft is usually secured with a pad dressing, which is removed 6–7 days after surgery. Usually remucosalization can be expected, and complete healing is obtained in about 4 weeks. The restriction to the skin graft is related to the difficulty to maintained it insetted due to its exposition to swallowing movements.

The advantage to let the defect to granulate by itself is the shortest time of the procedure; however, it usually takes up to 3 weeks to obtain a complete healing, implying some minor disturbances for the patient including pain and difficulty to swallow. The disadvantage of the graft is the secondary scar of the donor site but is offsetted by the result in the zone of resection and a shortened time of recovery.

4.1.2 Medium defects

For FOM defects up to 6 cm which may include a limited bone exposure, a regional pediculate flap can be employed to reconstruct; the most used are the

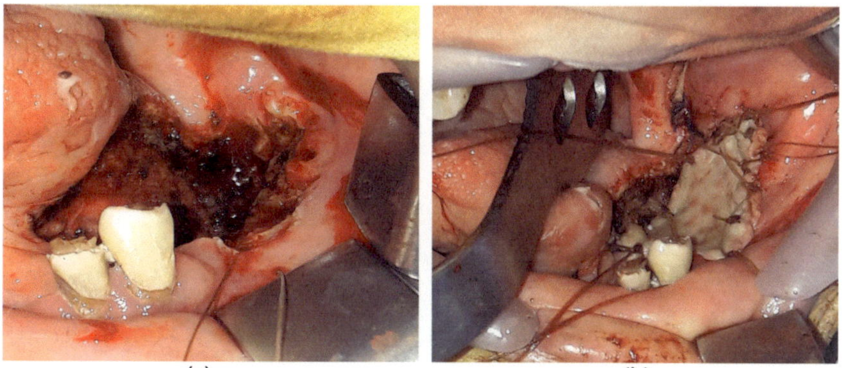

(a) (b)

Figure 1.
(a) FOM resection and (b) skin graft.

submental (SMF) and the supraclavicular flap (SCF). Additionally, in that kind of defects, especially when postoperative radiotherapy is projected, a pediculate flap must be planned if possible.

4.1.2.1 The submental pediculate flap

The submental pediculate flap is vascularized by the submental artery, a branch of facial artery. It must include a segment of the anterior belly of digastric to perfuse the overlying skin through perforants. The amount of tissue available to harvest depends on the pitching test that predicts the possibility of primary closure of the donor site. This flap entails to avoid sacrifice of its vascular pedicle so the clue is that it should be planned and harvested at the beginning of neck dissection [5] (**Figure 2a–c**). Sometimes nodal disease levels Ia and Ib limit the ability to harvest the submental flap without impairing the oncological resection. The main advantage of this flap is the proximity between the donor site and the floor of the mouth so it can be insetted easily; the main problem is that if it is harvested with a big amount of muscle, the result once insetted may be a bulky flap resulting on swallowing and speaking problems.

4.1.2.2 The supraclavicular pediculate flap

The supraclavicular pediculate flap is an alternative to the submental flap particularly when a larger amount of skin is needed and in cases of huge nodal

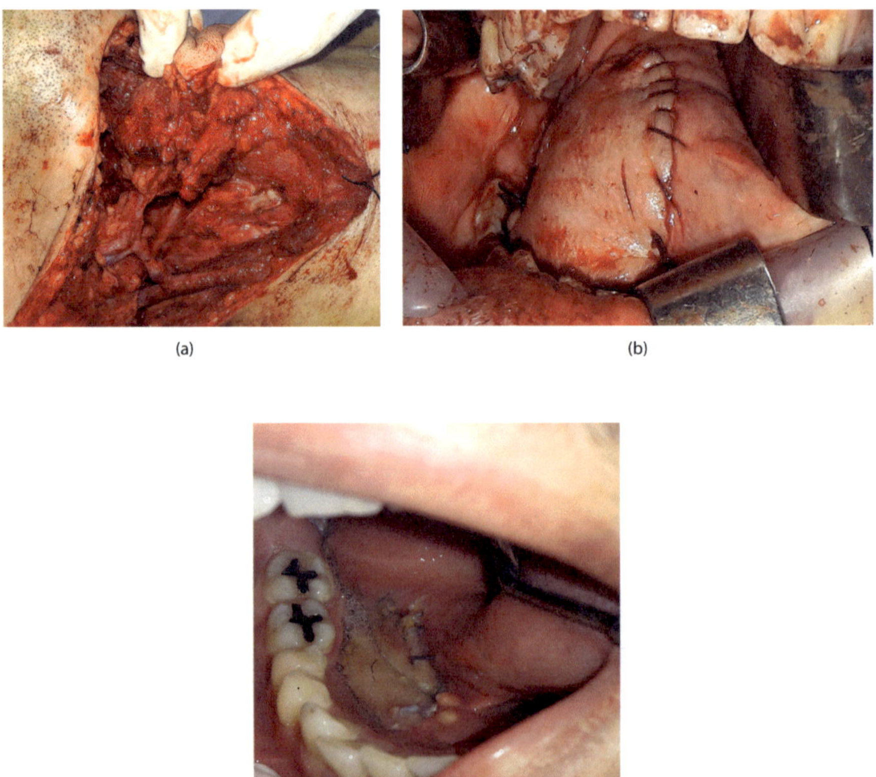

(a) (b) (c)

Figure 2.
(a) Submandibular flap harvest, (b) submandibular flap insetting, and (c) final result.

disease in level I. The flap can be raised if there are no bulky nodes in the neck in the level IV. The SCF is based on axial circulation from the supraclavicular artery which arises from the transverse cervical artery and in a small percentage of cases from the suprascapular artery. It can be used to reconstruct soft tissue defects measuring up to 20 cm in size after tumor excision, being an advantage over the SMF in FOM defects. As well as the submandibular flap, usually there is low donor site morbidity permitting its primary closure, and of course the main restriction is related to neck dissection in level IV due to the possibility to injure the cervical transverse pedicle impairing its vascularization [6]. Another advantage is that it can be raised at the end of the surgery after neck dissection or in cases when you do not plan to dissect level IV or there is no doubt about the probability to alter its vascularization; it can be harvested at the beginning of neck dissection once you have defined the size of the defect you need to reconstruct (**Figure 3a–b**).

The main complication for both flaps is the loss of the flap due to arterial or venous ischemia. To prevent that fatal complication, a meticulous dissection is needed to preserve its vascularization during harvesting and trying to avoid tension during insetting. When only venous congestion is present, the flap may recover without additional intervention, but if ischemia is established, the lost flap must be retired to avoid infection and systemic complication, and if possible, a new way of reconstruction must be considered.

4.1.3 Large defects

In a bigger or composite defect of FOM, the reconstruction can be a challenge, especially when the bone, tongue, and skin are involved. It is important to assess preoperatively the degree of bone invasion to suitably plan possible mandibulectomy requiring additional bone tissue for reconstruction. If only soft tissue is required, a radial forearm free flap (RFFF) or an anterolateral free flap (ALT) can be harvested, but if the bone required a fibula free flap (OCFF), the iliac crest flap (VICF) or the scapula free flap (SFF) are the main options.

4.1.3.1 The radial forearm free flap

The radial forearm free flap based on the radial artery provides a pliable and thin skin that makes the RFFF an ideal choice for reconstruction of the floor of the mouth; in few cases if a small marginal segment of the bone is required, a composite radial free flap including a limited segment of radial bone can be obtained [7]; if furthermore the tongue is compromised, the RFFF can be insetted with a bilobed design allowing one lobe to restore the volume of the tongue and the second one to

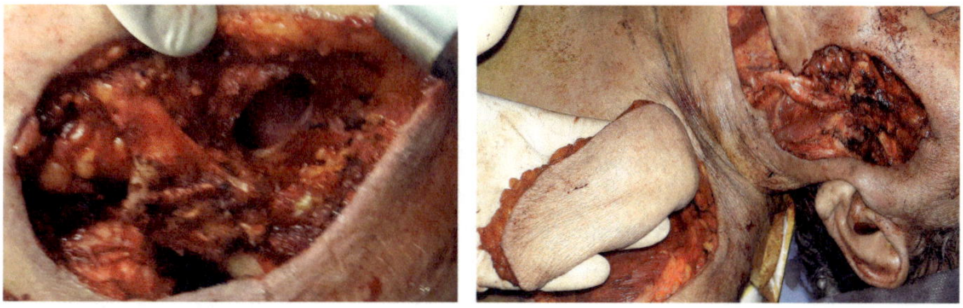

(a) (b)

Figure 3.
(a) Yugal mucosa resection and (b) supraclavicular flap harvest.

resurfaces the FOM [8]. The RFFF is considered the battle horse in microvascular reconstruction due to the skin quality, the length of the pedicle, the size of the vessels, and the easy preoperative assessing since it does not require vascular images just the Allen test to evaluate distal perfusion of the hand provided by palmar arch, and additionally, it is easily harvested. Its limit is usually referred to the size in cm that can be harvested (up to 20 × 12 cm), but it almost never applies as an exception in oral cavity reconstruction. The principal risk and disadvantage of the osteocutaneous radial free flap is the risk of fracture when a segment of the bone is included in the RFFF, so prophylactic fixation of the radius with the appropriately sized 2.4-mm locking reconstruction plate is performed to avoid fracture of the donor site [9]. The disadvantages of this flap are the hairy non-mucosalizing skin paddle, the cosmetic deformity of the donor site due to skin grafting that sometimes let an ugly scar and, in some cases, a bulky dysfunctional flap. The hairy skin can atrophy after radiation, or it can be treated with laser peeling, so in most of the cases, the final reconstruction result is excellent. To improve the cosmetic result of the donor site, any effort must be done to preserve the paratenon over the flexor tendons; setting a 4 mm better than a 2 mm skin graft over the donor site with an appropriate plaster bandage for temporal immobilization is also suggested. This usually ends in a better cosmetic result. Finally, to avoid a bulky dysfunctional flap, planning an adequate design of the size and form of the flap before harvesting is advisable.

4.1.3.2 The ALT flap

The ALT flap is also proposed as an excellent recourse when only the skin and soft tissue are required, especially in thin patients; it is advocated by many as a first choice to avoid the donor site morbidity. This flap pending on a septocutaneous branch coming from the lateral circumflex femoral artery involves a more difficult dissection due to the smaller diameter of the vessels [10]. It can be harvested thinner (supra fascial) or thicker (subfascial) depending on specific needs of skin and soft tissue. One important advantage is that can be raised even bigger allowing primary closure. The disadvantage of a hairy non-mucosalizing skin paddle is like the RFFF, and in an obese patient the flap is unacceptably bulky. Another disadvantage occurs when the nerve branch to the vastus lateralis muscle is cut unnoticed causing knee instability. In rare occasions the donor site needs to be skin grafted.

4.1.3.3 The osteocutaneous fibula free flap

The osteocutaneous fibula free flap is considered by many, the gold standard when oncological resection includes a large segmental mandibular defect that may or no include skin and is generally the first choice [8, 11] and the iliac crest and scapula [12] are alternatives chiefly in segmental small defects. The osteocutaneous fibula free flap (OCFF) based on peroneal artery is a reliable, and versatile flap for mandibular reconstruction and is considered the gold standard in mandibular reconstruction. It usually offers enough length of bone and skin to reconstruct a partial or complete mandibular resection and allows to place bone-integrated implants. It is essential to plan its harvesting and design from the beginning at the outpatient clinic, since it is mandatory to perform limb vascular imaging studies to assess the normal vascular anatomy and avoid fatal vascular morbidity or ischemia of the donor limb after bone resection. It does not need to plate the remaining fibula that remains attached to the tibia, and if harvesting in the right way, it does not cause limb instability. As a norm, it is easy to harvest and one-stage reconstruction can be performed. There are some downsides to it; first the size of the skin paddle is limited just to permit primary closure of skin donor site; but if needed it also can be skin grafted. Second the hairy and non-mucosalizing skin paddle that is placed intraorally could end in an disturbing sensation, usually temporally if radiation is added to the treatment, and third in cases of arterial or venous disease in the lower extremities or previous surgery, there is a formal contraindication for flap harvesting [13].

4.1.3.4 The scapula free flap (SFF)

The scapula free flap (SFF) based on the circumflex artery arising from the subscapular artery, which is a branch of the axillary artery in the upper thorax, similarly provides acceptable bone length while supplying significantly larger skin and soft tissue paddles (up to double in overall area). It is an excellent alternative to small and wide to medium defects when wide bone is necessary. The main disadvantage of this flap is the need of repositioning during the surgical procedure restraining a double team approach [14].

4.1.3.5 The vascularized iliac crest bone flap (VICF)

The vascularized iliac crest bone flap (VICF) has also been proposed as a new approach to reconstruct a mandibular deformity, especially in lateral mandibular defects [15]. This flap is based on the deep circumflex iliac vessels and usually harbors consistent anatomy; the length of the vessel averages 8–10 cm, and its diameter averages 2–3 mm. Pending on specific reconstruction needs may be harvested as a full thickness bicortical or as a partial thickness unicortical bone, and its main advantage is the natural curved contour of the bone that is ideal for lateral mandibular reconstruction. It can be raised with skin or muscle when needed. The donor site morbidity is related to the local appearance deformity and the probability to develop a future hernia.

Nowadays three of the osteocutaneous free flaps previously mentioned could be combined with the use of a three-dimensional virtual technology to preoperatively plan the resection, the design of the plates for bone fixation, and the cutting guides to enhance the functional and cosmetic results. This new technology is proposed to optimize surgical outcome and as a safer way of modeling. It can also be implemented in mandibular or midface reconstruction using fibula free flap or iliac crest flap. It requires a preoperative CT scan planning design and preparation of the customized mandibular reconstruction plate and cutting guides providing a most precise reconstruction [16, 17]. Current communication between the resective surgeon, reconstructive surgeon, and team that supports the technology is necessary to assess all the information previous to surgery. The principal limits are the cost and access to the technology but usually are over headed by the benefit of a precise reconstruction. With this tendency to a more precise reconstruction and rehabilitation, one important aim of bone reconstruction is to restore the chewing function so dental implants are required to best accomplish that. The moment to inset them in the postoperative scenery usually takes up to 3 or 4 years waiting to finish healing and therapies including radiation and preventing osteoradionecrosis of the new mandible. With that in mind, there is a new trend to inset dental implants during the first reconstruction procedure and before radiation so that the chewing can be restored earlier [18]. To accomplish that goal, a preoperative consult with the maxillofacial surgeon is mandatory so can be involved in planning implants setting.

The additional fatal complications of the micro vascularized flaps are the arterial or venous ischemia. A strict postoperative care must be done for an early detection of venous or arterial suffering which may allow an appropriate reoperation in an intent of saving the flap. In the fatal case of flap loss, again it is crucial to retire the dead tissue and if possible cover the defect with a new pediculate or micro vascularized flap.

4.2 Tongue

In the oral cavity the more common defects requiring reconstruction are those from glossectomies. The tongue is a highly functional organ, with a complex muscle mobility that functions as a coordinate unit to articulate words, swallow, and push the bolus back, so the primary goal of reconstruction is to preserve the ability to move it intelligibly and not tethered with adequate soft tissue coverage, avoiding bulky flaps. The three-dimensional oncological resection needs adequate margins up to 1 cm, so the size of the defect may be variable, a quarter, half, near total, or total and can be simultaneously related or not with other structures like the floor of the mouth, cheek, skin, or bone. Based on that, reconstruction may be just a primary closure, a local or a pediculate flap, or a simple or composite free flap.

4.2.1 Small defects

In cases of small defects up to one-third of the tongue, primary closure could be done (**Figure 4a** and **b**), and if needed, due to a small floor of mouth resection, a skin graft is added in order to avoid a scar combined with tongue fixation. Usually the functional results are optimal, but sometimes skin graft contraction and hyperpigmentation can result, or graft fixation may be inadequate leading to shearing and wound dehiscence [19].

4.2.2 Larger defects

4.2.2.1 Pediculate flaps

In a bigger defect up to half of the tongue or particularly in a huge composite defect that may include the floor of the mouth, cheek, or both, a pediculate and free flap are the alternatives preferred. In a defect up to 6 or 7 cm, the pediculate submandibular flap can be harvested and is my first choice as long as the neck is N0 or N+ with no fixed nodes and small metastatic nodes (**Figure 5a** and **b**). It usually provides a non-bulky flap that can be harvested to cover the defect and can be tied to the tongue to allow mobility for swallowing and speech [20–21]. In cases of N2 neck with huge or fixed metastatic nodes that impacts the possibility of preserve the submandibular pedicle, a supraclavicular pediculate flap can be harvested specially

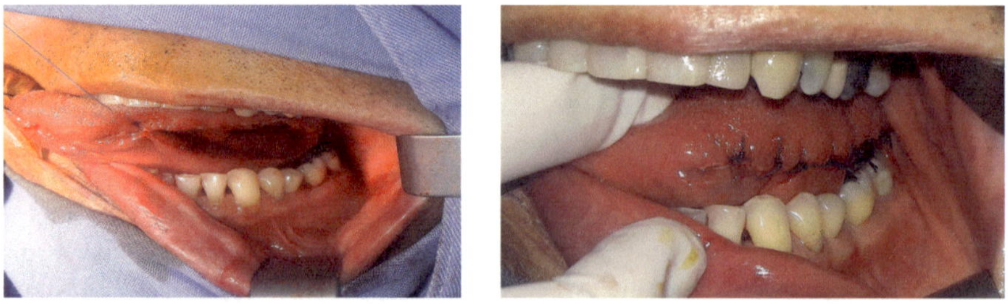

(a) (b)

Figure 4.
(a) Primary closure and (b) primary closure outcome.

DOI: http://dx.doi.org/10.5772/intechopen.91049

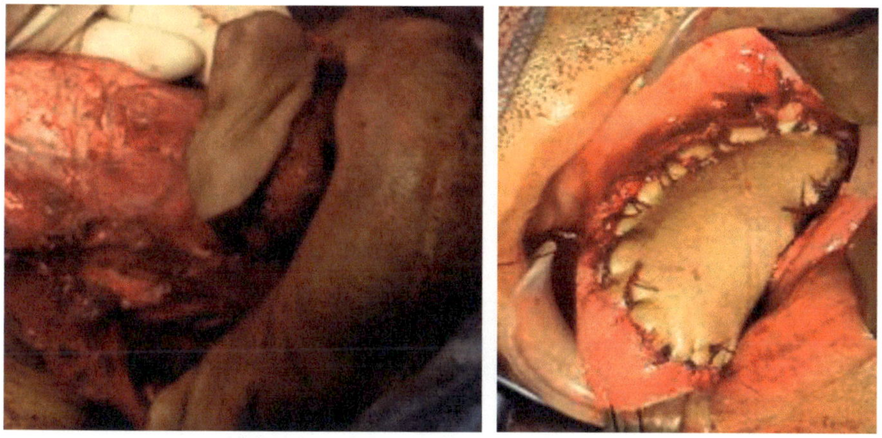

Figure 5.
(a) Submandibular flap harvest and (b) submandibular flap insetting.

to reconstruct tongue with a composite cheek defect [22]. This flap previously described, is also recommended in cases when a free flap cannot be performed due to any specific contraindication such as inexperience or lack of a reconstructive team in microvascular surgery or if the patient is in a poor physical condition and a shortened procedure is mandatory [23].

4.2.2.2 Free flaps

In cases of a near total or total glossectomy that frequently is associated with composite resections of the floor of the mouth, cheek, skin, or mandible, a free flap is required (**Figure 6a–c**). Speech and swallowing functions after reconstruction for those defects remain disappointing due to the reduced mobility of the flap and the poor functional muscle quality, therefore, the more tongue musculature left, the better rehabilitation of speaking and swallowing will be achieved, and of course, a better functional outcome. The reason for that is that the coordinate movement of the tongue cannot be replaced and the new tissue attached to the rest of the tongue relies on its mobility and just leaves a bulk. If sensation is attempted, a sensory nerve reconstruction provided by the free flap should be intended at the time of reconstruction. If a total glossectomy is performed, the main goal of reconstruction is to provide an adequate amount of soft tissue and bulky flap to allow the neo-tongue to get in touch with the palate to push food toward the hypopharynx and in some way to help in speech [24]. Nevertheless, normal movement will not be accomplished, fundamentally affecting speech and articulation. If only soft tissues are essential, a radial forearm free flap (RFFF) or an anterolateral thigh flap (ALTF) (**Figure 7a** and **b**) are the first option to reconstruct the defect, both of them provide a good amount of soft tissue that can be sentient, just to fulfill the objective mentioned before. The use of free flaps to transfer muscle to achieve motor innervation of the neo-tongue, like the latissimus dorsi or gracilis free flap has been intended with disappointing results in terms of function [25].

4.2.2.3 Alternative options

For selected patients in whom free tissue transfer is not an option, the pectoralis major myocutaneous flap offers a reliable reconstructive procedure following both

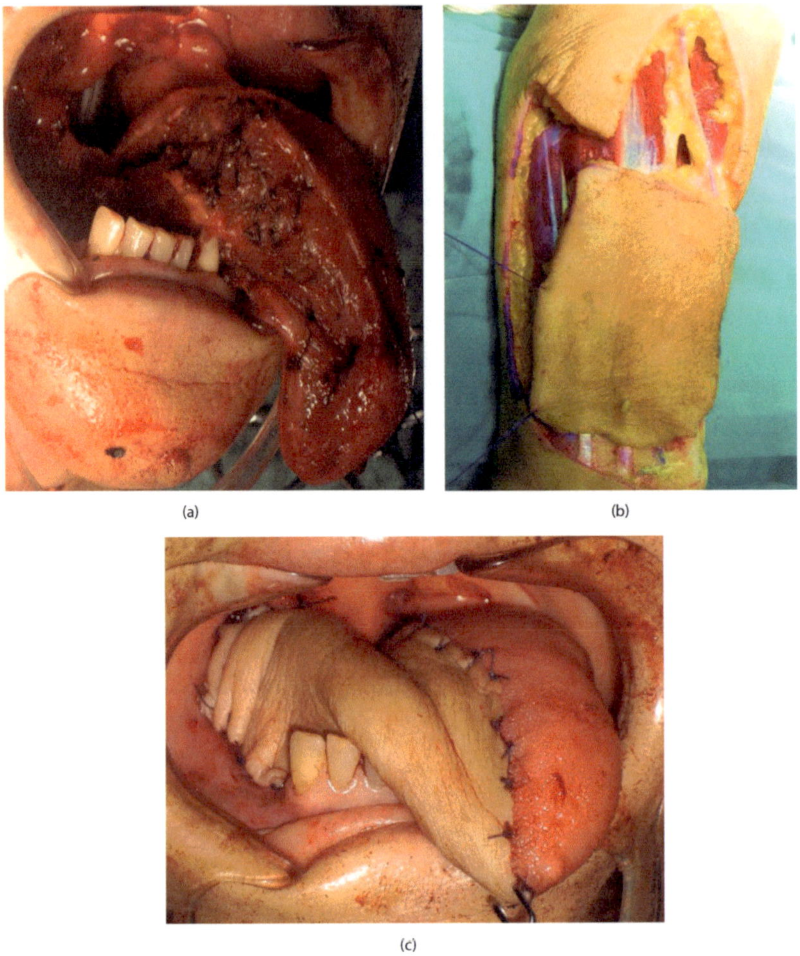

Figure 6.
(a) Tongue defect after resection, (b) RFFF harvest and (c) RFFF insetting.

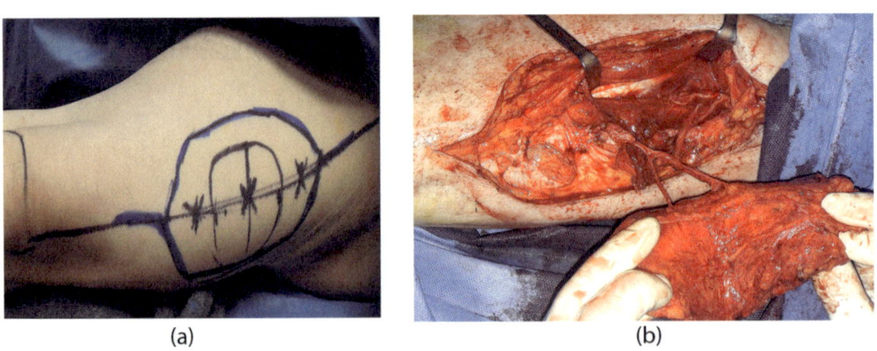

Figure 7.
(a) ALT flap design and (b) ALT flap harvest.

primary and salvage surgery (**Figure 8**). This flap based on the thoracoacromial artery can be raised as a myocutaneous or fasciocutaneous flap. It is reliable, robust, and easily harvested in terms to tongue reconstruction and can provide muscle and skin to fulfill the tongue and floor of the mouth and effectively separate the oral cavity from the neck. It must be suspended across the mandibular arch by either suturing

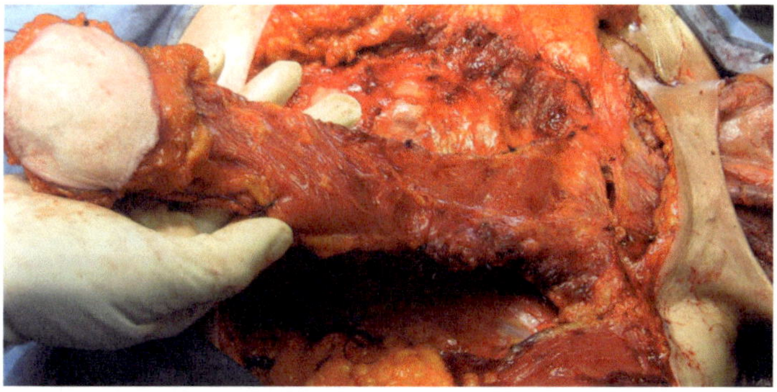

Figure 8.
Major pectoral flap harvest.

to the pterygoid musculature or securing to the mandible using drill holes to avoid and prevent the flap from falling [26]. This flap is considered a horse battle in rescue setting when a free flap fails. When the defect includes mandible, during the reconstruction it must have keep in mind that mandible contributes to airway stability, oral competence, speech, deglutition and mastication, so the goal of this reconstruction must include the preservation of the ability to open the mouth, occlusion, and the restoration of the inter arch continuity solutions to promote dental implants and restore chewing as mentioned in floor of mouth defects extended to mandibula. Not reconstructing the central defects will conclude in loss of the lip support with Andy Gump deformity, and not reconstructing the lateral defects will cause malocclusion and lateral shift in the position of mandible, so any intent must be done to reconstruct the mandible. Options in reconstruction include metal plates (**Figure 7**), non-vascularized bone grafts, osteomyocutaneous pedicled flaps, and osteocutaneous free flaps. Fixing soft tissues just with plates was widely used in the past and usually results in extrusion intraorally, external exposure or fracture of the plate up to 60% of the cases with a worst defect and a very poor functional outcome [27]. Autogenous bone grafts from iliac crest, scapula, or calvarium usually end in no vascularization of the new bone and its atrophy even more if radiation is added to the treatment, and finally similar results as the plating alone are obtained, so similarly they are no more used.

Currently the gold standard in mandible reconstruction is the osteocutaneous free flaps (**Figure 9a–c**) and carries the same consideration as mentioned in floor of mouth reconstruction with a trend to perform a first time micro vascularized bone reconstruction with dental implants mainly in a previous dentulous young patient [28]. In an aged edentulous patient in the reconstruction setting, there is most likely no need to be aware for dental implants unlike dentulous young patient. Again, in selected patients with poor clinical condition and not suitable for a long procedure, a osteocutaneous pediculate flap such as a osteomyocutaneous trapezius flap [29] or a bicortical parietal osteofascial pedicled flap [30] can be perform providing a better functional result compared with just soft tissue coverage. Both flaps require experience, skills, and anatomic knowledge to harvest them in a short period of time but are an excellent alternative when needed.

4.3 Cheek

The cheek resection is done less frequently except in some countries like India, where cheek cancer is frequent and as a consequence of chewing tobacco; usually its oncological resections leave a complex defect that includes skin and mucosa in an area where a functional lip is required to avoid food spillage. The consequent

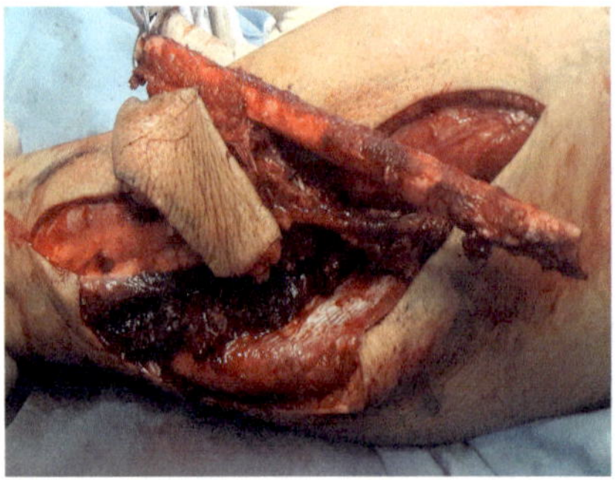

(a)

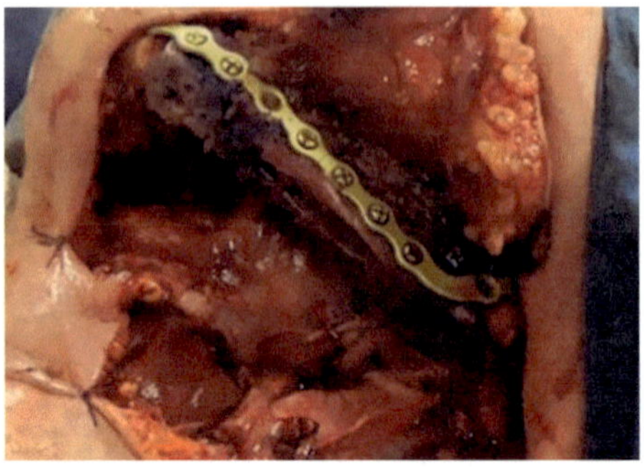

(b)

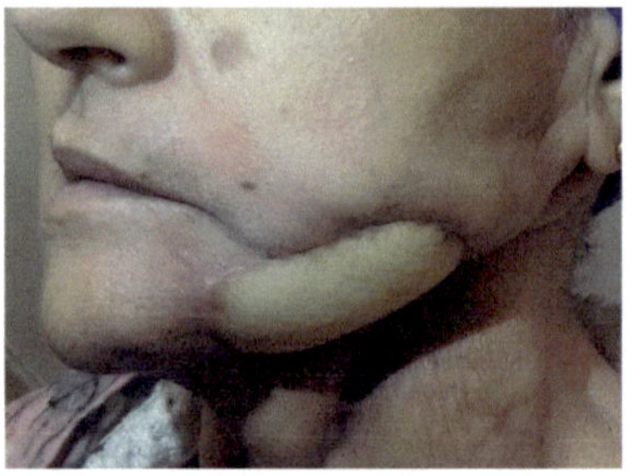

(c)

Figure 9.
(a) FFF harvest, (b) FFF insetting and (c) FFF early postoperative outcome.

defect may be small or big and simple or composite associated to another oral cavity subsite resection. Small lesions of the cheek could be let alone to epithelize, but a bigger one will end in a scar and retraction, so a reconstruction must be done. In most of the cases a facial artery mucomucosal flap (FAMM) could be used. This flap based on a branch of the facial artery is elevated in the layer underneath the facial artery including the overlying buccinators muscle and a small portion of orbicularis oris muscle close to the oral commissure; it is rotated to cover the defect commonly restoring it, and the donor site could be primary closed or let it to heal secondarily without impairing its final functional result. A huge defect might need a pediculate flap such as submandibular or supraclavicular flap or even a microvascular free flap. Some encourage for the supraclavicular pediculate flap as the first option in this scenery, which usually provides a good amount of a non-bulky tissue without affecting oncological resection of node neck dissection in level Ia and Ib, and adducing that submandibular flap is too bulky to placed it in this specific region.

4.4 Hard palate

The extent of resection of hard palate is crucial to define the type and modality of reconstruction. The defect may be small and involve any portion of the hard palate, the premaxilla, or any portion of the maxillary alveolus with or without tooth-bearing or may be as huge as more than 50% of the hard palate. Many of the times, it is associated with partial or total maxillectomy so ending in a complex defect. Small defects can be let just to re-epithelize with excellent results. For a bigger one, a skin graft can be used; the problem is to support it long enough to achieve its integration to the hard palate; sometimes, the flap is detached and lost in which case healing by second intention is required. Small to medium defects may demand to harvest a palatal mucoperiosteal flap (PMPF). This flap is based on the greater palatine artery; preserving this vascular pedicle allows to rotate it to resurface the mucosal defect [31]. Its limit is related to the amount of tissue needed, and up to 3 cm can be covered with this flap. In a bigger 3–5 cm hole, also a submandibular pediculate flap could be used to cover it. In as much as in this location, there are no specific needs for muscle or for a thicker soft tissue; any attempt should be done to assemble it with just enough muscle behind that guarantees skin perfusion by perforants preventing necrosis and providing a flat new tissue. A composite defect that includes the maxillary alveolus with tooth-bearing or partial to total maxillectomy will end in oroantral communication (**Figure 10a** and **b**). This type of reconstruction needs special considerations that are not the subject of this chapter and are best described in midface reconstruction; in general terms the main goal of the reconstruction is to restore chewing and solve the oroantral communication, so options for small include lesions and the use of an obturator that covers the opening avoiding leaks through the paranasal sinus and improving chew. As the aperture gets bigger, soft tissue flaps like a radial forearm free flap or an anterolateral thigh free flap are needed [32], and if dental implants are planned, microvascular osteocutaneous flaps obtained from fibula free flap or iliac crest free flap must be designed.

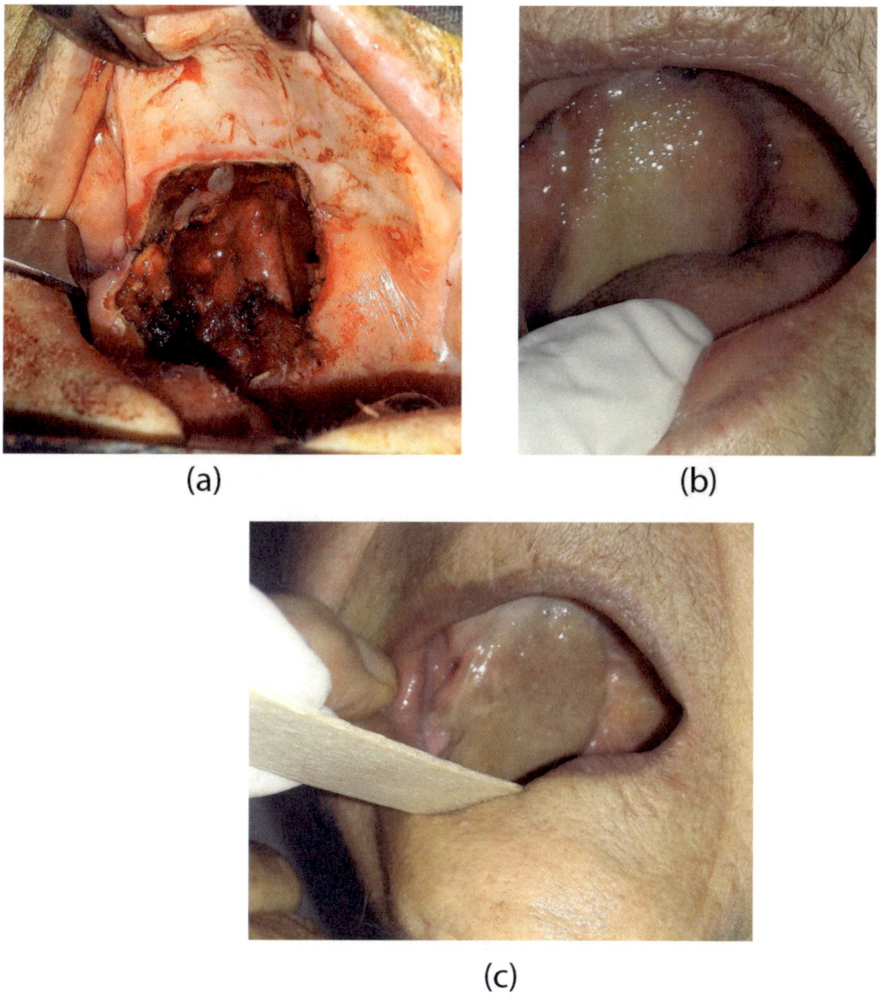

Figure 10.
(a) Hard palate defect after resection, (b) hard palate outcome after 1 month reconstruction and (c) hard palate outcome after 2 years of reconstruction.

5. Care of flaps and donor site

The use of flaps in reconstruction requires special care in terms of surveillance of perfusion and integration. The pediculate flaps usually do not jeopardize the perfusion, but sometimes a minor venous congestion can be expected. As a preventive measure, any intent must be done to avoid tension or compression of the vessel that perfuses the flap. The free flaps require special attention due to the risk of arterial or venous thrombosis and flap failure. Strict vigilance during the first 72 h after surgery and searching for signs of an early venous congestion or arterial occlusion can detect early failure of the flap and may permit in many cases a successful intervention to preserve the flap. The use of Doppler monitoring may help to reach that goal.

The donor site when skin grafted may be left secured and covered with wet gauze up to 8 days to reach adherence of the tissue. Sometimes small bleeding is expected with no need of a revision surgery. If the donor site is primary closed, surveillance of a compartment syndrome is necessary especially if it is closed is under tension.

6. Future directions

Reconstruction has been evolving during the last 20 years. Access to technology is assisting the planning of the resection and reconstruction. Additionally, 3D printers will better permit in the future to mimic tissue, so almost a perfect design of the tissue to reconstruct will be performed. Even that, function of some organs like tongue jet cannot properly be replaced, so much work is still necessary to reach that goal. New techniques in surveillance in microvascular perfusion like specific measurement of flap perfusion zones with heat chambers are being developing.

7. Tips in oral reconstruction

- In oncological resection, patient survival must be guaranteed being the main goal to take a decision in terms of reconstruction.
- Satisfactory reconstruction favors rehabilitation and quality of life.
- The best reconstruction is the less invasive and time consuming that could achieve the aim of adequate function, esthetics, and rehabilitation.
- Clinical condition of the patient, comorbidities, and status performance may limit a long-time procedure, so a local or pediculate flap must be choose.
- Whenever possible a local or pediculate flap is preferred if reconstruction outcomes are going to be as similar as to a free flap reconstruction.
- Free flap reconstruction when indicated must be done to restore or improve function and cosmetic end and needs a team with skills in microvascular reconstruction.
- Adequate knowledge of different alternatives in reconstruction provides the best comprehensive approach to reconstruct defects based on the location, size, color match, function, and complexity of structures involved.
- **Figures 11** and **12** show a rational approach in oral reconstruction.

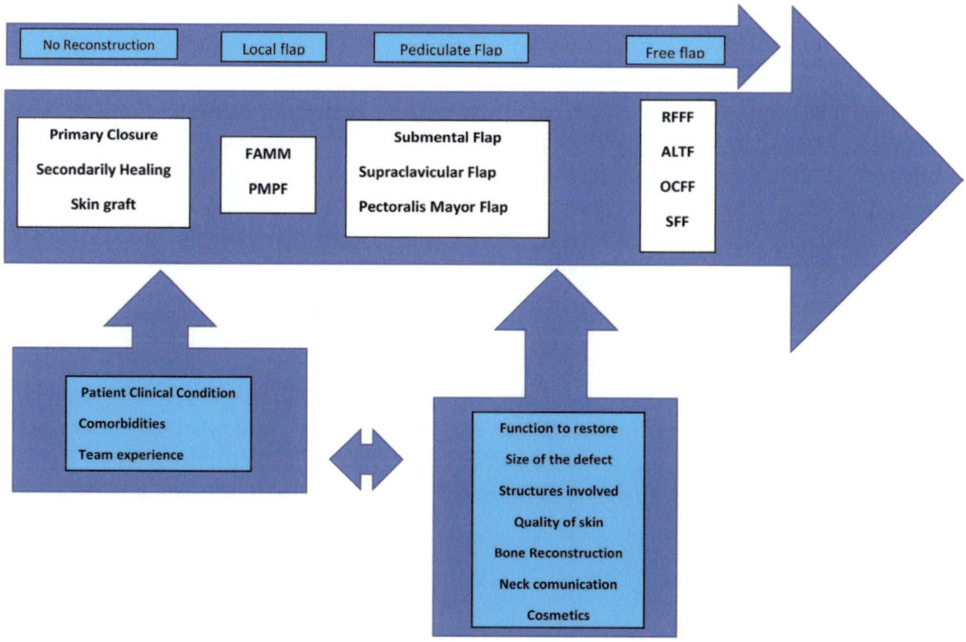

Figure 11.
Reconstruction based on patient status.

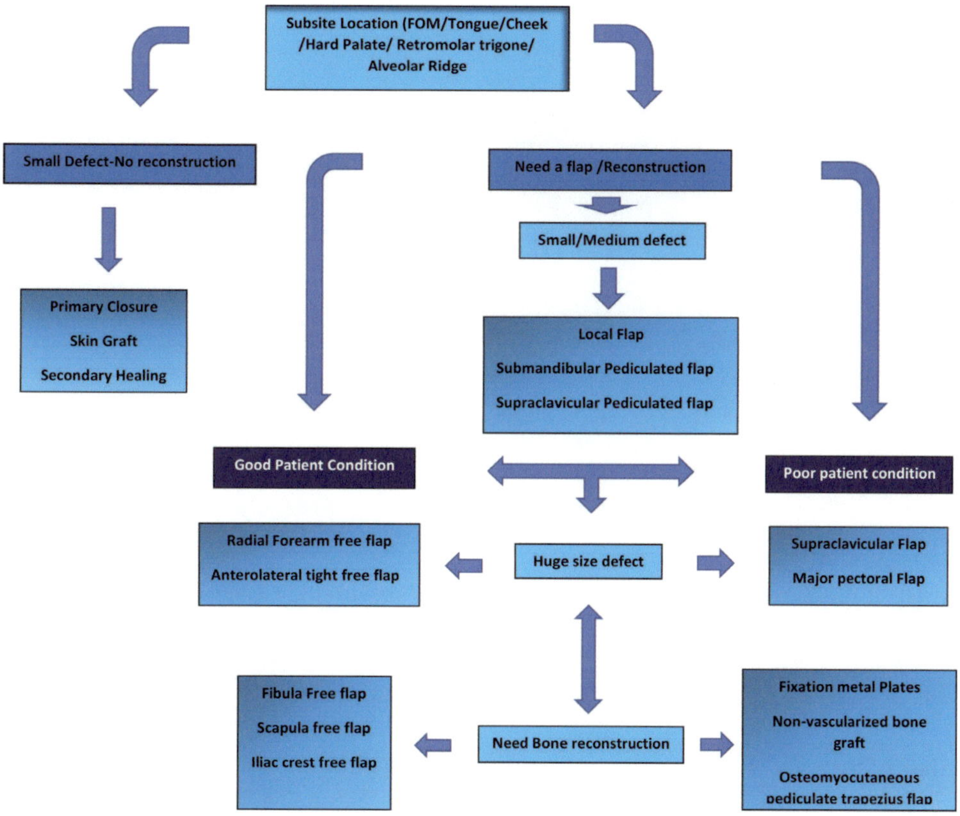

Figure 12.
Reconstruction based on size of the defect.

8. Conclusions

Head and neck cancer requires a multidisciplinary approach to face diagnosis, treatment, and rehabilitation. Oral cancer is one of the most frequent sites in which functional disturbance due to the primary tumor invasion or destruction of normal tissue or its treatment like extensive surgery, chemotherapy, radiation, or the combination of them ends in functional and cosmetic disturbance that impacts quality of life. Especially surgery creates a defect that alter function in terms of deglutition, swallowing, speech, breathing, and esthetics. Immediate reconstruction is necessary and must be intended to restore or improve rehabilitation.

Reconstruction calls to assay factors related to the patient, to the tumor defect, and to the team expertise. The best and simplest reconstructive option must be offered to refurbish as similar as possible to a new normal functional tissue, as well as guaranteeing patient survival with low morbidity, without neglecting the reasonable employment of technical and economic resources. Critical analysis must be done in every case to decide from a primary close to escalate up to a micro vascularized free flap.

Conflict of interest

The author declares no conflict of interest.

Author details

Andres Chala
Surgical Department, Head and Neck Service, Caldas University,
Manizales (Caldas), Colombia

*Address all correspondence to: andreschalag@hotmail.com

References

[1] Ferlay J, Bray F, Pisani P, Parkin DM. GLOBOCAN. Cancer Incidence, Mortality and Prevalence Worldwide. IARC Cancer Base No. 5, Version 2.0. Lyon: IARC Press; 2004

[2] Gurney T, Eisele D, Orloff L, Wang S. Predictors of quality of life after treatment for oral cavity and oropharyngeal carcinoma. Otolaryngology–Head and Neck Surgery. 2008;**139**(2):262-267

[3] Hiatt J, Gardnmer L. Textbook of Head and Neck Anatomy. 4th ed.: Lippincott Williams and Wilkins; 2010. pp. 31-34

[4] Dupoirieux L, Plane L, Gard C, Penneau M. Anatomical basis and results of the facial artery musculomucosal flap for oral reconstruction. The British Journal of Oral & Maxillofacial Surgery. 1999;**37**(1):25-28

[5] Genden EM, Buchbinder D, Urken ML. The submental island flap for palatal reconstruction: A novel technique. Journal of Oral and Maxillofacial Surgery. 2004;**62**:387-390

[6] Sanghoon L, Hye-Min C, Jin-kyu K, Nam W. The supraclavicular artery island flap: A salvage option for head and neck reconstruction. Maxillofacial Plastic and Reconstructive Surgery. 2018;**40**:25

[7] Evans GR, Schusterman MA, Kroll SS, Miller MJ, Reece GP, Robb GL, et al. The radial forearm free Xap for head and neck reconstruction: A review. American Journal of Surgery. 1994;**168**:446-450

[8] De Bree R, Rinaldo A, Genden E, Suárez C, Rodrigo JP, Fagan J, et al. Modern reconstruction techniques for oral and pharyngeal defects after tumor resection. European Archives of Oto-Rhino-Laryngology. 2008;**265**:1-9

[9] Villaret DB, Futran NA. The indications and outcomes in the use of osteocutaneous radial forearm Xap. Head & Neck. 2003;**25**:475-481

[10] Ross GL, Dunn R, Kirkpatrick J, Koshy CE, Alkureishi LW, Bennett N, et al. To thin or not to thin: The use of the anterolateral thigh flap in the reconstruction of intraoral defects. British Journal of Plastic Surgery. 2003;**56**:409-413

[11] Urken ML. Composite free Xaps in oromandibular reconstruction. Review of the literature. Archives of Otolaryngology—Head & Neck Surgery. 1991;**117**:724-732

[12] Shpitzer T, Neligan PC, Gullane PJ, Boyd BJ, Gur E, Rotstein LE, et al. The free iliac crest and fibula flaps in vascularized oromandibular reconstruction: Comparison of long-term evaluation. Head & Neck. 1999;**21**:639-647

[13] Erovic BM, Lercher P. Manual of Head and Neck Reconstruction Using Regional and Free Flaps. Springer-Verlag Wien; 2015. pp. 225-238

[14] Urken ML, Bridger AG, Zur KB, Genden EM. The scapular osteofasciocutaneous Xap: A 12-year experience. Archives of Otolaryngology—Head & Neck Surgery. 2001;**127**:862-869

[15] Zho M, Shao Z, Zhu Y, Liu B, Wu T. Comparison of complicated and simple guiding templates in mandibular reconstruction using vascularized iliac crest flap. BioMed Research International. 2019:7. DOI: 10.1155/2019/7496538. Article ID 7496538

[16] De Maesschalck T, Courvoisier D, Scolozzic P. Computer-assisted versus traditional freehand technique in fibular free flap mandibular reconstruction:

A morphological comparative study. European Archives of Oto-Rhino-Laryngology. 2017;**274**:517-526

[17] Succo G, Berrone M, Battiston B, Tos P, Goia F, Appendino P, et al. Step-by-step surgical technique for mandibular reconstruction with fibular free flap: Application of digital technology in virtual surgical planning. European Archives of Oto-Rhino-Laryngology. 2015;**272**:1491-1501

[18] Barbier L, Pottel L, Lamoral F, Duyck J, Jacobs R, Abelos J. Evaluation of quality of life after mandibular reconstruction using a novel fixed implant-supported dental prosthesis concept: A pilot study. The International Journal of Prosthodontics. 2019;**32**:162-173

[19] Schramm VL, Myers EN. Skin grafts in oral cavity reconstruction. Archives of Otolaryngology. 1980;**106**:528-532

[20] Uppin SB, Ahmad QG, Yadav P, Shetty K. Use of the submental island flap in orofacial reconstruction—A review of 20 cases. Journal of Plastic, Reconstructive & Aesthetic Surgery. 2009;**62**:514-519

[21] Sebastian P, Thomas S, Varghese BT, Iype EM, Balagopal PG, Mathew PC. The submental island flap for reconstruction of intraoral defects in oral cancer patients. Oral Oncology. 2008;**44**:1014-1018

[22] Fang S, Zhang D, Chen WL, Wang YY, Fan S. Reconstruction of full-thickness cheek defects with a folded extended supraclavicular fasciocutaneous island flap following ablation of advanced oral cancer. Journal of Cancer Research and Therapeutics. 2016;**12**:888-891

[23] Giordano L, Di Santo D, Occhini A, Galli A, Bertino G, Benazzo M, et al. Supraclavicular artery island flap (SCAIF): A rising opportunity for head and neck reconstruction. European Archives of Oto-Rhino-Laryngology. 2016;**273**:4403-4412

[24] Yu P. Oral cavity reconstruction. In: Reconstructive Plastic Surgery of the Head and Neck. Current Technics and Flap Atlas. 1st ed. Thieme Medical Publishers, Inc.; 2016. pp. 18-39

[25] Yousif NJ, Dzwierzynski WW, Sanger JR, Matloub HS, Campbell BH. The innervated gracilis musculo-cutaneous flap for total tongue reconstruction. Plastic and Reconstructive Surgery. 1999;**104**(4): 916-921

[26] Su W, Hsia Y, Chang Y, et al. Functional comparison after reconstruction with a radial forearm free flap or a pectoralis major flap for cancer of the tongue. Otolaryngology and Head and Neck Surgery. 2003;**128**:412-418

[27] Mariani PB, Kowalski LP, Magrin J. Reconstruction of large defects postmandibulectomy for oral cancer using plates and myocutaneous flaps: A long-term follow-up. International Journal of Oral and Maxillofacial Surgery. 2006;**35**(5):427-432

[28] Chang YM, Santamaria E, Wei FC, et al. Primary insertion of osseointegrated dental implants into bula osteoseptocutaneous free flap for mandible reconstruction. Plastic and Reconstructive Surgery. 1998;**102**(3):680-688

[29] Gallego S, Herrera JO, Ruiz A, Cárdenas YA. Clinical experience with the vertical trapezius myo-cutaneous flap in head and neck reconstruction. Cirugía Plástica Ibero-Latinoamericana. 2014;**40**:63-72

[30] Gálvez F, Luaces R, Patin B, Pombo M, Collado J, López JL. Mandibular reconstruction with the bicortical parietal osteofascial pedicled

flap: Our experience in 9 cases. Revista Española de Cirugía Oral y Maxilofacial. 2017;**39**:72-79

[31] Batra H, Jindal G, Kaur S. Evaluation of different treatment modalities for closure of oro-antral communications and formulation of a rational approach. Journal of Maxillofacial and Oral Surgery. 2010;**9**(1):13-18

[32] Moreno MA, Skoracki RJ, Hanna EY, Hanasono MM. Microvascular free flap reconstruction versus palatal obturation for maxillectomy defects. Head & Neck. 2010;**32**(7):860-868

Section 3

Endodontics

Chapter 12

Applications of CBCT in Endodontics

Jesús Mena Álvarez and Álvaro Zubizarreta Macho

Abstract

There are many articles published in recent years on the use of CBCT in endodontics and this diagnostic technique is increasingly required in order to have a more accurate prognosis of the teeth to be treated. The purpose of this chapter is to discuss the use of Conical Beam Computed Tomography (CBCT) in the field of endodontics. This issue is controversial at the moment because of the increase in the radiation to which patients are being subjected; however, we know that sometimes the X-rays taken with different angles in relation to some teeth depending on the different cases are incompatible in form and density, which does not allow us to make an exact diagnosis. The use of CBCT would have provided an image of greater diagnostic value in those cases. In addition, the use guidelines published by the American Endodontics Association and the American Radiology Association jointly mark the way forward and the use we can give the CBCT for the diagnosis of complex cases.

Keywords: CBCT, endodontics, tomography, root canal treatment

1. CBCT description

CBCT is the technique that allows three-dimensional reconstruction, but using a conical beam to decrease the dose for the patient compared to conventional CT. For almost a century, dentists have been studying a 2D representation of a 3D structure, that structure is the tooth. This simplification of the information produces inherent disadvantages, among which the anatomical structures in the plane of the roots and apices of the teeth studied mask many details, which occur mainly in the area of the upper molars, where the zygomatic arch or the breast can complicate the detail of the posterior anatomy of the roots of the teeth, which entails a complicated diagnosis and treatment [1]. In practice this means that radiolucent areas may not be identified, being able to find difficulties in relating the position of the apex in proximity to vital structures and not being able to detect the exact situation of the calcifications of the teeth. The correct identification of the morphology and anatomy of the root canals can be difficult, as well as the identification of root fractures and root resorption [2].

We can rule out a series of milestones in the history of CBCT and radiology beginning in 1895 when Wilhelm Roentgen discovered X-rays in Germany, but it is not until 1896 when the first intraoral radiography is performed by Edmond Kells in New Orleans. Already in 1967 Godfrey Hounsfield developed the first CT scanner and in 1971 it was introduced in medical examination. In 1990 Tachibana and Matsumoto reported the first use of CT in endodontics and in 1997 Quantitative

Radiology produced the first CBCT, the New Tom 9000, for dental use after Arai's pioneering work in Japan and in Mozzo in Italy, obtaining in 2001 the first CBCT licensed for use in the US [3].

2. How does a CBCT work?

The process begins with an emitter that directs a very fine beam of X-rays through a collimator (system that from a divergent beam forms a parallel beam). This beam affects the object under study which is crossed or irradiated by a percentage of lightning. This radiation, which has not been absorbed by the object, in the form of a spectrum, is collected by detectors. The detectors depending on the CBCT are of different materials, they can be silicon or selenium or a CCD sensor (digital analog converter) the X-ray source and the detector are connected in such a way that they have a synchronous movement.

The function of the CCD sensor is to convert the information obtained from analog to digital that transforms the electrical signal produced by the interaction of the detector with the patient's emerging X-rays, into a binary signal suitable for processing by software specially designed for each brand of CBCT.

The source-detector assembly rotates and performs the X-ray shot, obtaining a projection or cut of the tooth under study. The team performs several rotations to obtain 360 images or cuts corresponding to each degree of rotation that are reconstructed, thus achieving a three-dimensional image of the skull. This 2D data is then converted through conical beam algorithms [4] into a 3D volume of data for a PC in any of the 3D planes or a 3D image. Normally, transverse images are generated in the three orthogonal planes from the CBCT scan. The professional selects the position and thickness of the cut inside the data volume. The three views can be evaluated simultaneously, since the modification of the cut in one of the planes modifies the rest of the planes displayed. This can be manipulated by PC software to provide more detail of specific areas of interest [5].

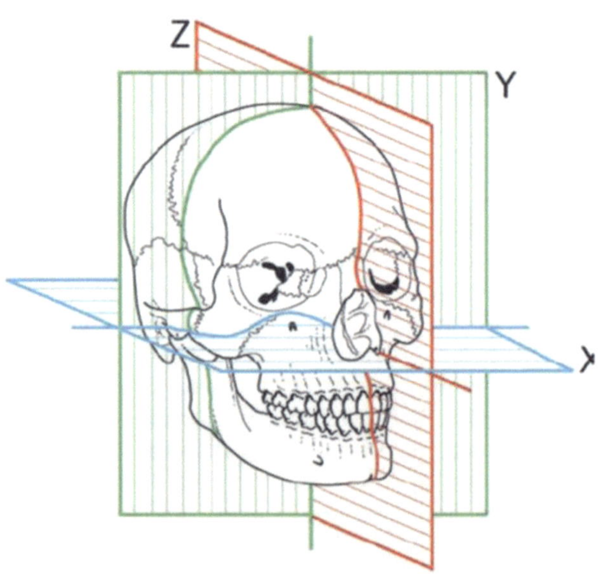

Figure 1.
Illustration of the 3-dimensional planes.

Sagittal plane: Perpendicular to the ground and parallel to the middle sagittal plane, which divides the body into left and right halves (Z).

Axial plane: Perpendicular to the longitudinal axis of a body (X).

Coronal plane Divide the skull into a ventral part and another dorsal part (Y) (**Figure 1**).

Axial and proximal views are of particular value since they are generally not seen on a conventional periapical radiograph [6].

Thanks to the cone-beam technology and algorithmic calculations it is possible to overcome the distortions produced by the patient's breathing [7].

3. Essential CBCT concepts related to endodontics

The most important concepts in the use of CBCT in endodontics are the field of vision and the spatial resolution of the machine.

The visual field to be studied or Field of View (FOV) is directly related to the area to be scanned which will be digitally represented on the computer. The FOV measurement for face studies in dentistry with conical beam tomography is 14 cm. what determines the quality of the tomographic image (the size of the pixel and the voxel) is the division between FOV and the matrix. Roughly speaking, CBCT systems can be classified into two categories: limited (dental or regional) or complete (ortho or facial). The limited range FOV is 40–100 nm, while the field of view of the full range is 100–200 nm. A typical FOV consists of millions of voxels [8].

In endodontics, the FOV can be small or "focused" (5 cm by 5 cm or less) because the root canal treatment generally involves one tooth in an arch. This reduction in FOV reduces the amount of effective radiation dose [9]. Other advantages of a small FOV field of view are decreased time to process and read the image, better ability to avoid metallic structures that can cause interference, greater spatial resolution and improved diagnostic potential [10]. Most small FOV machines produce an effective radiation dose in the same order of magnitude as a panoramic radiograph or a periapical series [11].

The degree of spatial resolution is determined by the voxel size, it is desirable that the resolution of a CBCT machine used for endodontics should not exceed 200 μm, the average width of the periodontal space. Otherwise no pathological changes will be identified.

4. Uses of small-field CBCT in endodontics

Possible applications in endodontics include the diagnosis of endodontic pathology and its origin, root canal system morphology, root evaluation (fractures and traumas), analysis of external or internal root resorption, invasive cervical resorption, presurgical planning, lesion extension, complicated anatomies, location of calcified root canals, endodontic retreatment, evaluation of iatrogenies such as perforations, separate instruments or extrusion of sealing material [12–14].

4.1 Definitive diagnosis of the periapical radiolucent areas

Endodontic treatment aims to preserve the tooth with normal function and prevent or cure apical periodontitis. However, periapical radiographs provide a two-dimensional view of a three-dimensional object. Therefore, periapical radiographs cannot detect lesions such as apical periodontitis confined within the spongy bone.

Bender et al. in 1961 demonstrated in vitro that bone lesions cannot be diagnosed effectively by X-rays unless cortical bone is perforated [15, 16].

Goldman et al. showed that there was considerable disagreement among professionals in the diagnosis of radiolucent areas with radiographs. The reasons for these inconsistencies are the 2D nature of the radiographic image and anatomical distortion that can mislead the professional. Increasing the number of X-rays, taken at different angles improves diagnostic accuracy [17].

Conical beam tomography results in 3D images that eliminate the overlap of anatomical structures. The use of CBCT helps detect periapical radiolucent lesions or areas and make a differential diagnosis with a non-invasive technique that is very accurate (**Figure 2**).

According to Levin et al., the etiology of irreversible pulpitis could be caries or deep restorations, pulp exposure, cracks or any irritating pulp among others [18]. Radiographic visualization of teeth with irreversible pulpitis on conventional periapical radiographs can be normal except for the presence of the etiological cause. Occasionally, if the inflammatory process has spread to the periapical area, a thickening of the periodontal ligament space may be visible [12].

However, the use of 2D radiography still has serious limitations. The studies carried out by Estrela et al. in 2008 evaluated apical periodontitis (AP) in 1508 teeth by 3 methods (panoramic, periapical radiographs and CBCT) concluded that the diagnostic accuracy was significantly higher with periapical radiographs (54.5%) than with panoramic radiographs (27.5%) using the CBCT as a gold standard reference about diagnostic accuracy; apical periodontitis was correctly identified with conventional radiography only when it was sufficiently advanced. Estrela concluded that prevalence of AP was significantly higher with CBCT, overall sensitivity was 0.55 and 0.28 for periapical and panoramic radiographs, respectively and AP was correctly identified with conventional methods when showed advanced status. CBCT was proved to be accurate to identify AP [19].

Lofthag Hansen in 2007 compared the periapical state of 46 maxillary and mandibular molars with two angled periapical radiographs and CBCT scans. CBCT detected 38% more lesions than periapical radiographs [20]. Low et al. in 2008 [21] and Cotton et al. [22] in 2007 give us similar results. García-Silva de Paula in 2009 with an in vivo study examined the periapice of 83 teeth in dogs

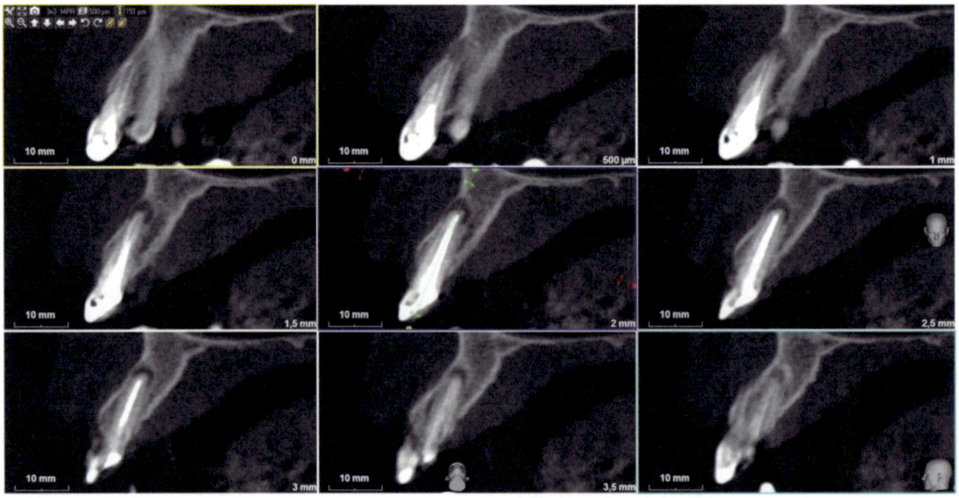

Figure 2.
Images of the CBCT scan.

with periapical radiography and CBCT using histological examination as a gold standard and the conclusions were that CBCT diagnosed healthy areas more accurately than radiography and was more sensitive in detecting apical periodontitis (AP). The AP was detected in 71% of roots with radiography, 84% with CBCT and 93% with histology [23, 24].

4.2 Visualization of root fractures

Vertical root fractures (VRF) are a type of fractures that extend along the major axis of the tooth. If the diagnosis is not carried out, progressive destruction of the periodontal ligament and alveolar bone occurs which can influence the prognosis of adjacent teeth and future restorations. However, VRF may not produce any signs or symptoms such as pain or discomfort from chewing. Therefore, it is important that VRFs be diagnosed as quickly as possible. The prevalence of VRFs in several populations has been reported between 2 and 5% and depending on the literature reviewed; the percentage of endodontic and fissured teeth varies between 3 and 30%. The highest incidence occurs between 40 and 60 years [25]. The most common teeth where it occurs are lower molars and upper premolars [26]. One third of the VRFs are radiographically detectable, usually when the beam is perpendicular to the fracture line or the granulation tissue separates fragments [27]. (**Figure 3a** and **b**).

Mesio-distal fractures are almost impossible to detect with normal radiography [28]. The most effective in vivo diagnostic method of an LRF is surgical exposure of the fracture, and visual inspection under magnification with the help of staining. Edlund et al. examined 32 teeth in 29 patients, which gave symptoms of a VRF, with CBCT and subsequent surgical exploration; the results showed a high correlation between the diagnosis through CBCT and direct visualization, which confirms numerous in vitro studies that support the validity of CBCT in the diagnosis of VRF [29].

4.3 Diagnosis and treatment of dento-alveolar trauma

Most maxillofacial traumatic injuries involve only teeth (50%) or teeth and adjacent soft tissue (36%) while those affecting the alveoli are 13.6% remaining [30]. Unfortunately, periapical radiography has low sensitivity for the diagnosis of minimal displacements of teeth, alveolar or root fractures, however CBCT has the advantage that it is more comfortable for the traumatized patient; extraoral scan generates a multidimensional image avoiding the need for multiple intraoral radiographs. Bernardes et al. in 2009 compared, retrospectively, conventional periapical radiographs and CBCT images in 20 patients with suspected root fractures and found that CBCT was able to detect fractures in 90% of patients, while radiography could only detect fractures in 30–40% of patients. In conclusion, they reported that CBCT was an excellent complement to conventional radiography in the diagnosis of root fractures [31].

4.4 Identification of the apices of the teeth in relation to anatomical structures

Conventional radiographs do not always allow for the evaluation of the spatial relationship of roots with their surrounding anatomical structures [32]. This is important in the context of surgical planning and treatment [21]. Radiological identification of the position of the roots and their apices against structures vitals such as the maxillary sinus or the dental canal is essential for pre-surgical evaluation for endodontic microsurgery and to prevent injury during root canal filling. Velvart et al. studied 55 patients with 44 lower molars and 6 lower premolars, which had been referred for apical surgery due to persistent periapical areas.

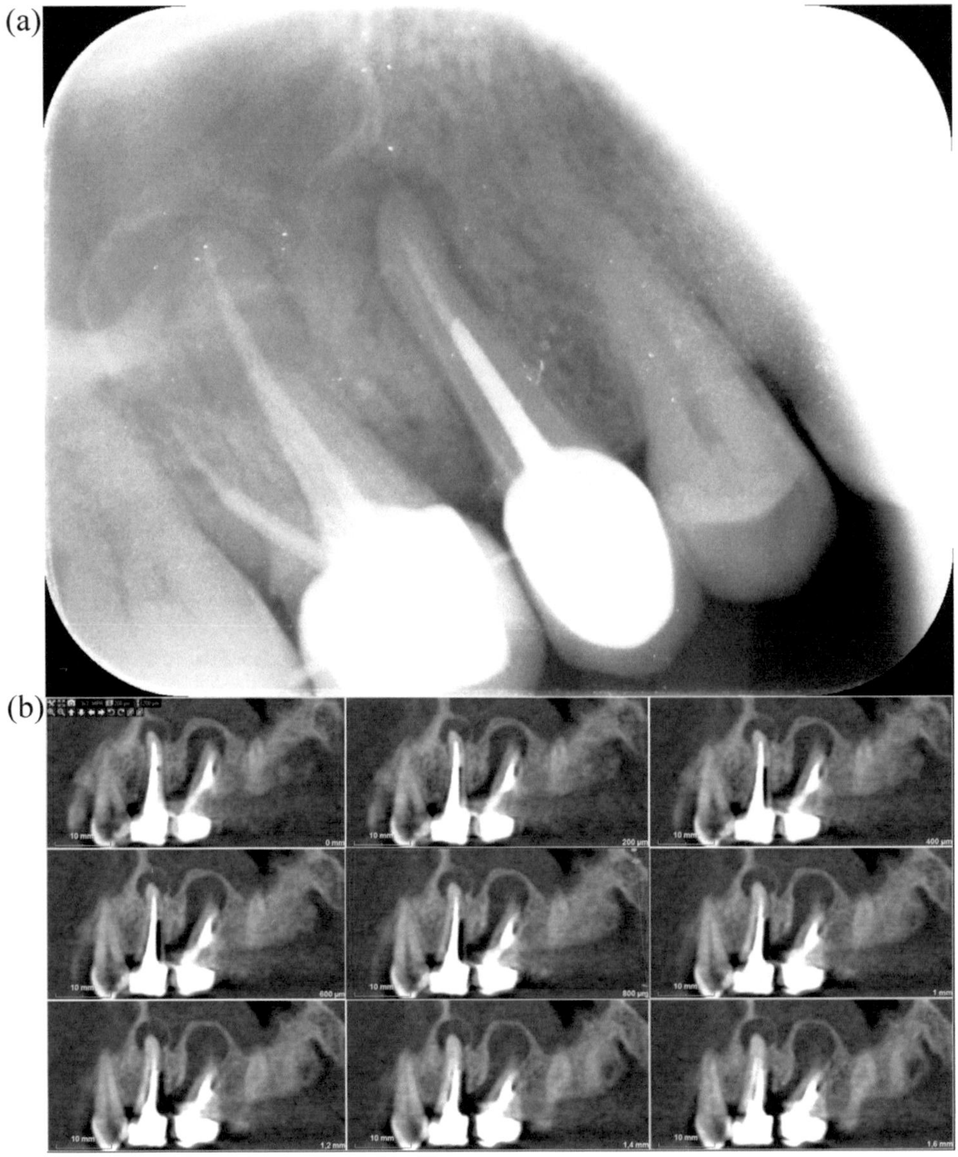

Figure 3.
(a) Periapical radiography and (b) CBCT scan of the same lesions.

CBCT and periapical radiography were performed to identify these lesions, and concluded that the root canal system could be identified in 3 cases with normal radiography, but it was identified in all cases with CBCT and CBCT was also able to quantify the amount of cortical and spongy bone and the three-dimensional extent of the lesion [33]. (**Figure 4a** and **b**).

Rigolone et al. studied 43 upper first molars using CBCT for a possible microsurgical treatment of the palatine root and concluded that this method could provide enough information for a minimally invasive microsurgical technique through a vestibular access instead of a palatal access approach [34]. Low et al. in 2008 evaluated 37 premolars and 37 molars, derived for endodontic surgery in the upper jaw and verified that CBCT was able to identify 34% more lesions than periapical radiography; this detection was influenced by the proximity of the apices to the floor of the maxillar sinus and it was more difficult in

(a)
(b)
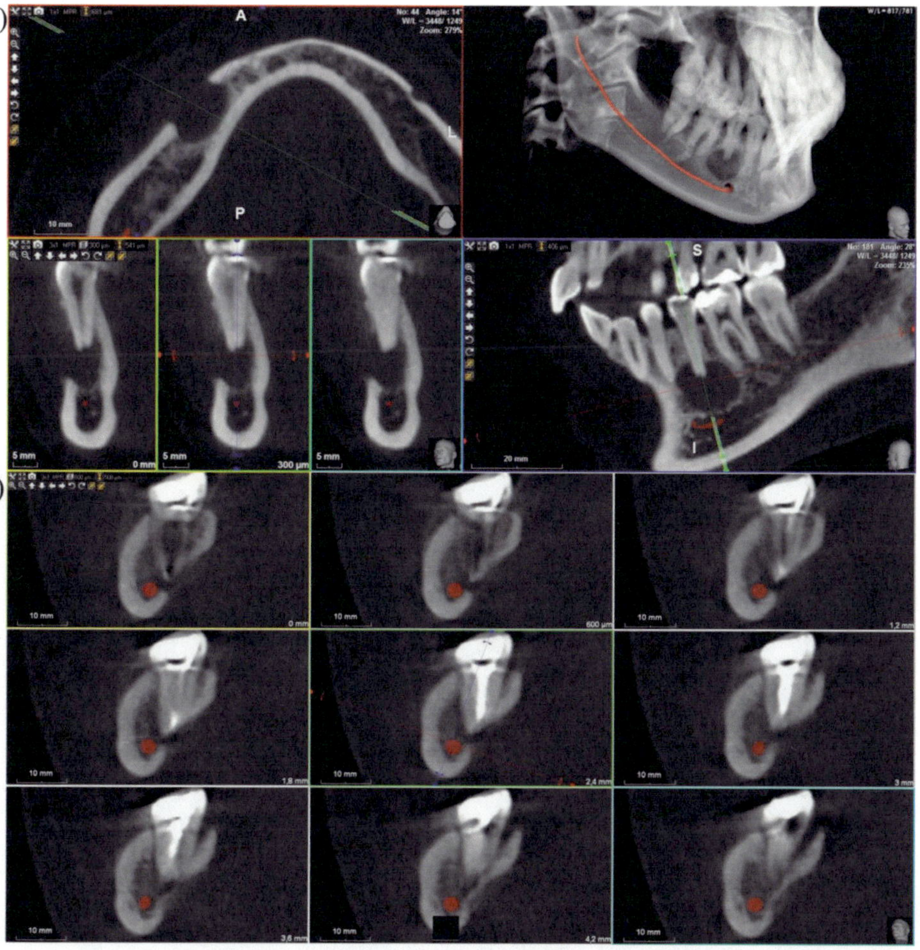

Figure 4.
The CBCT scan allows a diagnosis and treatment plan in all planes. (a) Sagital view and (b) Coronal view.

upper second molars. CBCT was also able to identify sinus membrane thickening, expansion of lesion in maxillary sinus, and apico-marginal communications while periapical radiographs not. These are important pre-surgical markers that may indicate possible surgical complications, oral antral fistula and vertical root fracture [21].

4.5 Identification of root resorption

Root resorption is the loss of dentin or cement as a result of osteoclastic activity. The resorption can be classified according to its location in internal or external. The cells responsible for resorption, whether internal or external, have been described as osteoclasts, odontoclasts and dentinoclasts.

Internal root resorption occurs exclusively as a result of pulp inflammation. Until very recently, the diagnosis of internal or external resorption defects has been limited to the information obtained from conventional radiography techniques. Currently, the use of CBCT is used in the planning of diagnosis and treatment of a case of resorption [35]. (**Figure 5a, b** and **c**).

Accurate identification is essential to ensure both correct treatment and management as it differs depending on the type of resorption. Gartner et al. described the guidelines to differentiate the types of resorption and the use of

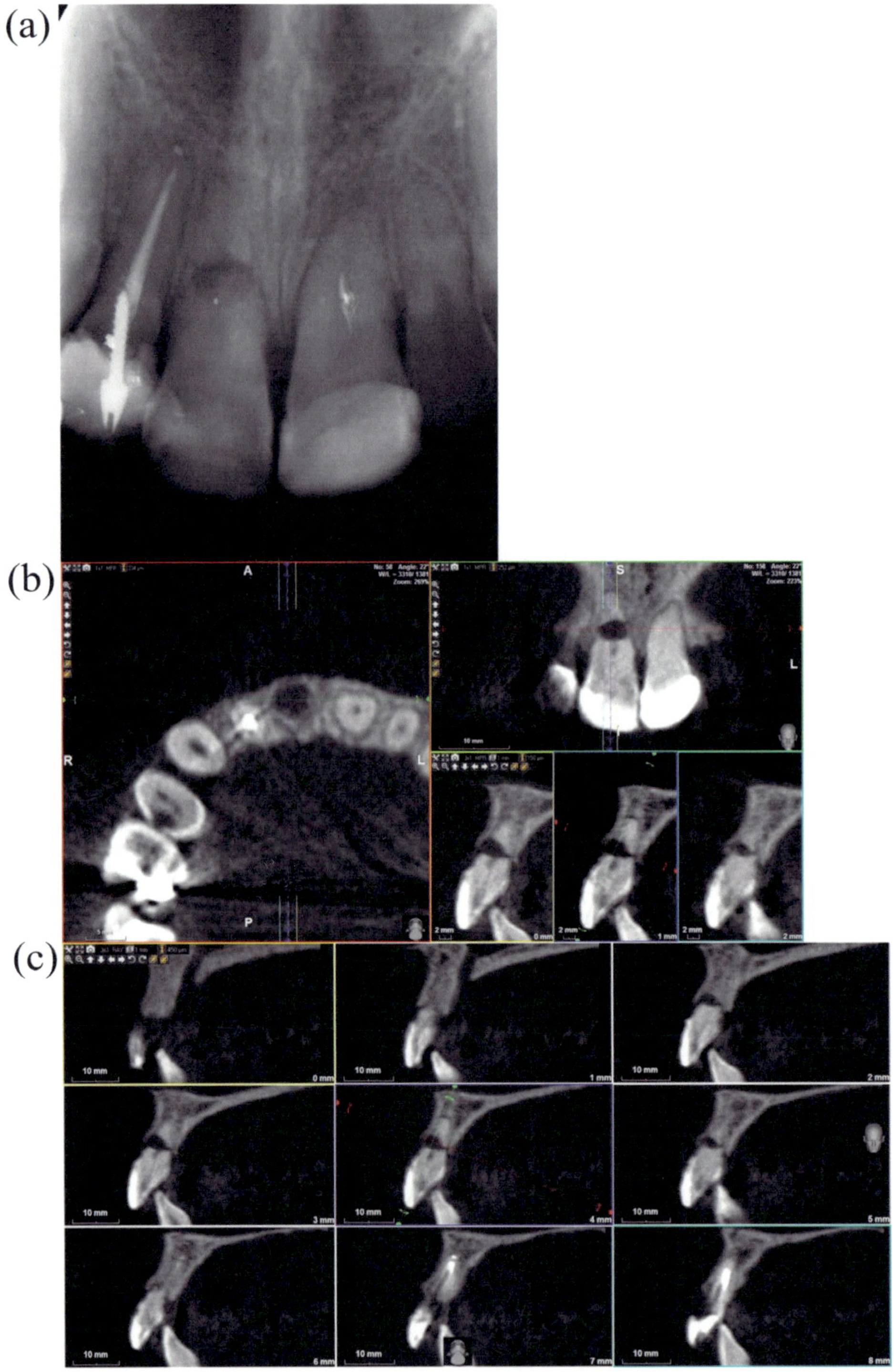

Figure 5.
(a) Periapical radiography of teeth affected by a root resorption, (b and c) CBCT scan of the teeth affected by a root resorption.

2D radiographic techniques with a parallelizer was postulated as the method to differentiate internal resorption from external. However, conventional radiography does not represent the lesion, being unable to identify its true size, location and access [36]. The diagnostic advantages of CBCT lie in the ability of its software to access the most favorable orthogonal views related to the specific spatial vision and the ability to reproduce an accurate three-dimensional image of the lesion in relation to the root anatomy. Cohenca et al. in 2007 concluded that CBCT was extremely useful for diagnosing the degree of root resorption, determining subsequent treatment. Internal root defects, such as resorption, can perforate the external surface, and this may not be detectable by conventional radiographic techniques. The test should be done during diagnosis and treatment planning. The main limitation of conventional radiographic techniques is that a two-dimensional image can only provide limited clinical information regarding three-dimensional structures. The CBCT provides additional information about the location and nature of the root. With the low effective doses, and the relevant additional information provided, the use of CBCT scanners is justified in the management of complex endodontic problems. The results of images obtained by CBCT can modify the treatment planning, as well as the techniques that can be used during a surgical or non-surgical endodontics [37, 38].

4.6 The diagnosis of cystic lesions and non-endodontic pathology

The diagnosis of cystic lesions is very important because there is controversy about these lesions and the curation without surgical treatment, since cysts can only be diagnosed histologically, which needs surgical excision. Different studies have tried to differentiate between granuloma and cysts through radiographs, based on the different densities of the contents of the cavity. Simon et al. in 2006 using CBCT found that the diagnosis coincided with the histological examination in 13 of the 17 cases studied [39]. However, Rosenberg et al. in 2010 about 45 cases, concluded that the diagnosis did not could be confirmed with CBCT [40]. Other studies should be

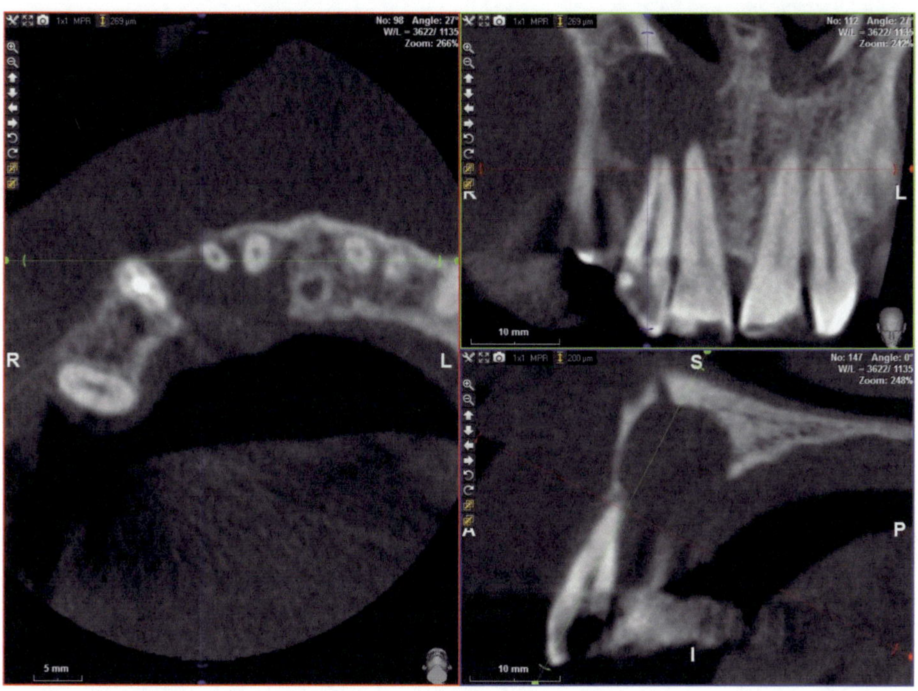

Figure 6.
Cyst lesion and adjacent tissues affected.

carried out to determine the diagnostic capacity of CBCT in these cases. Successful endodontic treatment depends on the correct identification of all root canals; this allows shaping, cleaning and filling.

Non-identification of the anatomy is one of the main causes of endodontic failure. Matherne et al. in 2008 compared the ability of three board-certified endodontists to detect the number of root canals on intraoral digital radiographs and CBCT images on 72 teeth extracted in 3 equal groups of upper molars, lower premolars and mandibular incisors. The observers could not detect at least one of the root canals in 40% of the teeth using 2D images, which demonstrate the advantage of CBCT over conventional radiology [41]. (**Figure 6**).

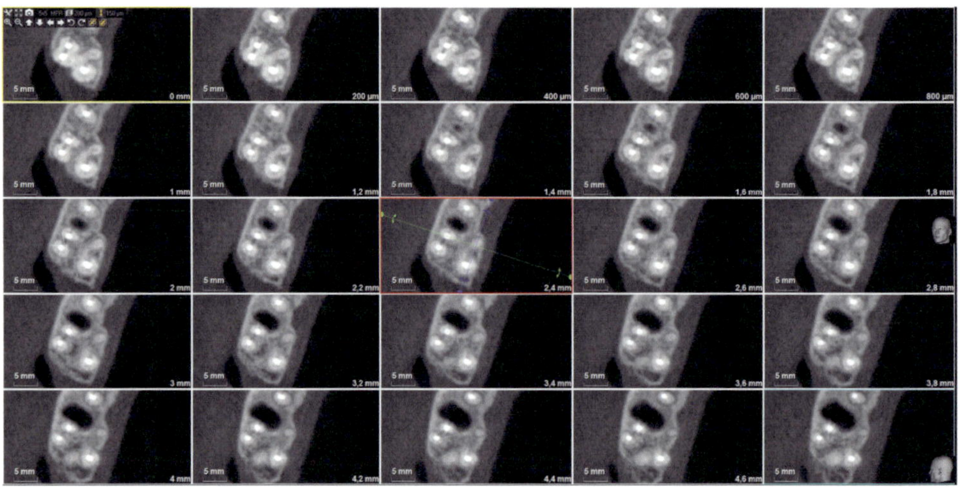

Figure 7.
Patient with second untreated palatine canal.

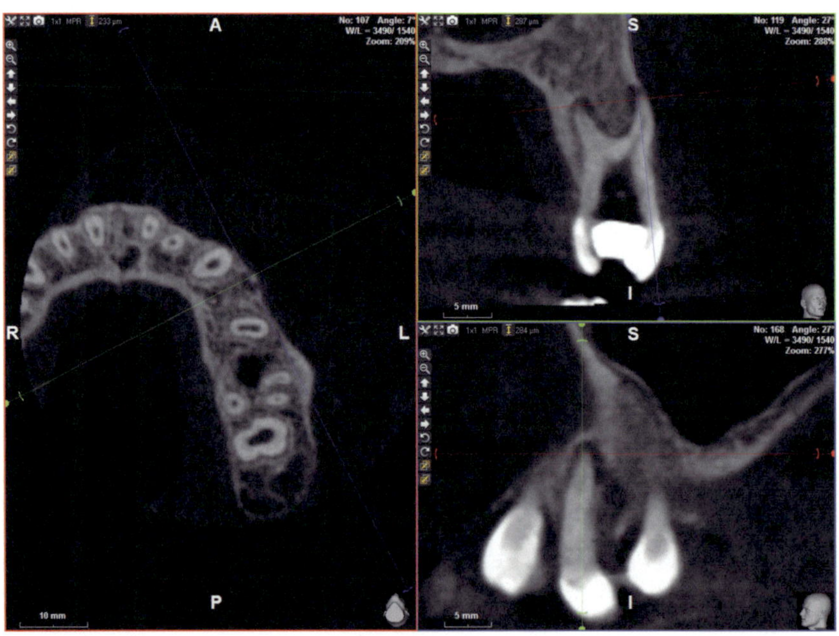

Figure 8.
Upper premolar with presence of taurodontism.

4.7 Recommendations

Following the consensus documents prepared by the American Association of Endodontics and the European Society of Endodontics, some recommendations are established for the use of CBCT in endodontics. The first recommendation states that intraoral radiography should be the choice for endodontic treatment, while a small field CBCT would be recommended for those patients with confused or nonspecific signs with untreated teeth or with previous endodontic treatments (**Figure 7**). They also recommend that CBCT could be considered for those teeth that are more likely to have complex anatomies or accessory root canals, (**Figure 8**) also if a CBCT has not been taken before, it could be considered to locate calcified root canals. However, for postoperative follow-up, the treatment of choice should be intraoral radiography. When the possibility of a vertical fracture is suspected if the need for CBCT can be considered, the same as when an injury does not heal and we have to consider the possibility of periapical surgery and when we find perforations or separate instruments before carry out a retreat; it is also recommended when we need to assess the proximity of delicate anatomical areas as well as for the management of dento-alveolar trauma in the absence of soft tissue damage or maxillofacial involvement [42, 43].

5. Conclusions

The help of CBCT technology in the diagnosis of endodontics either in the knowledge of the morphology and pathologies of the root canal system, in the evaluation of root and alveolar fractures, in the analysis of resorption, in the identification of pathologies of non-endodontic origin and in pre-surgical assessment, it is a very valuable method. Exact data lead to better treatment planning decisions giving more predictable results.

When comparing medical CT with CBCT it is verified that the accuracy has been increased, a higher resolution is obtained, the reduction of the exposure time, a reduction of the radiation and a lower cost for the patient is achieved.

Compared to conventional periapical radiography, CBCT eliminates the overlapping of surrounding structures by providing additional clinically relevant information.

Conventional two-dimensional radiographs remain the most accepted and used in endodontics imaging modality. These limitations arise mainly due to the inherent projection of a three-dimensional anatomy, which leads to geometric distortions and, consequently, misinterpretation.

Despite the obvious advantages of CBCT technology offered in the field of dentistry, there are some drawbacks and limitations as there is a growing concern among radiologists and maxillofacial about the increase in radiation on patients, in addition to the interpretation of these images require extensive knowledge of various structures. Because accurate diagnostic information leads to better clinical results, CBCT could prove to be a very valuable tool in modern endodontic practice [44].

CBCT's relatively modern technology has added another dimension to dental radiography and is rapidly becoming the gold standard for radiographic inspections in dentistry. At present, it cannot replace periapical radiography due to cost reasons and the degree of effective radiation [45]. However the techniques will improve to reduce the radiation dose and costs. CBCT currently has a reference place in endodontics, where the increase in the number of complex cases justifies the use of technology and the benefits to the patient are greater than the risks.

Author details

Jesús Mena Álvarez* and Álvaro Zubizarreta Macho
Faculty of Health Sciences, Alfonso X El Sabio University, Madrid, Spain

*Address all correspondence to: jmenaalvarez@gmail.com

References

[1] Tamse A, Kaffe I, Fishel D. Zygomatic arch interference with correct radiographic diagnosis in maxillary molar endodontics. Oral Surgery. 1980;**50**:563-565

[2] Patel S, Kanagasingam S, Mannocci F. Cone beam computed tomography (CBCT) in endodontics. Dental Update. 2010;**37**(6):373-379

[3] Farman AG, Levato CM, Scarfe WC. 3D X-ray: An update. Inside Dentistry. 2007;**3**(6):70-74

[4] Feldkamp LA, Davis LC, Kress JW. Practical cone beam algorithm. Journal of the Optical Society of America. A. 1984;**1**(6):612-619

[5] Scarfe WC, Levin MD, Gane D, Farman AG. Use of cone beam computed tomography in endodontics. International Journal of Dentistry. 2009;**2009**:634567. DOI: 10.1155/2009/634567. Epub 31 March 2010

[6] Kiarudi AH, Eghbal MJ, Safi Y, Aghdasi MM, Fazlyab M. The applications of cone-beam computed tomography in endodontics: A review of literature. Iranian Endodontic Journal. 2015;**10**(1):16-25

[7] Tyndall DA, Rathore S. Cone-beam CT diagnostic applications: Caries, periodontal bone assessment, and endodontic applications. Dental Clinics of North America. 2008;**52**(4):825-841

[8] Durack C, Patel S. Cone beam computed tomography in endodontics. Brazilian Dental Journal. 2012;**23**(3):179-191

[9] Moshiri M, Scarfe WC, Hilgers ML, Scheetz JP, Silveira AM, Farman AG. Accuracy of linear measurements from imaging plate and lateral cephalometric images derived from cone-beam computed tomography. American Journal of Orthodontics and Dentofacial Orthopedics. 2007;**132**:550-560

[10] Pauwels R, Beinsbergera J, Collaert B, Theodorakou C, Rogerse J, Walker A, et al. Effective dose range for dental cone beam computed tomography scanners. European Journal of Radiology. 2012;**81**(2):267-271

[11] Ludlow JB, Davies-Ludlow LE, Brooks SL, Howerton WB. Dosimetry of 3 CBCT devices for oral and maxillofacial radiology: CB Mercuray, NewTom 3G and i-CAT. Dento Maxillo Facial Radiology. 2006;**35**(4):219-226

[12] Abella F, Patel S, Durán-Sindreu F, Mercadé M, Bueno R, Roig M. Evaluating the periapical status of teeth with irreversible pulpitis by using cone-beam computed tomography scanning and periapical radiographs. Journal of Endodontics. 2012;**38**(12):1588-1591

[13] Ball RL, Barbizam JV, Cohenca N. Intraoperative endodontic applications of cone-beam computed tomography. Journal of Endodontics. 2013;**39**(4):548-557

[14] Bhuva B, James JJ, Patel S. The use of limited cone beam computed tomography in the diagnosis and management of a case of perforating internal root resorption. International Endodontic Journal. 2011;**44**:777-786

[15] Bender IB, Seltzer S. Roentgenographic and direct observation of experimental lesions in bone. Part I. Journal of the American Dental Association (1939). 1961;**62**:152-160

[16] Bender IB, Seltzer S. Roentgenographic and direct observation of experimental lesions in bone. Part II. Journal of the

American Dental Association (1939). 1961;**62**:708-716

[17] Goldman M, Pearson AH, Darzenta N. Endodontic success - Who's reading the radiograph. Oral Surgery. 1972;**33**:432-437

[18] Levin LG, Law AS, Holland GR, Abbott PV, Roda RS. Identify and define all diagnostic terms for pulpal health and disease states. Journal of Endodontics. 2009;**35**:1645-1657

[19] Estrela C, Bueno MR, Leles CR, Azevedo B, Azevedo JR. Accuracy of cone beam computed tomography and panoramic and periapical radiography for detection of apical periodontitis. Journal of Endodontics. 2008;**34**(3):273-279

[20] Lofthag-Hansen S, Huumonen S, Gröndahl K, Gröndahl H. Limited cone-beam CT and intra oral radiography for the diagnosis of periapical pathology. Oral Surgery, Oral Medicine, Oral Pathology, Oral Radiology, and Endodontics. 2007;**103**:114-119

[21] Low K, Dula K, Bürgin W, von Arx T. Comparison of periapical radiography and limited cone-beamtomography in posterior maxillary teeth referred for apical surgery. Identification of root morphology and canal anatomy. Journal of Endodontics. 2008;**34**(5):557-562

[22] Cotton TP, Geisler TM, Holden DT, Schwartz SA, Schindler WG. Endodontic applications of cone-beam volumetric tomography. Journal of Endodontics. 2007;**33**(9):1121-1132

[23] Garcia de Paula-Silva F, Hassan B, Bezarra da Silva L, Leonardo M, Wu M. Outcome of root canal treatment in dogs determined by periapical radiography and cone-beam computed tomography scans. Journal of Endodontics. 2009;**35**(5):723-726

[24] de Paula-Silva FW, Santamaria M Jr, Leonardo MR, Consolaro A, da Silva LA. Cone-beam computerized tomographic, radiographic, and histologic evaluation of periapical repair in dogs' postendodontic treatment. Oral Surgery, Oral Medicine, Oral Pathology, Oral Radiology, and Endodontics. 2009;**108**(5):796-805

[25] Tamse A, Fuss Z, Lustig J, Kaplavi J. An evaluation of endodontically treated vertically fractured teeth. Journal of Endodontics. 1999;**25**:506-508

[26] Cohen S, Berman LH, Blanco L, Bakland L, Kim JS. A demographic analysis of vertical root fractures. Journal of Endodontics. 2006;**32**:1160-1163

[27] Hannig C, Dullin C, Hülsmann M, Heidrich G. Three-dimensional, non-destructive visualization of vertical root fractures using flat panel volume detector computer tomography: An ex vivo in vitro case report. International Endodontic Journal. 2005;**38**(12):904-913

[28] Rud J, Omnell K. Root fractures due to corrosion. Diagnostic aspects. Scandinavian Journal of Dental Research. 1970;**78**(5):397-403

[29] Edlund M, Nair M, Nair U. Detection of vertical root fractures by using cone-beam computed tomography: A clinical study. Journal of Endodontics. 2011;**37**(6):768-772

[30] Gassner R, Bosch R, Emshoff R. Prevalence of dental trauma in 6000 patients with facial injuries: Implications for prevention. Oral Surgery, Oral Medicine, Oral Pathology, Oral Radiology. 1999;**87**:27-33

[31] Bernardes RA, de Moraes IG, Hungaro Duarte MA, Azevedo BC, de Azevedo JR, Bramante CM. Use of cone-beam volumetric tomography in

the diagnosis of root fractures. Oral Surgery, Oral Medicine, Oral Pathology, Oral Radiology, and Endodontics. 2009;**108**(2):270-277

[32] Cotti E, Vargiu P, Dettori C, Mallarini G. Computerized tomography in the management and follow-up of extensive periapical lesion. Endodontics & Dental Traumatology. 1999;**15**:186-189

[33] Velvart P, Hecker H, Tillinger G. Detection of the apical lesion and the mandibular canal in conventional radiography and computed tomography. Oral Surgery, Oral Medicine, Oral Pathology and Endodontology. 2001;**92**:682-688

[34] Rigolone M, Pasqualini D, Bianchi L, Berutti E, Bianchi SD. Vestibular surgical access to the palatine root of the superior first molar: "low-does cone-beam" CT analysis of the pathway and its anatomic variations. Journal of Endodontics. 2003;**29**:773-775

[35] Shemesh H, Cristescu RC, Wesselink PR, Wu M. The use of cone-beam computed tomography and digital periapical rediographs to diagnose root perforations. Journal of Endodontics. 2011;**37**(4):513-516

[36] Gartner AH, Mack T, Somerlott RG, Walsh LC. Differential diagnosis of internal and externalrootresorption. Journal of Endodontics. 1976;**2**:329-334

[37] Cohenca N, Simon JH, Roges R, Morag Y, Malfaz JM. Clinical indications for digital imaging in dento-alveolar trauma. Part 1: Traumatic injuries. Dental Traumatology. 2007;**23**:95-104

[38] Cohenca N, Simon JH, Marhtur A, Malfaz JM. Clinical indications for digital imaging in dento-alveolar trauma. Part 2: Root resorption. Dental Traumatology. 2007;**23**:105-113

[39] Simon JH, Enciso R, Malfaz J-M, Roges R, Bailey-Perry M, Patel A. Differential diagnosis of large periapical lesions using cone-beam computed tomography measurements and biopsy. Journal of Endodontics. 2006;**32**:833-837

[40] Rosenberg PA, Frisbie J, Lee J, Lee K, Frommer H, Kottal S, et al. The Journal of Endocrinology. 2010;**36**(3):423-428

[41] Matherne RP, Angelopoulos C, Kulild JC, Tira D. Use of CBCT to identify root canal systems in vitro. Journal of Endodontics. 2008;**34**:87-89

[42] AAE and AAOMR Joint position statement: Use of cone beam computed tomography in endodontics 2015 update. Journal of Endodontics. 2015;**41**(9):1393-1396. DOI: 10.1016/j.joen.2015.07.013

[43] Patel S, Durack C, Abella F, Roig M, Shemesh H, Lambrechts P, et al. European society of endodontology position statement: The use of CBCT in endodontics. International Endodontic Journal. 2014;**47**(6):502-504

[44] Kaya S, Yavuz I, Uysal I, Akkus Z. Measuring bone density in healing periapical lesions by using cone beam computed tomography: A clinical investigation. Journal of Endodontics. 2012;**38**(1):28-31

[45] Martin Palomo J, Rao PS, Hans MG. Influence of CBCT exposure conditions on radiation dose. Oral Surgery, Oral Medicine, Oral Pathology, Oral Radiology, and Endodontics. 2008;**105**:773-782

Chapter 13

Bioceramic Cements in Endodontics

Viviane Ferreira Guimarães Xavier, Luiz Felipe Moreira, Daniel Guimarães Xavier, Juliana Guimarães Xavier and Whyrllene Steine

Abstract

New bioceramic calcium silicate endodontic cements have been recently introduced in the market. They are biocompatible materials that stimulate mineralization. Its dimensional stability is similar to the Fillapex MTA with greater thickness and solubility than AH Plus (Dentsply, DeTrey, Konstanz, Germany) as it is water based. Stored in dispensed syringe, it has a pre-mixed consistency. They are used with the single cone obturation technique because they have properties that are changed when heated. They were developed by inducing bioactivity on the surface of the material when in contact with tissue fluids. An improvement in the osteoblastic differentiation of the cells of the periodontal ligament, induction of remineralization of the dentin, and excellent antimicrobial properties have also been associated with these cements. These properties make these cements an excellent alternative in the attempt to obtain a three-dimensional obturation of the Root Canal System (SCR).

Keywords: endodontics sealers, bioceramics, biocompatibility, bioactivity, MTA, calcium silicate, root canal obturation

1. Introduction

Recently introduced in the form of sealant cements, bioceramic endodontic cements are biocompatible compounds obtained by various chemical processes. They exhibit excellent biocompatibility properties due to their similarity to the biological process of hydroxyapatite formation and to the ability to induce a regenerative response from the periapical tissues [1]. In endodontics, bioceramic materials are mainly found as repair cement [2] and endodontic cement [3], for these materials showed interaction with and response to the stimulation of living tissues, they reached relevance to be studied.

According to Cheng et al. [4], bioceramics exhibit remarkable biocompatibility properties due to their similarity to the biological process of hydroxyapatite formation and the ability to stimulate a regenerative response. They present osteoinductive capacity as they absorb osteoinductive substances when in contact with bone healing process.

First-generation bioceramic cements known as MTA became popular in endodontics and were initially indicated as a retrobuturing material. Later, new indications for its use were developed such as direct pulp capping of permanent teeth, pulpotomy of deciduous teeth, specification, and repair of surgically and non-surgically root perforations. In addition to these indications, MTA can be applied in other clinical situations such as the coronal plug after endodontic obturation; in the repair of vertical root fractures; prior to the internal bleaching of the dental element, as temporary restorative material; repair of root perforations. Its properties have been modified in order to obtain the excellent properties already well established of the MTA such as biocompatibility, high pH, no reabsorption, increase of root resistance, low cytotoxicity, non-contracting, and chemical stability in an endodontic sealant cement of root canal that is easy to work inside the root canals [5].

Bioceramics are currently represented through restorative materials in the field of oral health, more precisely in endodontics. These bioceramic nanoparticulate cements have three presentations: the EndoSequence Root Putty Putty (ERRM Putty), in dense form; EndoSequence Root Repair Material Paste (ERRM Paste), which comes arranged in a syringe by having fluid constitution; and more recently, EndoSequence Root Repair Material [6–9].

For the closure of dentinal tubules, the use of bioceramic cements has been widely indicated. This material homogeneously seals the voids between the obturator material and the dentin walls. Its bioactivity favors bone repair and neoformation by interacting with periapical tissues.

2. Clinical properties

Among the clinical properties of endodontic cements are the endodontic repair capacity, and for this reason, it must be biocompatible, radiopaque, antibacterial, dimensionally stable, easy to handle, and should not be affected by blood contamination [11]. Some of the favorable properties of bioceramics in endodontics are their physical chemical properties, such as the release of Ca^{2+}, pH, and radiopacity [12]. The bioceramic sealing ability is excellent, as it promotes satisfactory sealing [13, 14], as well as the capacity to increase the resistance of the sealed teeth [15]. It shows a greater adhesion to the root canals, which can be seen when the endodontic retreatments are present in the longer residues [16], requiring longer clinical work time [17].

According to manufacturers' specifications, bioceramics have antibacterial activity, alkaline pH, radiopacity, and excellent biocompatibility. Its physical, chemical, and biological properties are the main characteristics for its application in dentistry. It is a biocompatible material, non-toxic, and chemically stable in biological environment. This material also has the advantage of bioactivity, that is, it is capable of forming hydroxyapatite during the hardening or prepping process, exerting influence on the bond between the dentin and the obturator material. Besides, it hardens when exposed to a humid environment, making the local dentinal tubules ideal, since the water from inside the tubules causes the cement to hydrate, promoting the reduction of the solidification time that results in the formation of hydroxyapatite [1].

According to Trope et al. [8], the various forms of bioceramics are similar in composition (calcium silicates, zirconium oxide, tantalum oxide, and monobasic calcium phosphate), having excellent mechanical, biological, and manipulative properties. In addition to being hydrophilic, they are also insoluble, radiopaque, and aluminum free. The working time is over 30 min and the holding time is around 4 h under normal conditions, depending on the amount of moisture available. EndoSequence BC RRM Fast Set Putty cement has been recently launched presenting all the properties of the original product, but with a formula that promotes a faster setting time (approximately 20 min).

3. Biocompatibility

During endodontic obturation, the cements come into contact with the periradicular tissues, which lead to the risk of a possible systemic toxicity [12], hence the great importance of biocompatibility. The materials EndoSequence Root Repair Material (ERRM) [11, 12], BioAggregate and iRoot [18], ProRoot MTA and MTA-Angelus [12], and EndoSequence BC sealer [19, 20] showed acceptable biocompatibility, not having induced critical cytotoxic effects [21].

Giacomino et al. [10] conducted a study to compare the biocompatibility and osteogenic potential of EndoSequence BC Sealer (Brasseler, Savannah, GA) and ProRoot ES (Johnson City Dental Specialties, Johnson City, TN) compared to Roth (Roth International, Chicago, IL) and AH Plus (Dentsply DeTrey). A precursor murine osteoblast lineage (IDG-SW3) was exposed to various concentrations of each of the cements for 7 days. Biocompatibility was determined by luminescence assay based on the quantification of adenosine triphosphate (Cell-Titer-Glo [Promega, Madison, Wisconsin]). The osteogenic potential was determined by fluorescence microscopy of the expression of DMP-1. Data were analyzed with bidirectional analysis of variance or univariate analysis of variance with the post hoc Bonferroni test. Both bioceramic cements have excellent biocompatibility even at high concentrations. On the other hand, cell death was detected when Roth and AH Plus were used in concentrations 100× lower than the bioceramic groups. It is important to note that both bioceramic cements significantly increased osteoblastic differentiation, although greater responses were observed with the EndoSequence BC Sealer. Concerning these results, DMP-1 expression, robust increase of osteogenic gene expression, and superior mineral deposition were shown. Osteoblastic differentiation and function were significantly impaired when Roth cement or AH Plus was used. Therefore, they concluded that the EndoSequence BC Sealer and ProRoot ES were significantly more biocompatible and promoted osteoblastic differentiation, a bioactivity not found in AH Plus and Roth cements.

4. Bioactivity

Bioactive materials can be used to repair diseases or damage to bone tissue and can remain in place indefinitely. An indication of bioactivity is the ability to develop a stable binding with living tissues in contact with simulated body fluid solution [22] via deposition of hydroxyapatite on the surface of a substrate [23].

The bioactivity of endodontic bioceramic materials was confirmed in the Bioaggregate [21], EndoSequence Root Repair Material [21], Pro RootMTA [21], and iRoot SP [24].

After the SCR closure, direct contact between the obturator material and the periapical tissues occurs, such as the periodontal ligament (PDL) and the bone, making a three-dimensional hermetic sealing to prevent recurrent infections of the periapical space, both of endodontic or coronal origin. This seal may be mechanical with materials that provide an airtight seal, but may also be of biological origin. In this case, the filling material induces the formation of hard tissue through the cells of the periodontal ligament, isolating the root canal from the surrounding tissues and stimulating the healing processes of damaged apical tissues [25].

According to Camps et al. [26], tricalcium silicate-based materials have a recognized bioactivity property, that is, the ability to induce hard tissue formation in both the dental pulp in the periapical region. In this regard, interactions of newly developed tricalcium silicate (BioRoot, Septodont, Saint Maur Des Fosses, France) with apical tissue were compared with a standard zinc oxide-eugenol cement (Pulp Channel Sealer [PCS]; SybronEndo Orange, CA). Cell viability was investigated by direct contact between human periodontal ligament (PDL) cells and BioRoot or PCS. For this, the extracted human incisors were sectioned at the enamel-cement junction; root canals were prepared, sterilized, and filled with lateral condensation with both materials. The root apexes were submerged in the culture medium for 24 h. These conditioned media were used to investigate their effects on human PDL cells. BioRoot had less toxic effects on PDL cells than PCS and induced a higher secretion of angiogenic and osteogenic growth factors than PCS. Given the results of the present study, it is suggested that calcium silicate cement (BioRoot) has a higher bioactivity than zinc oxide eugenol cement (PCS) in human PDL cells.

According to Niu et al. [27], a particularity of tricalcium silicate-based materials is their potential to express bioactivity, which is considered an important property for bone binding capacity. In this sense, Moinzadeh et al. [28] conducted a study to evaluate the interaction of EndoSequence BC RRM (Brasseler USA, Savannah, GA) in contact with simulated blood and tissue fluids, as these materials come into direct contact with the periapical region. These materials are hydrophilic; therefore, its properties improve in the presence of moisture, either from the periodontal ligament or dentinal tubules. However, specific environmental conditions may modify the material configuration. The reaction of tricalcium silicate with tissue fluids led to the formation of calcium hydroxide, and this was evident in the mass in contact with water and Hank's balanced salt solution. In this case, there was also the formation of globular crystals synonymous with hydroxyapatite formation. The material in contact with blood had a non-crystalline surface with additional peaks of calcium, phosphorus, and chlorine. However, in vitro material evaluation may not be representative of the clinical situation, because carbon dioxide present in the bloodstream leads to the formation of calcium carbonate rather than hydroxyapatite reported in in vitro studies.

5. Cytotoxicity

All endodontic treatment will be impaired if the sealing cement is irritating to the tissues of the periapical region, causing larger inflammation or promoting large tissue necrosis, which may lead to reduction in apical repair capacity. Hence, the great importance of knowing the biocompatibility and cytotoxicity of obturator cements [21]. The cytotoxicity of endodontic cements can cause cell degeneration and delay healing due to the direct contact of the cements with the periapical tissues [29]. Cements with satisfactory biocompatibility must have low or no toxicity to the periapical tissues.

When compared to their cytotoxicity, some bioceramic cements exhibit minimal levels of cytotoxicity (EndoSequence Root Repair Material) and Mineral Trioxide Aggregate (MTA) [11]. In a study by Fayyad [30] that compared cytotoxicity, some bioceramic cements exhibited minimal levels of cytotoxicity (EndoSequence Root Repair Material) and Mineral Trioxide Aggregate (MTA) of two materials, BioAggregate and iRoot (Innovative Bioceramix, IBC, Vancouver, Canada) on human fibroblast MRC-5 cells found that both showed acceptable biocompatibility and that the cytotoxic effect of the materials was concentration dependent.

According to Candeiro et al. [12], comparing the characteristics of biodegradable EndoSequence sealer with AH Plus, bioceramic cement presented lower cytotoxicity and was unlikely to damage the genetic information inside a cell compared to AH Plus.

The results involving the biological response of MTA Fillapex (Angelus, Londrina, Brazil) seem to be conflicting. This cement showed high cytotoxicity and genotoxicity, shortly after the manipulation. Another study reported that when implanted into subcutaneous tissue in rats for a period of 90 days, it remained toxic [31]. However, another study has shown that despite these initial toxic effects in the early stage the cytotoxicity of Fillapex MTA decreases over time, exhibiting activity adequate to the stimulation of the formation of hydroxyapatite crystals in cultured human osteoblast cells [29].

According to Damas et al. [2], bioceramic cements have several applications and some studies have shown that cytotoxicity levels are identical.

6. Antimicrobian activity

Much research has been conducted proving the relationship between microorganisms and periodontitis, as well as the presence of endodontic biofilm in the process of periapical diseases. Thus, during root canal treatment, the main objective is sanitation through chemical-mechanical preparation [32], which may be associated with intra-canal medication, ending with the three-dimensional obturation. As is known, the total eradication of bacteria in all root spaces is not always achieved due to the limitation of the mechanical action of the instruments. Ideally, the obturator materials should have an antimicrobial component to assist in the process of eliminating residual microorganisms within the dentinal tubules [33].

Bukhari and Karabucak [34] carried out a study to test the antibacterial activity of bioceramic cement compared to AH Plus (Dentsply International Inc., York, PA) in a biofilm composed of 8-week-old *Enterococcus faecalis* adhered to surfaces using a model of dentin infection. The surfaces of the unirradicular intact extracted canals were infected by *E. faecalis* biofilm. Cement AH Plus and EndoSequence BC Sealer (Brasseler USA, Savannah, GA) were placed on the wall of the root canal of the specimens during a period of 24 h and another of 2 weeks in humid conditions at 37°C. Infected samples incubated without shutter cement for similar periods were used as negative controls. In order to test the sealing cements, the specimens were labeled with fluorescence viability staining and confocal laser scanning microscopy to evaluate the proportions of dead and living bacteria in the canal walls during the determined periods. The EndoSequence BC Sealer significantly killed more *E. faecalis* in biofilm bound to channel surfaces when compared to AH Plus and control at both time points (P, 0.05–0.0005). In this sense, they concluded that the EndoSequence BC Sealer exhibited significant antimicrobial ability in the presence of dentin for up to 2 weeks in an 8 week old *E. faecalis* biofilm, compared to the AH Plus cement.

7. Color change

The aim of endodontic interventions is to prevent and treat apical periodontitis. However, the esthetic result is equally important, especially in the anterior region. Pulpal therapy procedures, such as direct pulp capping, repair of perforations, and regenerative endodontics involve the placement of materials in the coronal third of the tooth, which may have potential for discoloration [35]. In this sense, Kohli et al. [36] carried out a study with the objective of evaluating the in vitro tooth discoloration induced by bioceramic materials, EndoSequence RRM and BD in comparison with other materials used during endodontic treatment, such as gray MTA (GMDTA, Dentsply, York, PA, USA). The aim of this study was to evaluate in vitro the biomarker-induced coronal tooth discoloration, EndoSequence RRM and BD, in comparison with other materials used during endodontic treatment, such as gray MTA (GMTA); MTA white (WMTA, Dentsply), triple antibiotic paste

(TAP), and AH Plus sealant (AH+, Dentsply). Visual discoloration was observed in all specimens in the GMTA, WMTA, and TAP groups over 7 days, which increased over time. Significant coronary tooth discoloration was caused by TAP, GMTA, and WMTA, but not by BD, RRM or RRMF at the end of the experiment.

Discoloration of the crown such as the one present in the MTA is one of the disadvantages of restorative cement used in dentistry. This has to be taken into account when repairing furcation injuries or in cases where pulp protection is required. According to the literature, the bismuth oxide present in the MTA composition reacts with the residual sodium hypochlorite that remains inside the dentinal tubules after mechanical chemical preparation, resulting in dark precipitations and staining of the tooth. In the composition of the EndoSequence, the zirconia oxide is the opacifier used, preventing the unwanted darkening [37].

According to Kholi et al. [36], the bio-based materials Biodentine (Septodont, Saint-Maur-des-Fosses, France), ERRM, EndoSequence, ERRM putty (Brasseler, Savannah, GA), RMF, EndoSequence ERRM fast set paste (Brasseler), and AH+, AH Plus sealer (Dentsply), when left in the pulp chamber for periods of up to 6 months do not induce color change in the tooth structure. Alsubait et al. [37] compared the potential for discoloration of the Endosequence Bioceramic Root Repair Material Fast Putty Set (ERRM) and ProRootMTA (PMTA) by placing them on the crown of extracted human teeth for a period of 4 months and found progressive discoloration in teeth when treated with PMTA, whereas those with ERRM had no change in color stability.

8. Mechanism of action

The bioceramic cement is hydrophilic; therefore, it uses water present in the dentin tubules to initiate the firming reaction. The hydration of the material decreases the working time, consequently the amount of water mixed can reduce the time required; but the bioceramics only harden when present in a humid environment. After hydration, the calcium silicate gel and the calcium hydroxide are produced by the calcium silicate present in the mixture. Calcium hydroxide reacts with phosphate ions and produces hydroxyapatite and water. The continuous interaction of calcium silicate and water leads to the formation of hydrated calcium silicate [38]. The amount of water in the reaction is a critical factor in controlling the rate of hydration. The pH is similar when compared to the reaction time of calcium hydroxide. As this is highly alkaline, it reaches a value of 12.8 during the placement time, decreasing progressively over a period of 1 week [2]. The pH is affected by the release of calcium ions and by alkalinizing the medium, a condition that can influence the repair, besides promoting the mineralization process and its concentration. The release of hydroxyl ions can alter the dissociation [12].

Candeiro et al. [12] carried out a study with the purpose of evaluating the physicochemical properties of a bioceramic. Radiopacity, pH, calcium ion release, and flowability were studied and compared with AH Plus® cement (resin-based cement). The radiopacity and flow were evaluated by using ISO 6876/2001 standards. For the analysis of the radiopacity, metal discs with 10 mm diameter and 1 mm thickness were used and were covered with sealer cement. The flowability test was performed with 0.005 ml of cement on a glass plate. The release of calcium ions and pH were evaluated in periods of 3, 24, 72, 180, and 240 h with a spectrometer and pH meter, respectively. Radiopacity was then found to be significantly lower than AH Plus®, pH analysis, and calcium ion release were significantly higher than AH Plus®, and it was demonstrated that there were no significant differences in flowability. Thus, the bioceramics present values of radiopacity and fluidity within the limits of ISO standards and the other physicochemical properties analyzed show very favorable values for a sealant cement.

9. Marginal adaptation/sealing capacity

According to Shokouhinejad et al. [39], the marginal adaptation of the EndoSequence Root Repair Material (ERRM) was similar to that of the MTA. However, bioceramic-based cements when compared with resin-based cements (AH PLUS) exhibited more regions containing gaps. Bioceramic endodontic cements also showed infiltration results similar to MTA. In relation to sealing and its ability, the Bioceramic Root-end Repair (BCRR) is equivalent to the MTA [13]. Antunes et al. [14] reported that MTA and BioCeramic Root Repair Material (BC-RRM) showed similar sealing ability.

To what concerns bioceramics and the hydration of the material during the setting process, the formation of hydroxyapatite crystals occurs between the surface of the material and the dentin wall, which can provide adequate sealing and marginal adaptation in this region [19, 40, 41].

Antunes et al. [14] evaluated the sealing capacity of MTA cement and EndoSequence BC RRM-Fast Set Putty in an ex vivo study, in roots of 60 instrumented lower central incisors, which were sectioned in the apical region and ultrasonic tip retroinstruments, and using a new model of bacterial nutrient infiltration. Retrograde obturation was performed with the MTA and BC-RRM Putty in two sets of teeth. In the MTA group, 50% of viable species were detected while in the Putty BC-RRM group, 28% of the samples were positive for cultured bacteria. However, in the comparison analysis of the quantitative or presence/absence of bacteria, no significant difference was identified between the groups, leading the authors to conclude that the cements studied have similar sealing capacity.

10. Resistance of union

The ability of a root canal sealer to adhere intra-radicular dentin through micromechanical retention or resistance to friction is advantageous in maintaining the integrity of the sealant interface and dentin during mechanical stresses caused by flexion of the teeth, surgical procedures or preparation of the space for intra radicular retainers [42]. It has been shown that the release of calcium and hydroxyl ions from calcium silicate-containing material results in the formation of a layer of hydroxyapatite when it comes in contact with the fluids of the dentinal tubules. The formation of this interfacial layer develops a chemical bond between calcium and dentin walls [43]. Therefore, it is expected that the bioceramic cements, which are based on a calcium silicate composition, have the potential to chemically adhere to the dentin.

Shokouhinejad et al. [44] conducted an investigation to compare the bond strength of bioceramic (EndoSequence BC Sealer) and resin cement AH Plus in the presence and absence of smear layer. Uniradicular ex vivo specimens were used in this experiment using 5.25% sodium hypochlorite and 17% EDTA protocols for smear layer removal and in the other specimens no debris removal protocol, only 5.25% sodium hypochlorite irrigation. The modes of adhesion strength and failure were evaluated. No statistically significant differences were found between the groups filled with gutta percha and AH Plus sealant and gutta percha and bioceramic sealant. The presence or absence of smear layer does not appear to significantly affect the bond strength of filler materials.

Shokouhinejad et al. [45] evaluated the bond strength of EndoSequence BC endodontic cement (Brasseler USA, Savannah, GA) when used with gutta-percha in the presence or absence of moisture within root canals. The mean bond strength of EndoSequence BC sealant and filler in the wet channels was significantly higher than that of the dry 1 week. In contrast, there was no significant difference between dry and wet root canals at 2 months. In the dry channels, the adhesion strength increased significantly over time, while in the wet, the difference was not significant. The presence of moisture inside the root canals increased the bond strength of EndoSequence BC cement in 1 week. However, no difference was found between the bond strength of EndoSequence BC cement in the presence or absence of moisture in the root canals at 2 months.

11. Endodontic reintervention

According to Oltra et al. [16], recently new bioceramic sealant cements have been marketed and are being used in endodontic practice. However, these bioceramic cements have limited research related to their removal ability during endodontic re-interventions.

Uzunoglu et al. [46] evaluated the removal capacity of three different endodontic cements iRoot SP (bioceramic cement), MTA Fillapex (sealant based on MTA), and AH-26 (epoxy resin) from the root canal system. Channel filler was removed with ProTaper Universal Retreatment PTR. The time to reach the working length has been recorded. The roots were sectioned longitudinally and each half was evaluated using a stereomicroscope. Three observers scored every third of all specimens. In the GP/MTA Fillapex single cone group, the time required to reach working length was significantly shorter. The remaining filler material in the apical and middle thirds of the groups was similar. None of the tested cements can be completely removed from the root canal system.

Oltra et al. [16] analyzed the ability to remove two BC sealer endodontic sealants compared to AH Plus using microcomputer tomographic analysis. Computed tomography was performed before and after obturation and retreatment and then analyzed for residual material volume. The specimens were sectioned longitudinally and the digitized images obtained with the microscope. In the present experiment, significant differences were found, since less root canal filling material was associated with the AH Plus group when using chloroform as a solvent when compared with the others. BC Sealer samples represented using chloroform as the solvent had better results than those removed without chloroform. The results of the present experiment demonstrate that the BC Sealer group presented significantly more residual obturator material than the AH Plus group, regardless of whether the two cements were associated with the use of solvent for their removal.

Zuolo et al. [17] evaluated the effectiveness of the TRUShape system (Dentsply Tulsa Dental Specialties, Tulsa, OK) compared to Reciproc (VDW, Munich, Germany) in unblocking channels filled with two different sealants and the working time required to achieve working length. A tomographic microcomputer was used to evaluate the removal of obturation material. The average volume of remaining obturator material was similar when comparing the two file systems. However, in the groups filled with bioceramic, the percentage of remaining obturator material was higher than in the groups filled with Pulp Canal Sealer. The clearance was faster in the groups that were filled with Pulp Canal Sealer when compared with bioceramics. There was no difference in the percentage of remaining shutter material when comparing file systems. However, Reciproc was faster than TRUShape.

12. Fracture resistance

It is commonly believed that endodontically treated teeth are more fragile and more prone to fracture than vital teeth [47]. There are several factors that affect the strength of endodontically treated teeth: excessive tooth loss due to caries or trauma, dentin dehydration, access cavity preparation, instrumentation, excessive pressure during root filling, and preparation of intraradicular pins [48]. Reinforcement of the remaining tooth structure after endodontic procedures is one of the main objectives of rehabilitation. It has been suggested that the bioceramic cements may adhere to the dentinal surface of the root canal, strengthening the remaining dental structure, contributing to the long-term success of an endodontically treated tooth [49].

Topçuoğlu et al. [15] analyzed the strength of the values necessary to induce root fracture of teeth filled with three different endodontic sealants. Each specimen was then subjected to fracture testing using a universal testing machine at a speed of 1.0 mm/min (−1) until the root was fractured. The force required to fracture each specimen was recorded, and the data were statistically analyzed. The fracture values of the groups filled with bioceramic and gutta percha, and sealant based on epoxy resin and gutta percha, were significantly higher than those of group MTA and gutta percha. No significant differences were found between the bioceramic and epoxy resin groups, the Endosequence BC and AH Plus cements increased the strength of the values required to induce a root fracture of uniradicular premolars.

13. Conclusion

Based on the literature, it can be concluded that the bioceramic cements have satisfactory working properties, are easy to handle, and have excellent antimicrobial action and alkaline pH. They demonstrate ability to release calcium ions promoting adaptation and marginal sealing, shorter setting time, biocompatibility, acceptable cytotoxicity, and induce the osteoblastic differentiation of the cells of the periodontal ligament and remineralization of the dentin. They can also be used in humid environment and are easily removed in cases of reintervention, have good dentin adhesion, increasing root resistance to fracture, and do not cause coronary discoloration. All of these properties show that bioceramic cements are favorable to their use.

However, new research and studies are necessary so that further answers and alternatives about the product may be found in order to favor their use in dentistry.

Author details

Viviane Ferreira Guimarães Xavier[2*], Luiz Felipe Moreira[2], Daniel Guimarães Xavier[1], Juliana Guimarães Xavier[1] and Whyrllene Steine[2]

1 School of Professional Improvement-EAP, Association of Class, Brazilian Association of Dentistry - ABO, Brazil

2 Universidade Vale do Rio Doce - UNIVALE University, Brazil

*Address all correspondence to: vi.xavier@hotmail.com

References

[1] Zhang WLZ, Peng B. Assessment of a new root canal sealer's apical sealing ability. Oral Surgery, Oral Medicine, Oral Pathology, Oral Radiology, and Endodontology. 2009;**107**(6):79-82

[2] Damas BA, Wheater MA, Bringas JS. Hoen MM cytotoxicity comparison of mineral trioxide aggregates and EndoSequence bioceramic root repair materials. Journal of Endodontia. 2011;**37**:372-375

[3] Koch KA, Brave DG. Bioceramics, part I: The clinician's viewpoint. Dentistry Today. 2012;**31**(1):130-135

[4] Cheng L, Ye F, Yang R, Lu X, Shi Y, Li L, et al. Osteoinduction of hydroxyapatite/beta-tricalcium phosphate bioceramics in mice with a fractured fibula. Acta Biomaterialia. 2010;**6**(4):1569-1574

[5] Lima NFF, Santos PRN, Pedrosa MS, Delboni MG. Bioceramic sealers in endodontics: A literature review. Revista da Faculdade de Odontologia. 2017;**22**(2):248-254

[6] Kakani A. A review on perforation repair materials. Journal of Clinical and Diagnostic Research. 2015

[7] Debelian G, Trope M. The use of premixed bioceramic materials in endodontics. Giornale Italiano di Endodonzia. 2016;**30**(2):70-80

[8] Trope M, Bunes A, Debelian G. Root filling material and techinis: Bioceramics a new hope? Endodontic Topics. 2015;**32**:86-96

[9] Jitaru S, Hodisan I, Timis L, Lucian A, Bud M. The use of bioceramics in endodontics - literature review. Clujul Medical. 2016;**89**(4):470

[10] Giacomino CM, Wealleans JA, Kuhn N, Diogenes A. Comparative biocompatibility and osteogenic potential of two bioceramic sealers. Journal of Endodontia. 2019;**45**:51-56

[11] Ciasca M, Aminoshariae A, Jin G, Montagnese T, Mickel A. A comparison of the cytotoxicity and proinflammatory cytokine production of EndoSequence root repair material and ProRoot mineral trioxide aggregate in human osteoblast cell culture using reverse-transcriptase polymerase chain reaction. Journal of Endodontia. 2012;**38**(4):486-489

[12] Candeiro GT, Moura-netto C, D'Almeida-couto RS, Azambuja-Júnio N, Marques MM, Cai S, et al. Cytotoxicity, genotoxicity and antibacterial effectiveness of a bioceramic endodontic sealer. International Endodontic Journal. 2015;**49**(9):858-864

[13] Leal F, De-Deus G, Brandão C, Luna AS, Fidel SR, Souza EM. Comparison of the root-end seal provided by bioceramic repair cements and white MTA. International Endodontic Journal. 2011; **44**(7):662-668

[14] Antunes HS, Gominho LF, Andrade-Junior CV, Dessaune neto N, Alves FR, Rôças IN, et al. Sealing ability of two root-end filling materials in a bacterial nutrient leakage model. International Endodontic Journal. 2016;**49**(10):960-965

[15] Topçuoğlu HS, Tuncay Ö, Karataş E, Arslan H, Yeter K. In vitro fracture resistance of roots obturated with epoxy resin-based, mineral trioxide aggregate-based, and bioceramic root canal sealers. Journal of Endodontia. 2013;**39**(12):1630-1633

[16] Oltra E, Cox TC, LaCourse MR, Johnson JD, Paranjpe A. Retreatability of two endodontic sealers, EndoSequence BC Sealer and AH

Plus: A micro-computed tomographic comparison. Restorative Dentistry & Endodontics. 2017;**42**(1):19-26

[17] Zuolo AS, Zuolo ML, da Silveira Bueno CE, Chu R, Cunha RS. Evaluation of the efficacy of TRUShape and Reciproc file systems in the removal of root filling material: An ex vivo micro-computed tomographic study. Journal of Endodontia. 2016;**42**(2):315-319

[18] De-Deus G, Canabarro A, Alves GG, Marins JR, Linhares ABR, Granjeiro JM. Cytocompatibility of the ready-to-use bioceramic putty repair cement iRoot BP Plus with primary human osteoblasts. International Endodontic Journal. 2012;**45**(6):508-513

[19] Loushine BA, Bryan TE, Looney SW, Gillen BM, Loushine RJ, Weller RN, et al. Setting properties and cytotoxicity evaluation of a premixed bioceramic root canal sealer. Journal of Endodontia. 2011;**37**(5):673-677

[20] Carvalho CN, Grazziotin-Soares R, Candeiro GTM, Martinez LG, Souza JP, Oliveira PS, et al. Micro push-out bond strength and bioactivity analysis of a bioceramic root canal sealer. Iranian Endodontic Journal. 2017;**12**(3):343-348

[21] Willershausen I, Wolf T, Kasaj A, Weyer V, Willershausen B, Marroquin BB. Influence of a bioceramic root end material and mineral trioxide aggregates on fibroblasts and osteoblasts. Archives of Oral Biology. 2013;**58**(9):1232-1237

[22] Czarnecka B, Coleman NJ, Shaw H, Nicholson JW. The use of mineral trioxide aggregate in endodontics. Dental Medical Problems. 2008;**45**:5-11

[23] Coleman NJ, Nicholson JW, Awosanya K. A preliminary investigation of the in vitro bioactivity of white Portland cement. Cement and Concrete Research. 2007;**37**:1518-1523

[24] Chen I, Karabucak B, Wang HG, Koyama E, Kohli MR, Nah HD, et al. Healing after root-end microsurgery by using mineral trioxide aggregate and a new calcium silicate-based bioceramic material as root-end filling materials in dogs. Journal of Endodontics. 2015;**41**(3):389-399

[25] Ricucci D, Rocas IN, Alves FR, et al. Apically extruded sealers: Fate and influence on treatment outcome. Journal of Endodontia. 2016;**42**:243-249

[26] Camps J, Jeanneau C, Ayachi I, Laurent P, About I. Bioactivity of a calcium silicate-based endodontic cement (BioRoot RCS): Interactions with human periodontal ligament cells in vitro. Journal of Endodontia. 2015;**41**:1469-1473

[27] Niu LN, Jiao K, Wang TD, et al. A review of the bioactivity of hydraulic calcium silicate cements. Journal of Dentistry. 2014;**42**:517-533

[28] Moinzadeh AT, Portoles CA, Wismayer PS, Camilleri J. Bioactivity potential of EndoSequence BC RRM Putty. Journal of Endodontia. 2016;**42**:615-621

[29] Gandolfi MG, Taddei P. Tinti A and Prati C apatite-forming ability of ProRoot MTA. International Endodontic Journal. 2010;**43**:917-929

[30] Fayyad DM. Cytocompatibility of new bioceramic-based materials on human fibroblast cells (MRC-5). Oral Surgery, Oral Medicine, Oral Pathology, Oral Radiology, and Endodontics. 2011;**112**(6):e137-e142

[31] Gandolfi MG, Siboni F, PRATI C. Chemical-physical properties of TheraCal, a novel light-curable MTA-like material for pulp capping. International Endodontic Journal. 2012;**45**:571-579

[32] Siqueira JF Jr, Rocas IN. Clinical implications and microbiology of

bacterial persistence after treatment procedures. Journal of Endodontia. 2008;**34**:1291-1301

[33] Peters OA. Current challenges and concepts in the preparation of root canal system: A review. Journal of Endodontia. 2004;**30**:559-567

[34] Bukhari S, Karabucak B. The antimicrobial effect of bioceramic sealer on an 8-week matured *Enterococcus faecalis* biofilm attached to root canal dentinal surface. Journal of Endodontia. 2019;**45**:1-6

[35] Belobrov I, Parashos P. Treatment of tooth discoloration after the use of white mineral trioxide aggregate. Journal of Endodontia. 2011;**37**:1017-1020

[36] Kohli MR, Yamaguchi M, Setzer FC, Karabucak B. Spectrophotometric analysis of coronal tooth discoloration induced by various bioceramic cements and other endodontic materials. Journal of Endodontia. 2015;**41**(11):1862-1866

[37] Alsubait S, Al-haidar S, Al-sharyan NA. Comparison of the discoloration potential for EndoSequence bioceramic root repair material fast set putty and ProRoot MTA® in human teeth: An in vitro study. Journal of Esthetic and Restorative Dentistry. 2016;**29**(1):59-67

[38] Yang Q, Troczynski T, Liu D. Influence of apatite seeds on the synthesis of calcium phosphate cement. Biomaterials. 2002;**23**:2751-2760

[39] Shokouhinejad N, Nekoofar MH, Ashoftehyazdi K, Zahraee S, Khoshkhounejad M. Marginal adaptation of new bioceramic materials and mineral trioxide aggregate: A scanning electron microscopy study. Iranian Endodontic Journal. 2014;**9**(2):144-148

[40] Ayatollahi F, Hazeri baqdad abad M, Razavi SH, Tabrizizadeh M, Ayatollahi R, Zarebidoki F. Evaluating the accuracy of two microleakage assessment methods for mineral trioxide aggregate and calcium-enriched mixture cement. Iranian Endodontic Journal. 2017;**12**(4):497-501

[41] Silva Almeida LH, Moraes RR, Morgental RD, Pappen FG. Are premixed calcium silicate–based endodontic sealers comparable to conventional materials? A systematic review of in vitro studies. Journal of Endodontia. 2017;**43**(4):121-123

[42] Huffman BP, Mai S, Pinna L, et al. Dislocation resistance of ProRoot Endo Sealer, a calcium silicate-based root canal sealer, from radicular dentine. International Endodontic Journal. 2009;**42**:34-46

[43] Sarkar NK, Caicedo R, Ritwik P, Moiseyeva R, Kawashima I. Physicochemical basis of the biologic properties of mineral trioxide aggregate. Journal of Endodontia. 2005;**31**:97-100

[44] Shokouhinejad N, Gorjestani H, Nasseh AA, Hoseini A, Mohammadi M, Shamshiri AR. Push-out bond strength of gutta-percha with a new bioceramic sealer in the presence or absence of smear layer. Australian Endodontic Journal. 2011;**39**(3):102-106

[45] Shokouhinejad N, Hoseini A, Gorjestani H, Raoof M, Assa-Dian H, Shamshiri AR. Effect of phosphate-buffered saline on push-out bond strength of a new bioceramic sealer to root canal dentin. Dental Research Journal. 2012;**9**(5):595

[46] Uzunoglu E, Yilmaz Z, Sungur DD, Altundasar E. Retrea- tability of root canals obturated using Gutta-Percha with bioceramic, MTA and resin-based sealers. Iranian Endodontic Journal. 2015;**10**(2):93-98

[47] Schwartz RS, Robbins JW. Post placement and restoration of

endodontically treated teeth: A literature review. Journal of Endodontia. 2004;**30**:289-301

[48] Tang W, Wu Y, Smales RJ. Identifying and reducing risks for potential fractures in endodontically treated teeth. Journal of Endodontia. 2010;**36**:609-617

[49] Onay EO, Ungor M, Ari H, et al. Push-out bond strength and SEM evaluation of new polymeric root canal fillings. Oral Surgery, Oral Medicine, Oral Pathology, Oral Radiology, and Endodontics. 2009;**107**:879-885

Section 4

Oral Surgical Procedures

Chapter 14

Flap Techniques in Dentoalveolar Surgery

Randa Abdulmoein AlFotawi

Abstract

Most dentoalveolar procedures involve the reflection of mucosal flaps. This step is crucial for exposure or removal of impacted teeth, implant bed preparation, exposure of the alveolar bone for augmentation, periodontal surgeries, and repair of mucosal soft tissue defects, such as oroantral fistula. Because of the rich vascularity of the oral mucosa, great freedom is allowed for flap design, but it tends to result in carelessness and lack of thoughtful planning, which may lead to uneventful outcomes or/and complications. In this chapter, we review oral anatomy, classification, indications, and complications of common oral flap techniques; common flap designs are illustrated, and their fundamental principles are highlighted. The review has covered various flap designs based on their indications. Yet the common flap's principles are fundamental for all types of flaps regardless of their application, namely, it should provide wide exposure, clear vision, good access, and assure rich vascularity and good final aesthetic outcome.

Keywords: flap principle, applications, classification, flap technique

1. Introduction

Oral surgical flap by definition is the operation in which a portion of the mucoperiosteal tissue is surgically detached from the underlying bone for better access and visibility. Common principles have been applied for all flap designs. First, the base of the flap should be broader than the free end to ensure adequate blood supply. Second, the incision should be performed at a right angle to the underlying bone, avoiding any anatomical structures, and it should provide adequate visualization. Third, the flap should be wider than the anticipated underlying bone defect and delicately handled without tension. Fourth, the vertical releasing incision should start from the buccal vestibule and end up mesial or distal to the interdental papilla. Different flaps have been proposed for various intraoral surgeries, that is, third molar surgery, canine exposure, various periodontal surgery, dental implant preparation, endodontic surgeries, and repair of oroantrual communications. The review will focus on oral anatomy, classification, indications, complications of common oral flap techniques; common flap designs are illustrated, and their fundamental principles are highlighted.

2. Third molar surgery

2.1 Background

The flap design has considerable effects on primary wound healing in lower third molar surgery [1]. When the conventional sulcular flap design is used, 56% of the patients develop a disorder in primary wound healing [1]. The envelope flap is fixed anteriorly with intersulcular sutures. Notably, dehiscence can take place inconspicuously and unnoticed by the patient and may heal secondarily. The secondary wound healing can cause wedge-shaped defects of the gingiva distal to the second molar or can lead to a loss of attachment distal to the second molar. This periodontal complication after lower third molar surgery has been investigated by several studies [2–5]. Dehiscence occurs in only 10% of cases of triangular flap design [1], and the triangular flap design decreases tension in the area distal to wound closure compared with the envelope flap technique. The vestibular triangular flap can be easily moved to the lingual, ensuring a wound closure that is almost tension-free. The mesial vestibular relieving incision, which is only adapted coronally by a single suture, allows depletion of the postoperative hematoma during masticatory movements. On the first postoperative day, a present hematoma is easy to relieve by spreading and compression. The advantage is that the release area has bone support. Such postoperative morbidity has important medical-legal and economic implications. Many surgical approaches, such as those with the use of surgical drains, different wound closure techniques, and various flap designs, have been tried to minimize the complications [6].

2.2 Envelope flap

An envelope flap with a sulcular incision from the first to the second molar and a distal relieving incision to the mandibular ramus is a widely used technique for lower third molar surgery (**Figure 1**).

The envelope flap is closed with two or three single button sutures distal to the second molar, with special attention to an exact repositioning in the area of the gingival margin. In addition, the flap is adapted with interdental sutures between the first and the second molars.

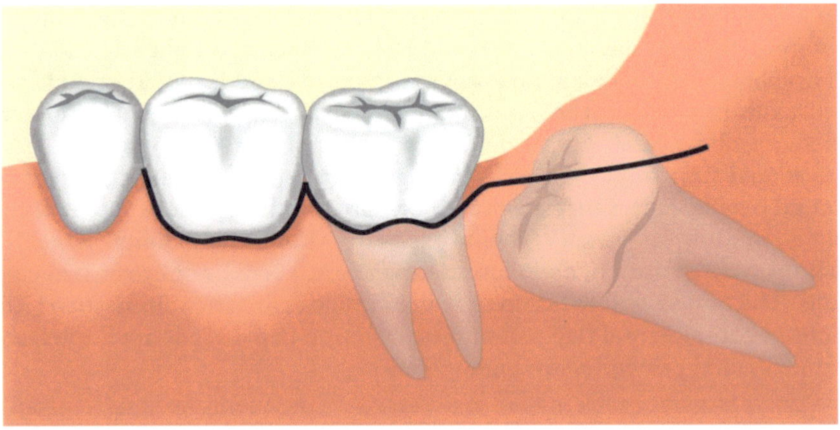

Figure 1.
Envelope flap for the removal of the third molar.

Advantages

- Good exposure during surgery
- Mesial cut could be extended if cystic surgery or endosurgery is required
- The envelope flap provides adequate soft tissues, covering for any bone defects
- The envelope flap has a wider base, assuring vascularity up to the wound margins

Limitations

- Inducing loss of the alveolar bone distal to the second molar probably due to wound dehiscence
- Sulcular incision may lead to periodontal damage
- The envelope flap leads to a total loss of the attached gingiva in this area after the operation, thus causing pocket formation and loss of attachment in the area of the second molar [1]
- Dehiscence to the second molar [7]
- Hypersensitivity in the area of the distally exposed root surface of the second molar
- Alveolar osteitis and soft tissue abscess are severe complications

2.3 Triangular flap design and modification (buccally based triangular flap)

This technique was described by Szmyd [6]. The incision is conducted from the mandibular ramus to the distobuccal crown edge of the second molar, followed by a perpendicular incision obliquely into the mandibular vestibulum, with a length of about 10 mm. In contrast, the modified incision extends over the mucogingival borderline, and the periodontium of the second molar is only touched at the dentofacial edge (**Figures 2** and **3**). The flap is lingually based on the triangular flap [8].

For suturing, the same suturing technique is used distally (envelop), whereas the perpendicular incision is only adapted with a single coronally placed suture. The main aim is exact repositioning of the gingival margin in the area of the second molar. The loose adaption in the apical portion allows easy relief of a hematoma.

Advantages

- Reduces the incidence of wound dehiscence
- A suitable choice for compromised cases of nicotine exposure
- This flap can be easily moved to the lingual, ensuring a wound closure that is almost tension-free [8]

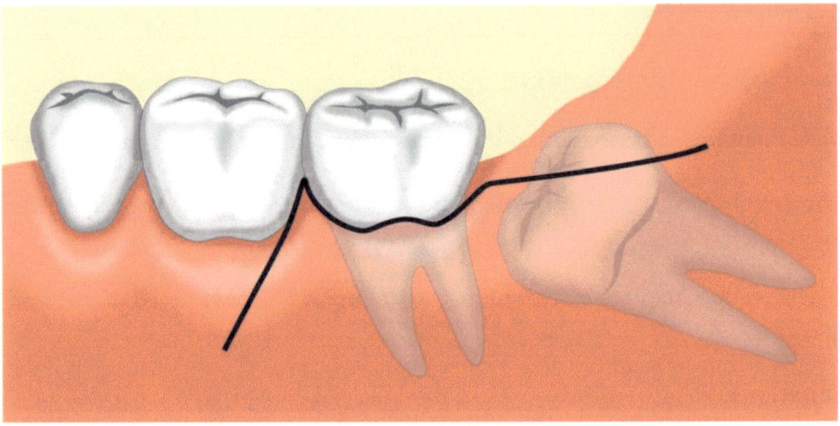

Figure 2.
Triangular flap for the removal of the third molar.

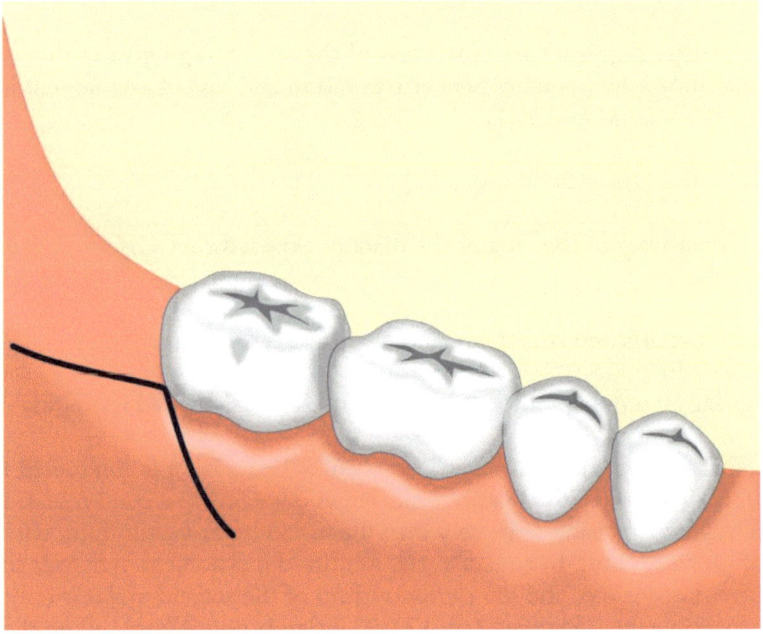

Figure 3.
Modified triangular flap for removal of the third molar.

Limitations

- Swelling and trismus
- Pain
- No significant difference in postoperative complications between the lingually based triangular flap and the traditional buccally based triangular flap after surgery of the third molar [8]

3. Flap techniques for canine exposure or removal

3.1 Background

Canines are among the most commonly impacted teeth after the third molar teeth. Different causes have been suggested and investigated in literature [9]. The impacted canines need to be either exposed or removed to avoid some possible complications. Untreated canines may cause tooth malalignment, root resorption of adjacent teeth, infections, and cystic changes.

The location of an impacted canine will determine the access for surgical exposure or removal. About one-third of the impacted maxillary canines are positioned labially or within the alveolus, while two-thirds are located palatally [10]. Kokich [11, 12] suggested that the following four criteria related to tooth position within the alveolar bone housing need to be carefully evaluated before exposing the impacted canine:

1. The first criterion looks at the labial-palatal position of the impacted canine. When there is labial impaction, the treatment of choice is an open technique (gingivectomy or apically positioned flap). While impaction in the mid-alveolus requires an open or closed technique, a palatal impaction is usually treated using a closed technique.

2. The second criterion evaluates the impaction position relative to the mucogingival junction (MGJ) in an apical-coronal dimension. When the majority of the impacted crown is positioned coronal to the MGJ, the gingivectomy open technique can be conducted. If the crown is located at the MGJ level, an apically repositioned flap is used. When the crown is apical to the MGJ, a closed technique is generally utilized.

3. The third criterion involves the evaluation of the amount of keratinized gingiva (KG) mainly with facial impactions. When there is an abundance of KG, the impacted canine is positioned relatively close to the MGJ, and a gingivectomy procedure is recommended. However, if there is inadequate KG, an apically repositioned flap or closed technique is suggested.

4. The fourth criterion evaluates the mesial-distal position of the canine relative to the lateral incisor. If the canine crown is positioned distal to the mesial aspect of the lateral incisor, an open technique is performed. If the crown is positioned mesial to the lateral incisor, a closed technique for the pataltal eruption of canine.

3.2 Labially impacted canine techniques

Labial canine impaction is usually difficult to approach because aesthetic outcomes of final soft-tissue healing are a challenge. An inappropriate surgical technique or flap design may lead to compromised aesthetic results [12]. During the process of uncovering a labially impacted maxillary canine, mucogingival problems, such as an immersed clinical crown, limited keratinized gingiva, gingival recession, and scarring, may occur if an inappropriate surgical intervention is employed [13]. In addition, the vertical and horizontal locations of the impacted canine also greatly affect orthodontic tooth movements and soft-tissue responses. Therefore, it is

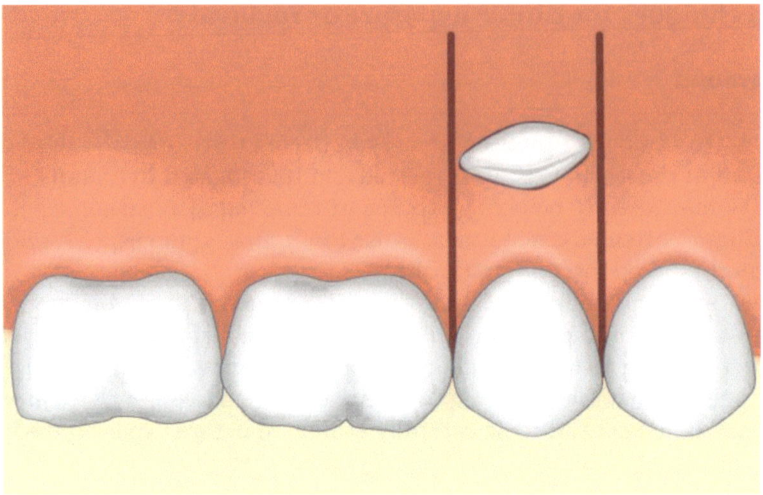

Figure 4.
Window excision at the labial soft tissue opposite to the crown of the impacted upper canine.

critical to make the right decision about the choice of a proper surgical technique to expose labially impacted teeth.

The proposed flap techniques include the window excision of the soft tissue (**Figure 4**), apically positioned flap, closed eruption technique, and sequential approach.

3.3 Window excision of the soft tissue

Figure 4 shows the window excision of the soft tissue when the canine crown is coronal to the mucogingival junction.

Advantages

- Directly expose the crown part
- Easy to perform

Limitations

- Sacrifice the gingival tissue
- Require wider attached gingiva

3.4 Apically positioned flap

Figures 5 and **6** show the apically positioned flap if there is insufficient attached gingiva.

Advantage

- Preserve attached gingiva

Limitation

- Not suitable in highly impacted canine

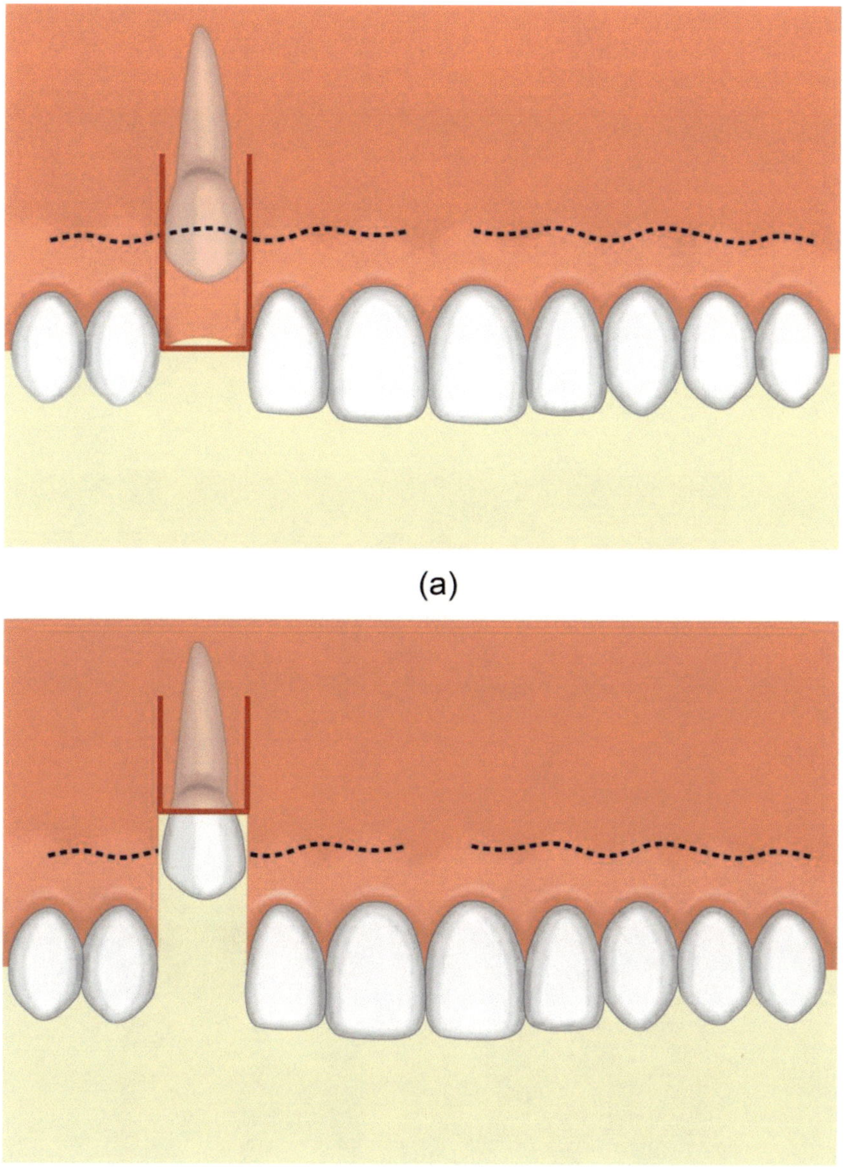

(a)

(b)

Figure 5.
An apically repositioned flap: (a) outline of the flap; (b) flap repositioned apically to provide a collar of the attached gingiva around the exposed tooth.

3.5 Closed eruption technique

Figure 7 shows that highly impacted canine and the crown tip are properly aligned mesiodistally.

Advantage

- The closed mucosal flap is more comfortable for patients

Limitation

- Uncontrollable orthodontic forces on the nonvisible tooth during orthodontic extrusion

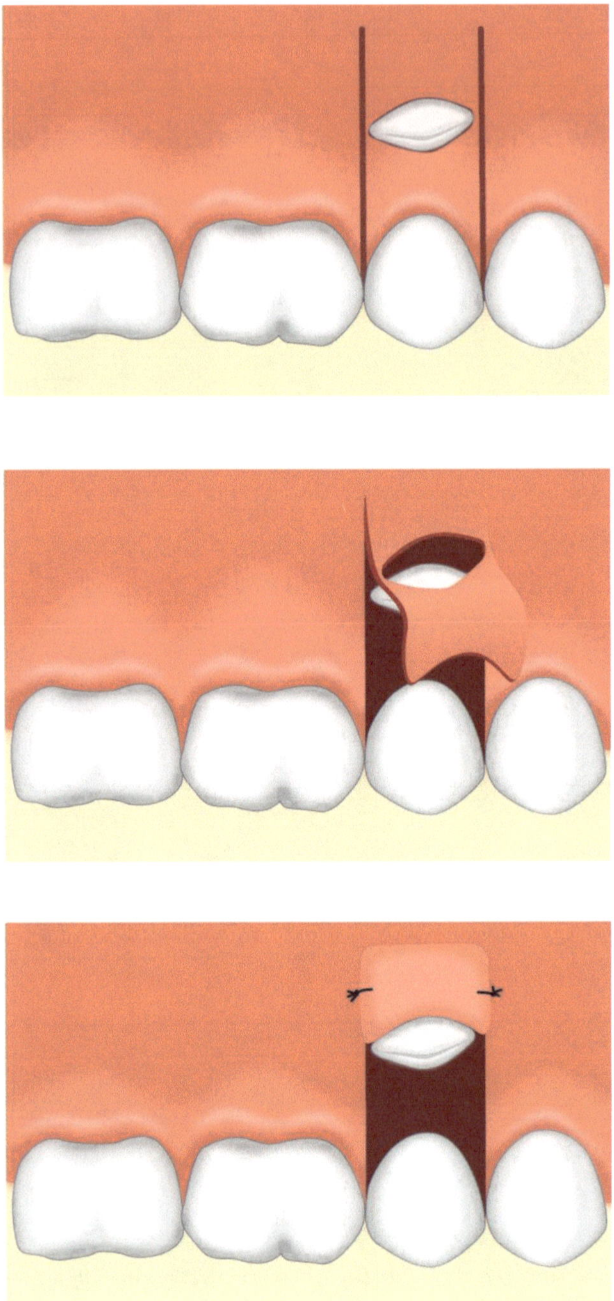

Figure 6.
Window is created (top image) labially opposite to the crown of the impacted canine, and (bottom image) the attached free gingival margin is placed apically.

3.6 A sequential approach

If a maxillary canine is highly impacted, its crown protrudes labially, or its cusp tip is displaced mesially (**Figure 8**), two-stage approaches may be indicated, in which exposure is carried out first (**Figure 6**) and mucogingival surgery such as gingivoplasty is performed at a later stage. Laterally sliding flap (**Figure 9**) provides additional keratinized tissue with natural color and consistency at the recipient site

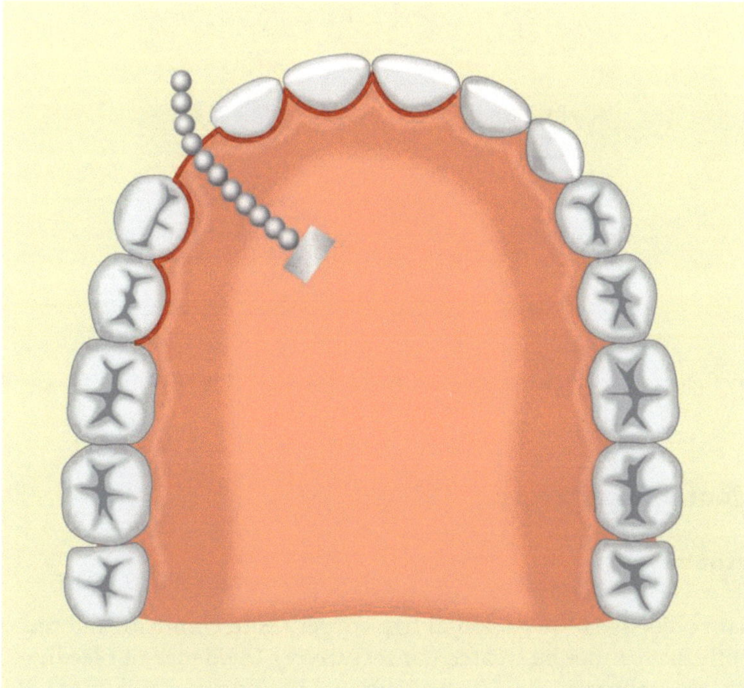

Figure 7.
Gingival margin flap with bracket and chain bond it to the crown of the impacted canine.

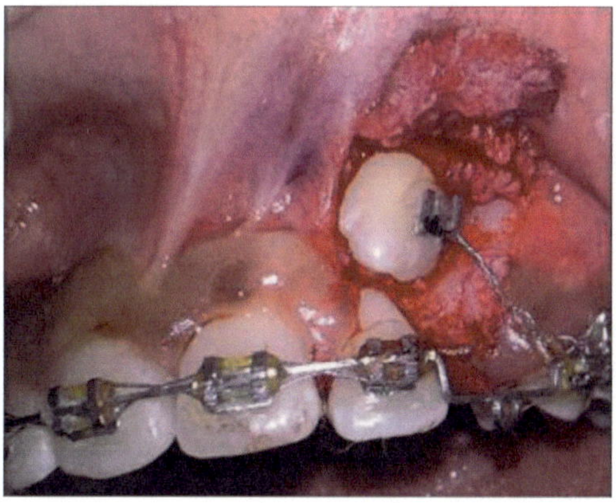

Figure 8.
Mesially exposed impacted canine that may require two-stage surgery to achieve minimal attached gingiva.

if adequate keratinized gingival is available over lateral incisor. Pedicle flap can be the second option and can be dissected from both the central and lateral incisor areas to transfer to cover the recipient bed (**Figure 9**).

Advantage

- Achieve 3–4 mm keratinized gingiva in highly impacted canine [9]

Limitations

- Two-stage surgery
- Donor site morbidity is expected

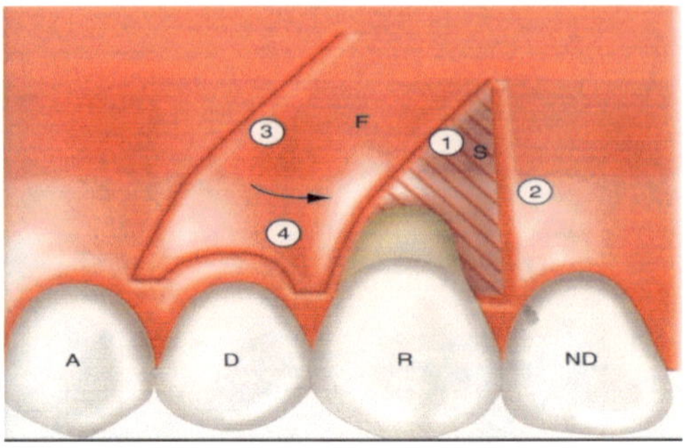

Figure 9.
The principle of lateral pedicle repositioned flap. R, recipient tooth; D, donor tooth; F, flap; S, split-thickness dissection.

4. Periodontal flap surgery

4.1 Background

The main objective of periodontal flap surgery is to eliminate and reduce the pocket depth that cannot be treated conservatively (evidence of bleeding, loss of attachment, or suppuration) with conventional periodontics treatment. Raising surgical flap facilitates removal of the inflamed tissue inside the pocket, provides access for tooth surface cleaning, and helps remove harmful plaque and calculus.

Indications

- Provide access to the tooth's root surface for instrumentation
- Correction of gingival overgrowth by gingivectomy
- Create new periodontal attachment
- Improve aesthetics and function following gingival recession by the root coverage technique

Contra-indications

- Poor plaque control
- Uncontrolled systemic disease
- Heavy smokers
- Teeth with poor long-term prognosis

4.2 Full-thickness periodontal flap

Raising full mucoperiosteum exposes the underlying bone. The modified Widman flap [14] is one example of this type of flap. It includes a scalloped incision 1 mm from the crevicular margin involving the interproximal area of the teeth, allowing the flap to be raised without releasing incision (**Figure 10**).

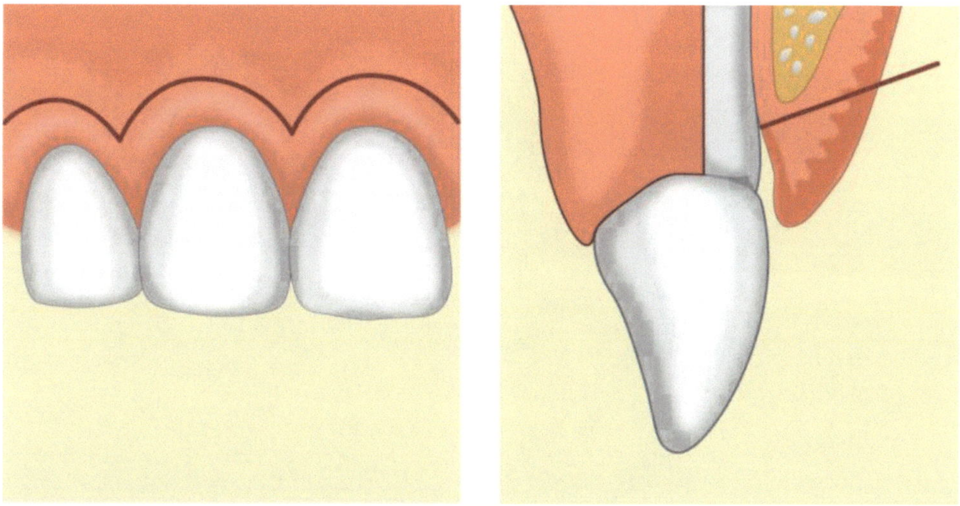

Figure 10.
Modified Widman flap technique. The image is adapted from The Hungarian higher education in dentistry in Hungarian, German, and English.

Advantages

- Allow close adaptation of soft tissues to the root surface with minimal trauma
- Less postoperative teeth sensitivity
- Better aesthetic results
- Allow root surface debridement
- The pocket reduction is achieved by long junctional epithelial attachment to the root surface

Limitations

- Not indicated if osseous surgery is planned
- Cannot be used for full pocket removal

4.3 The apically repositioned flap

Reverse bevel incision is made at the attached gingiva angled to excise the periodontal pocket in a scalloped fashion. Two releasing incisions are made mesial and distal to the defect. After the flap is elevated, pocketing tissues are discarded, osseous surgery can be performed, and the flap is then apically repositioned and sutured in position as illustrated above in the canine exposure section (**Figure 11**).

Advantages

- Expose the alveolar bone and allow osseous surgery to correct infrabony defects
- Allow excellent access to the root surface for debridement

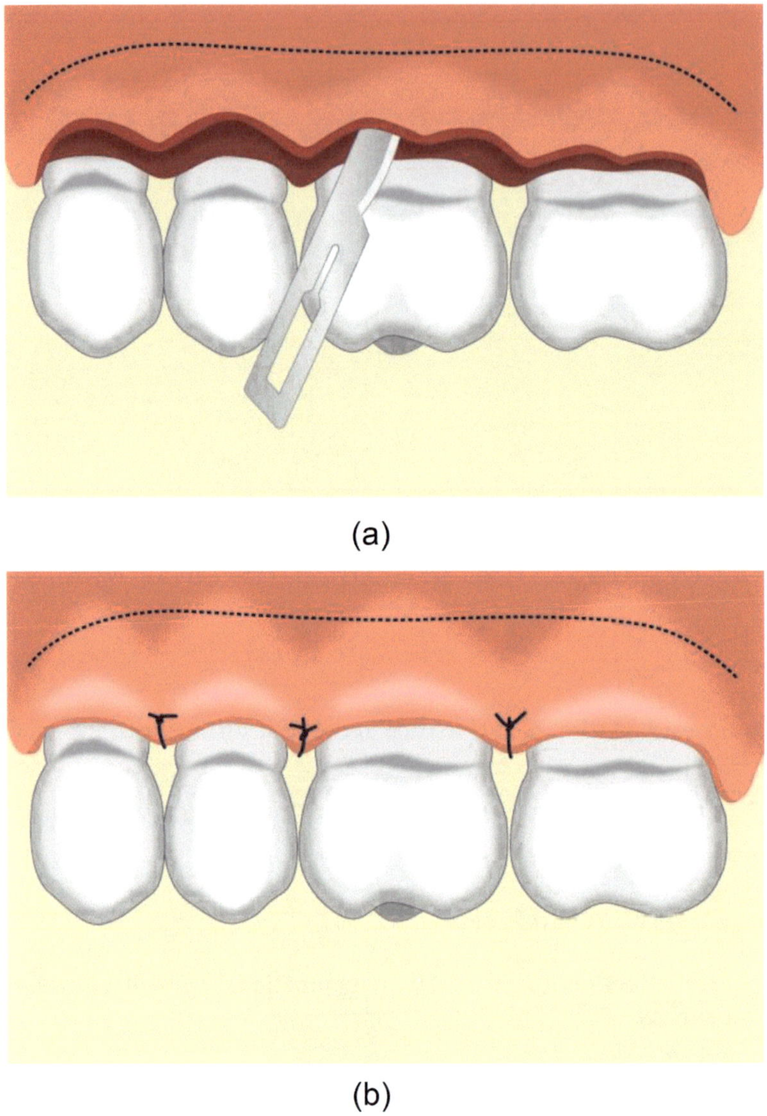

Figure 11.
Apically repositioned flap for periodontal surgery. (a) The bevel, scalloped incision for pocket elimination. (b) The flap positioned apically.

Limitation

- Not applicable in the palatal tissue

4.4 Gingivectomy

Beveled incision excises the supra-gingival pocket and allows for gingival re-contouring.

Advantages

- Suitable for gingival hypertrophy (supra-alveolar pocket)
- Re-contouring severely damaged gingival tissues

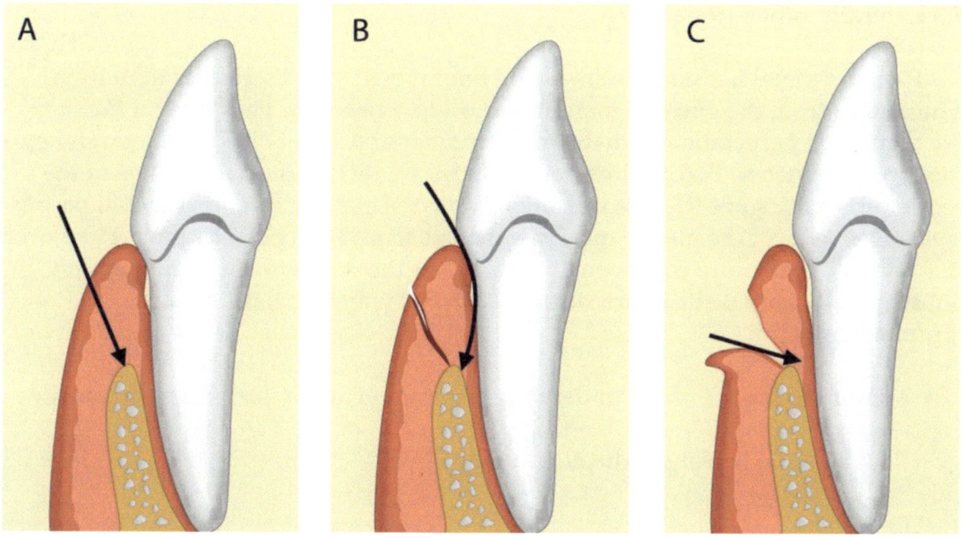

Figure 12.
The stages for crown lengthening. (A) Internal beveling; (B) sulcular incision; (C) removal of excess tissues to expose the crown or the gingival overgrowth.

- Crown lengthening (**Figure 12**)

Limitations

- Not indicated in case of deep "true" infrabony pocket
- Not suitable for removal of intrabone lesions
- Row wound exposes the root surface, making it sensitive and susceptible to caries
- Because of the loss of the attached gingiva, some bone remodeling may occur

5. Mucogingival graft surgery

5.1 Background

Mucogingival graft surgery aims at the correction of local gingival defects. It will be conducted if changing the morphology of gingival margin improves the plaque control, high frenal attachment, and severe gingival recession.

5.2 Split thickness flap

Raising partial soft tissues and leaving the mucoperiosteum attached to the bone are commonly used techniques to address such mucogingival problems. Moreover, pedicle flap includes either laterally, coronally, or double papilla repositioned flaps. The flaps are indicated in very narrow areas of isolated gingival recession or even in the presence of wide recession with adequate door tissues on either side [15].

5.3 Laterally repositioned flap

Two horizontal incisions are made on both mesial and distal sides of defects 1 mm away from the gingival margin of the adjacent tooth. Two vertical incisions are then made perpendicular to the initial incisions on either side, which extend into the alveolar mucosa. Partial-thickness pedicles are reflected on either side of the recession area (**Figure 9**). The reflection is carried out to a level that would permit free movements of the mesial and distal pedicle flaps. Both pedicles are rotated over the defect to make sure they would remain over the defect without any tension. Subsequently, both pedicles are sutured with 6-0 polypropylene sutures.

Advantages

- Minimal exposure of the underlying periosteum at the interdental donor sites
- Rapid wound healing at the donor site

Limitations

- Cannot be used in a generalized recession
- Cannot be used if there is an inadequate amount of keratinized tissues at donor sites

5.4 Coronally repositioned flap

A partial-thickness flap is raised around the defect with the help of two horizontal and two vertical incisions on either side of the defect without involving the marginal gingiva of adjacent teeth. To facilitate a tension-free coronal displacement, its base can be separated from the periosteum with the help of a periosteal releasing incision. The flap is then advanced coronally and sutured at the level of cementoenamel junction (CEJ) using 5-0 polypropylene sutures (**Figures 13** and **14**).

5.5 Free gingival grafts

This graft is a harvested tissue and is completely removed from the blood donor area, and it is used to augment the amount of the attached (keratinized) gingiva. This approach can be only used with the combination with another surgical approach.

5.6 Two-stage surgical techniques

Two-stage surgical techniques use double pedicle flap with a connective tissue graft, followed by coronally advanced flap.

Advantages

- Treatment for a severe localized gingival recession
- Excellent color matching and dual blood supply to graft

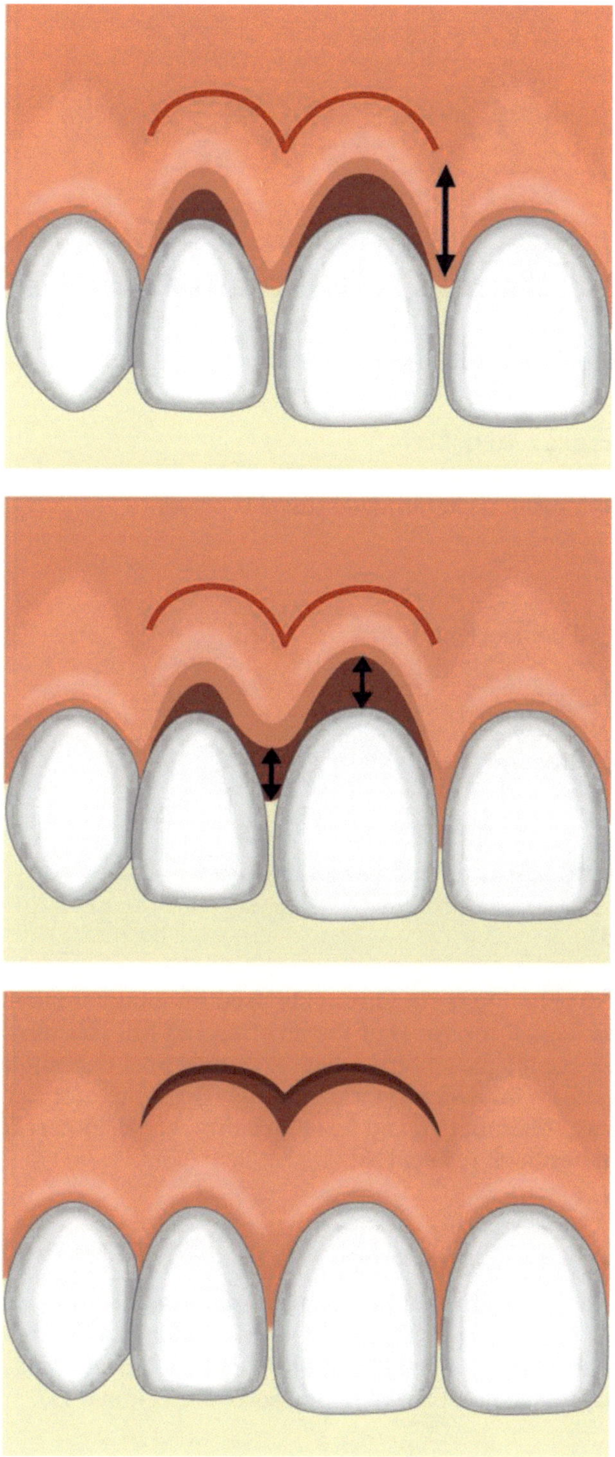

Figure 13.
Coronally repositioned flap used to cover localized recession. The top image shows the recession area, and the incision line is done 4–5 mm from the gingival margin; the bottom image shows that partial-thickness flap is raised and sutured coronally.

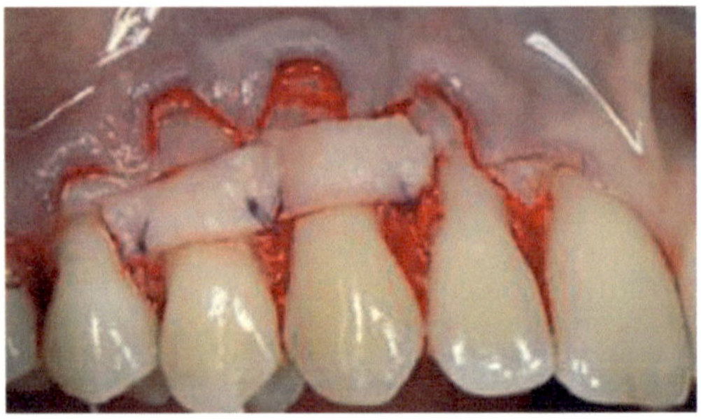

Figure 14.
Free gingival graft is applied to cover the root surface with less amount of attached gingiva.

- Very predictable results
- Can be used if minimal keratinized tissue is present

Limitations

- Requires good pedicel length
- Two-stage surgery
- A free graft is required

6. Flap for dental implant bed preparation

6.1 Background

Two-stage flap techniques are commonly used for dental implant surgery and include a flapless (e.g., Punch or Half Punch) flap and full-thickness flap, such as mid-crest, double papilla preservation flap. Full-thickness flap might be more suitable for immediate implantation; the flapless flap is superior to full-thickness flap in cases of less inflammation and less morbidity, has shallower biological width, and shows better aesthetic results [16].

6.2 Punch flap

A small hole in the keratinized mucosa is required to be present on the crest of the ridge at the area of interest (**Figure 14**). This punch can be created using a blade or punch drill. Precise placement of the cut can be obtained using the surgical guide with the help of the planning software (**Figure 15**).

Advantages

- Minimal surgery
- Minimal postoperative pain/discomfort
- Suitable for one-stage surgery

Limitations

- Simultaneous bone grafting is not possible
- Minimal exposure to the bone for thickness evaluation
- Require sufficient keratinized mucosa

6.3 Half punch

In the case of the presence of inadequate or deficient buccal tissues, half punch approach is used. Half punch flap is conducted with horizontal crestal incision and reflects full-thickness flap buccally. Subsequently, punch approach is used lingually or palatally to remove minimally required tissues for implant placement (**Figure 16**).

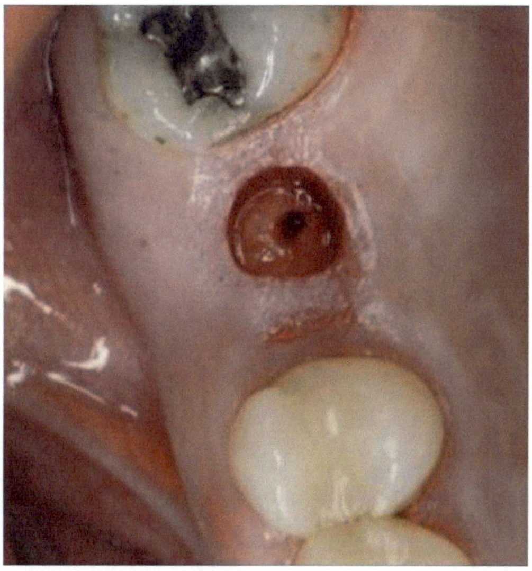

Figure 15.
Punch flap (flapless) at mid-crest of ridge.

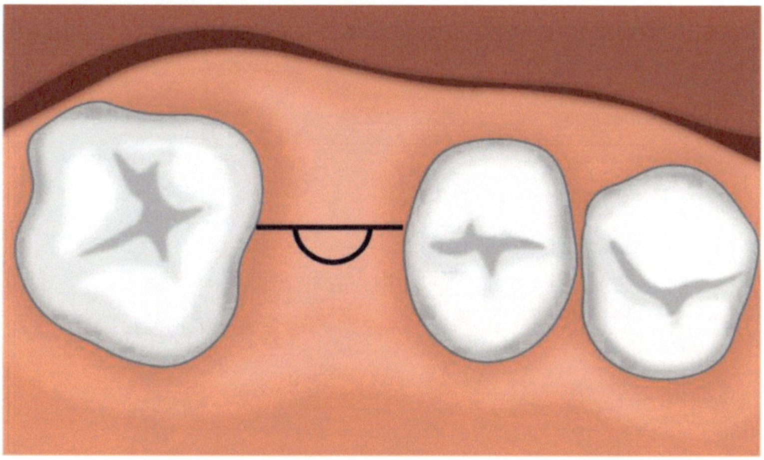

Figure 16.
Half punch flap used for implant bed preparation.

Advantage

- One-stage implant surgery with possible simultaneous bone grafting

6.4 Mid-crestal incision

Mid-crestal incision is performed at the middle of the ridge bone, and buccal and lingual/or palatal flaps are then raised to expose the full surgical site (**Figure 17**).

Advantages

- This flap can be used for both one- and two-stage implant surgery
- Buccal and palatal/lingual bone grafting is possible

Limitation

- Requires sufficient buccal and palatal tissues

6.5 Palatal/lingual crestal flap

The incision is similar to mid-crestal incision; however, it is made more toward the palatal side/lingual. The flap is then raised to perform the bone preparation (**Figure 18**).

Advantages

- Suitable in cases when there are less buccal tissues available to raise full-thickness flap
- Bone grafting can be performed buccally or palatally/lingually
- Suitable for both one- and two-stage implant surgery

6.6 Mesial papilla preservation flap

This flap is designed to maintain the interdental papilla for aesthetics in some cases.

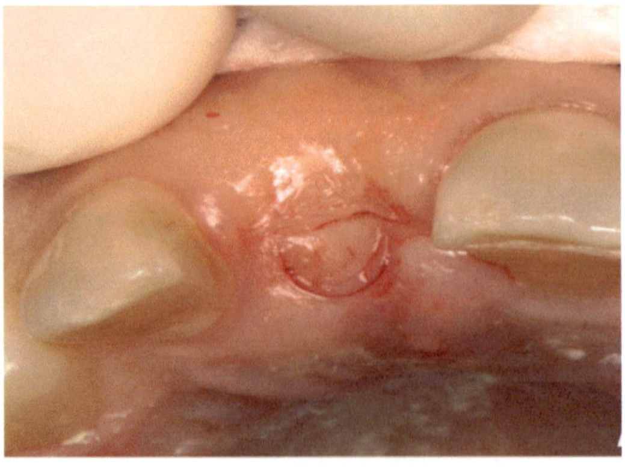

Figure 17.
The edentulous ridge with minimal attached gingiva. Half punch flap is performed.

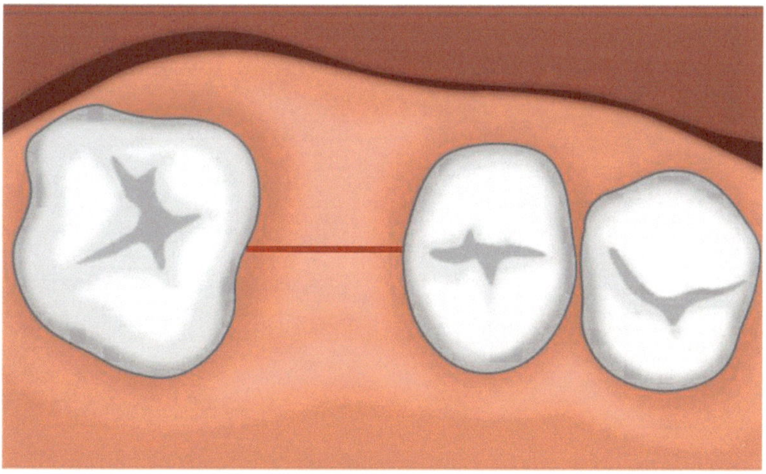

Figure 18.
Mid-crestal incision used during implant bed preparation.

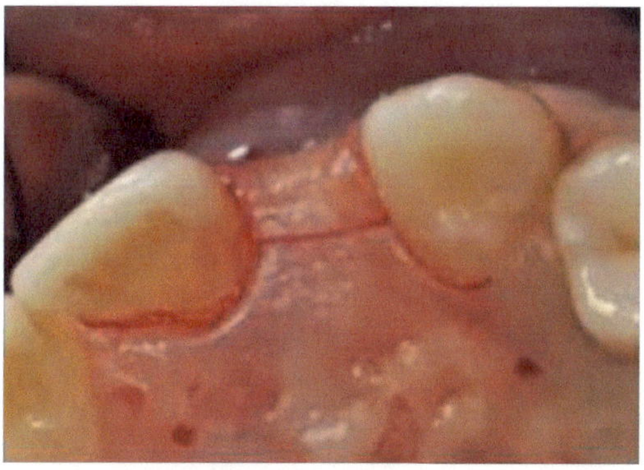

Figure 19.
Platatal crestal flap used for implant bed preparation.

In this flap, vertical releasing incision distal to the papilla is made and is connected to a crestal incision on the other side of the defect. An intrasulcular incision on the distal tooth is performed, and the flap is raised, followed by implant bed preparation (**Figure 19**).

Advantages

- Good aesthetic results
- Minimal surgery and soft tissue manipulation

Limitations

- Not suitable if bone grafting is required
- Used for the second stage of implant surgery to help get maximum aesthetic results by preserving the papilla

6.7 Distal papilla preservation

This flap is opposite to mesial preservation flap, and the aim is to preserve the distal side of the defect to allow bone grafting (**Figures 20** and **21**).

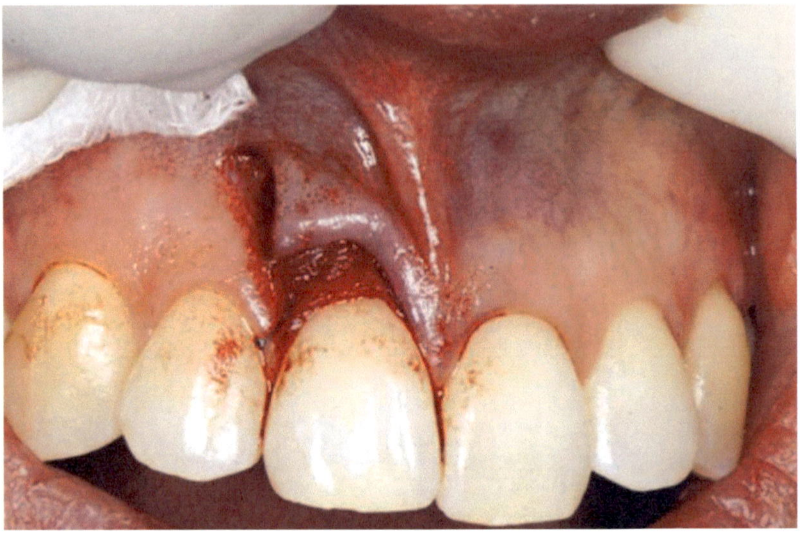

Figure 20.
Mesially papilla preserved incision for implant bed preparation.

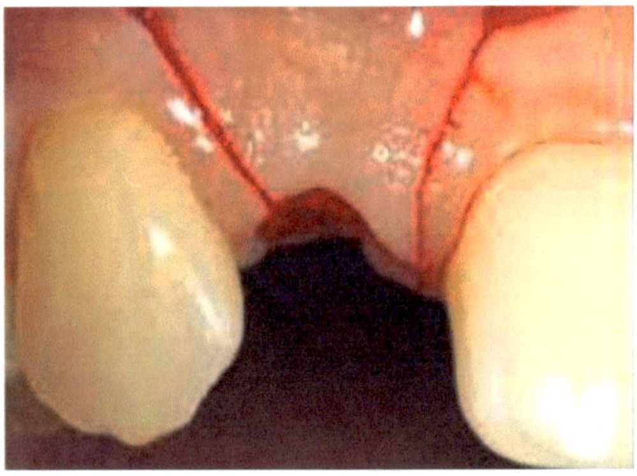

Figure 21.
Double papilla preservation with two vertical releasing incisions.

6.8 Double papilla preservation

This flap is designed to preserve both mesial and distal papilla at the defect area. Two vertical incisions are performed and connected with lingual or palatal crestal incision, thus allowing the release of the mucoperiosteal flap toward the buccal aspect.

Advantages

- More aesthetic results
- Suitable for the second stage of implant surgery where the mobilization of a good amount of tissues may be required

Limitation

- Vascularity may be compromised in the narrow space

6.9 Full-thickness flap reflection for large edentulous spaces (book flap)

The buccal or lingual mucoperiosteal flap can be reflected, allowing an alveolar split to be done using thin osteotomes for alveolar ridge expansion if required.

Advantages

- Wide exposure allows observing the undercut lingually or buccally
- Easy to lean and perform alveoloplasty
- Easy to perform bone cutting and splitting

Limitations

- Bone devitalization and subsequent remodeling resorption in narrow ridge [17].
- Less predictable outcomes

6.10 Partial-thickness flaps for ridge expansion

This is a minimally exposed osteoperiosteal flap to overcome the limitation of full-thickness flap for the wide edentulous area when the resulting vascularity may jeopardize the outcomes (**Figure 22**).

Advantages

- Maintain the integrity of periosteum
- Maintain bone vitality (vascularity)
- Alveolar width stability, that is, minimal postoperative resorption compared with full-thickness flap

Limitations

- The bone is cut blindly; therefore, the surgeon must have a good conceptualization of the alveolar anatomy to not miss the midpoint of the

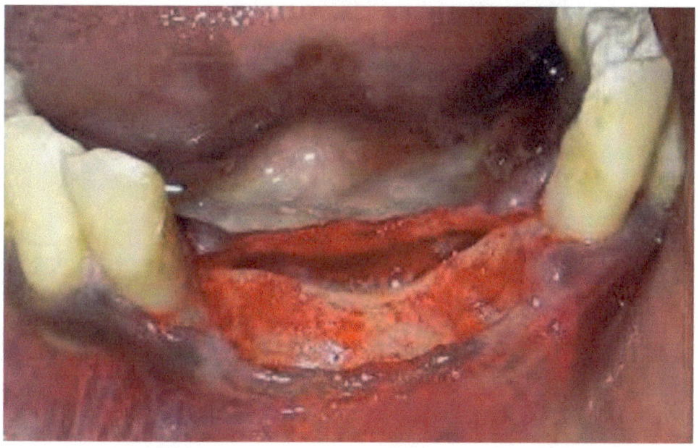

Figure 22.
Full ridge exposure using the full thickness flap buccally and lingually.

alveolus. The surgeon should avoid extending to the vestibular depth or palatally directed osteotomy

- Requires extensive flap dissection [17]

7. Endodontic surgery flap

7.1 Background

Flap design in periapical surgery should be adequate for the planned surgical procedure, offering good access to the zone surrounding the affected apexes without altering the soft-tissue circulation. The flap should be a firm continuous incision and not cross an underlying bony defect. If a vertical incision is needed, it should be in the concavities between bone eminences. The vertical incision should not extend into the mesiobuccal fold, and its termination of the gingival crest must be at the mesial or distal line angle of the tooth. Additionally, the base of the flap must be at least equal to the width of its free end. The most frequently used flap in periapical surgery is the Luebke-Ochsenbein flap involving submarginal incision, with semilunar or Partsch flap variants.

7.2 Luebke-Ochsenbein flap

A horizontal incision is made in the attached gingival tissue about 3–4 mm above the gingival margin, with two vertical releasing incisions on either side of the flap located one or two teeth distal to where the lesion is located (**Figure 23**).

Advantages

- This type of flap is easy to detach
- It is less aggressive with the gingival tissue than an intrasulcular incision flap

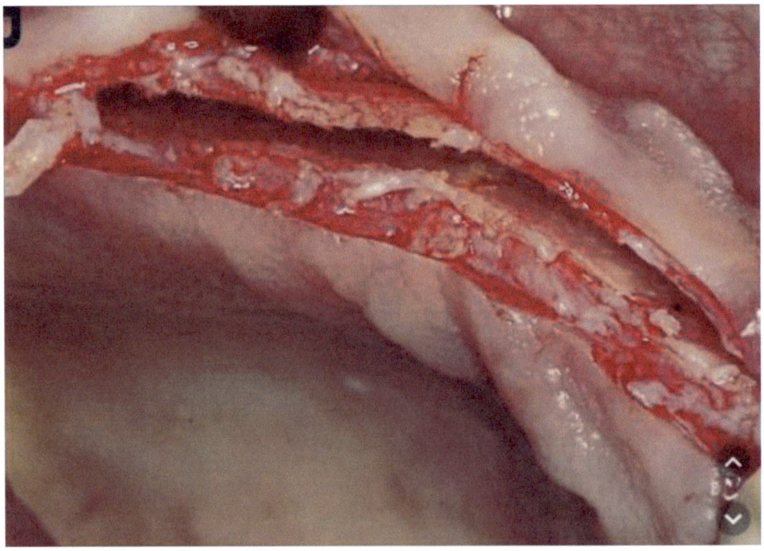

Figure 23.
Partial-thickness flap before ridge expansion for future dental implant insertion.

- It is useful in patients with fixed prosthesis restorations because of less recession of the gingival margin and interdental papillae [17–19]

Limitation

- It can leave a postsurgical scar if the repositioning sutures are not performed adequately [20]

7.3 Partsch flap

The semilunar (Partsch) flap is a variant involving a submarginal incision in the alveolar mucosa to form a crescent- or semilunar-shaped flap (**Figure 24**). The semilunar flap is almost exclusively used for the maxillary canines [21]. Care is required to avoid performing the incision above the bone defect.

Advantage

- Small incision suitable for upper canine surgery

Limitations

- Limited surgical access to the root apex
- Flap tension is high due to the presence of muscle fibers, making suturing difficult and increasing the risk of suture dehiscence [5, 22]

7.4 Neumann flap

This flap involves intrasulcular incision in its triangular and trapezoidal versions and offers perfect access for periapical surgery, with sufficient access to the affected bone and lesion-related roots. The intrasulcular incision may be triangular or trapezoidal (**Figure 25**). The most common intrasulcular flap involves a triangular incision with a single vertical releasing incision located one or two teeth distal to the lesion (**Figure 26**). This flap is characterized by increased tension, and the traction forces increase especially at the fixed extremity. This technique allows for easy flap repositioning after periapical surgery.

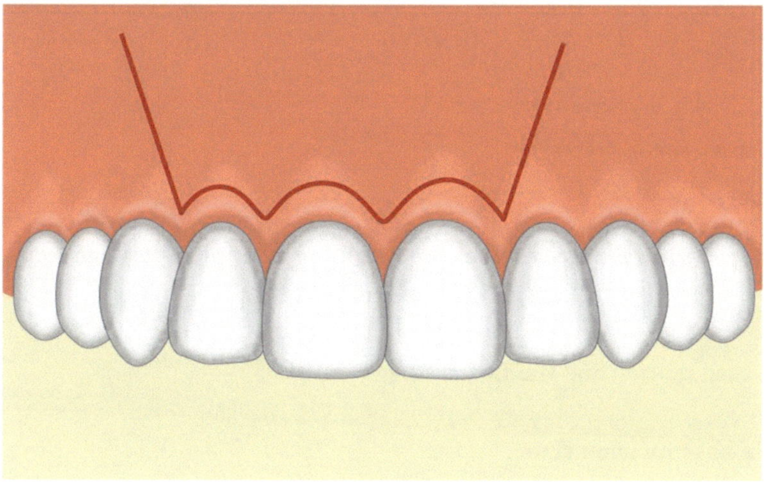

Figure 24.
Submarginal incision and two vertical incisions mesial and distal to the defect area.

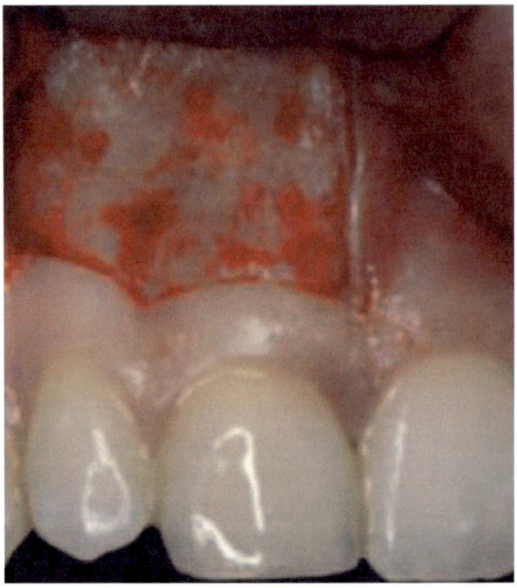

Figure 25.
Luebke-Ochsenbein flap is used clinically for periapical surgery.

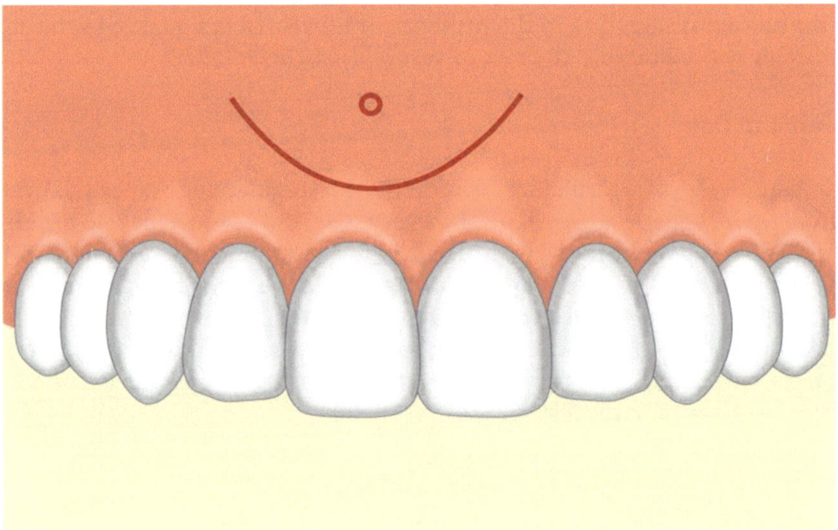

Figure 26.
Semilunar flap in a form of crescent.

Advantage

- This technique allows easy flap repositioning after periapical surgery

Limitation

- Increased tension and traction forces

7.5 Papilla base incision flap

This flap, which was originally described by Velvart, is characterized by a horizontal incision following the dental sulcus along the neck of the teeth and

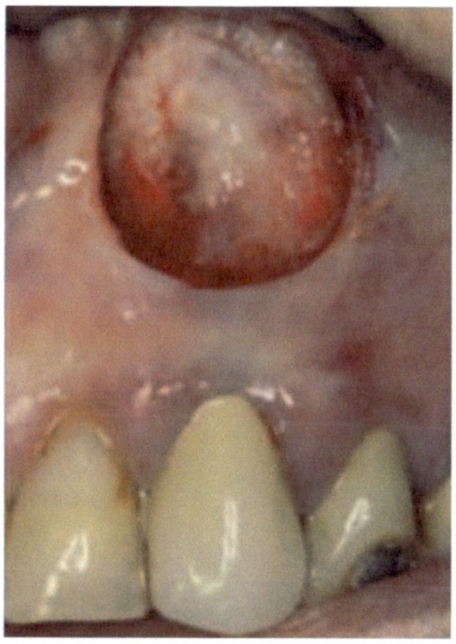

Figure 27.
Clinical application of Partsch flap for periapical surgery.

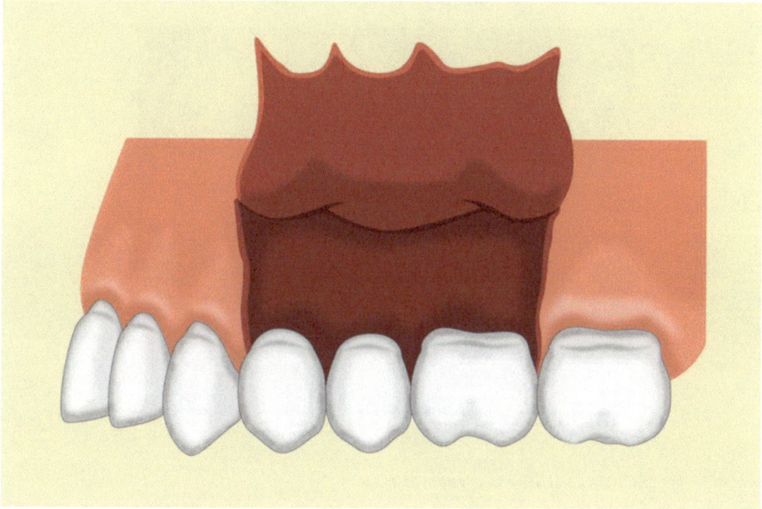

Figure 28.
Trapezoidal flap with two releasing incisions.

extending to the base of the papillae (**Figure 27**). The papillae adhere for posterior suturing of the flap. A vertical releasing incision is made to maximize the exposure.

Advantage

- Produces less recession at the interdental papillary level than a sulcular incision [23]

Limitations

- A surgically complicated flap requiring adequate surgeon experiences
- Requires the presence of enough healthy attached gingiva for suturing

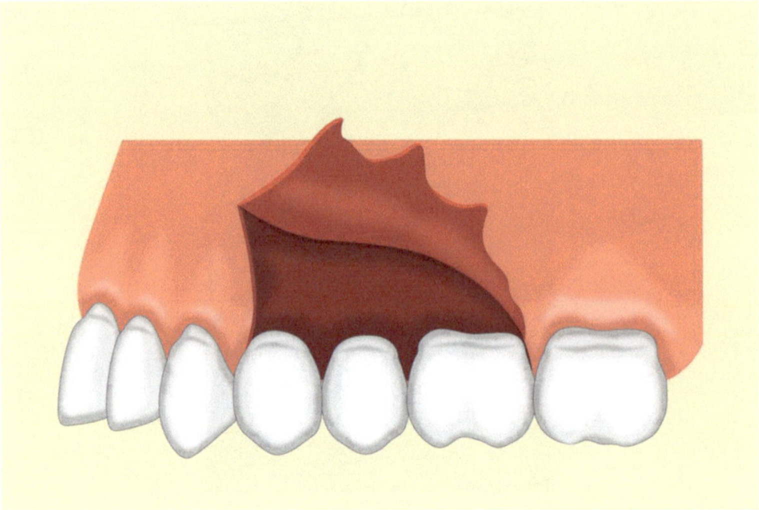

Figure 29.
Triangular flap with a single releasing incision.

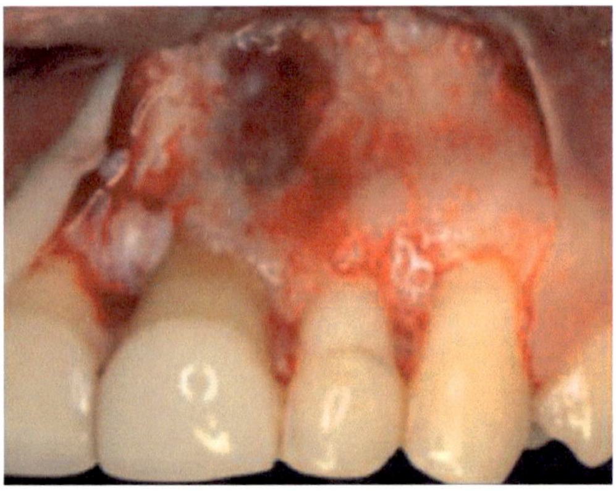

Figure 30.
Clinical application for the intrasulcular trapezoidal flap.

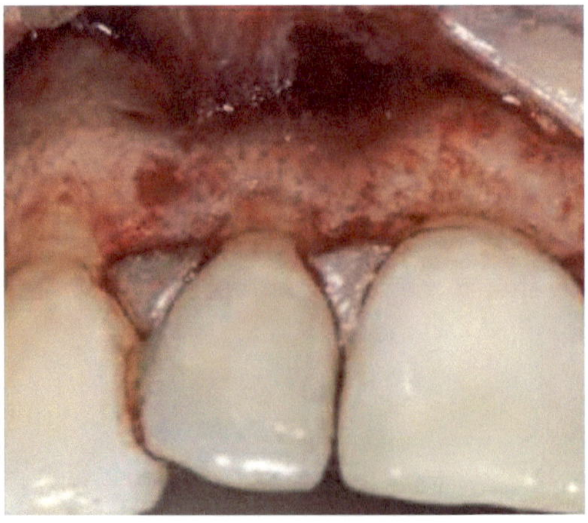

Figure 31.
The papilla adhered to the bone and the raised full mucoperiosteal flap.

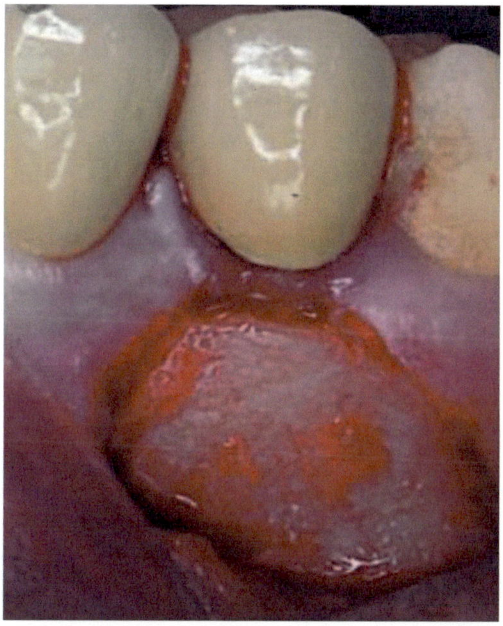

Figure 32.
The raised papilla preservation mucoperiosteal flap.

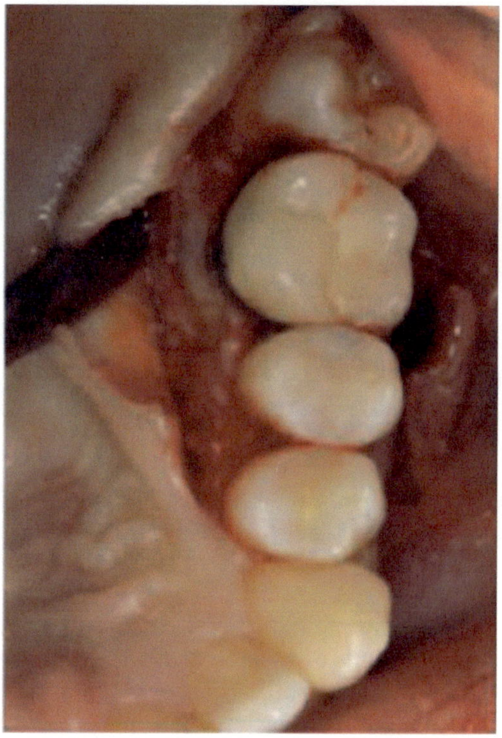

Figure 33.
The raised palatal full mucoperiosteal flap for palatal periapical surgery.

7.6 Papilla-preserving flap

A horizontal incision is made following the dental sulcus to the dental papilla, and the vertical releasing incision is seated away from the papilla (**Figures 28–33**) [19].

Advantage

- This flap is useful in teeth with a generous mesiodistal width, affording an adequate surgical field

Limitations

- The narrow neck needs careful releasing, careful adaptation, and suturing
- This flap may be not suitable in narrow mesiodistal distance between teeth

7.7 Palatal flap

A festoon flap is performed at the gingival margins on the palatal side. This flap is used in periapical surgery of the palatal roots of the maxillary molars. Palatal releasing incisions are not necessary. If any such incisions are made, they should be performed between the canine and premolar, representing the vascularization limit between the nasopalatine artery and the anterior palatine artery, or distal to the second molar behind the emergence point of the anterior palatine artery [24].

Advantage

- Useful in cases in which the palatal roots of molars or lateral incisors require exposure

Limitations

- If the flap needs to be expanded to gain greater visibility, the incision can be extended mesially to the canine
- This flap may cause pain and discomfort for the patient postoperatively
- Chance of hematoma formation may jeopardize the blood supply of the flap

8. Flaps for management of oroantral communication

8.1 Background

Oroantral communication/fistula is an unnatural communication between the oral cavity and the maxillary sinus. These complications occur most commonly during the extraction of upper molar and premolar teeth (48%). The major reason is the anatomic proximity or projection of the roots within the maxillary sinus [25]. Other causes of oroantral communication/fistula include tuberosity fracture, dentoalveolar/periapical infections of molars, implant dislodgement, maxillary sinus, trauma (7.5%), presence of maxillary cysts or tumors (18.5%), osteoradio-necrosis, flap necrosis, and dehiscence following implant failure [25, 26]. Two basic principles must be considered while operating for Oroantral communication/fistula. First, the sinus must be free of any types of infection with adequate nasal drainage. Second, closure must be tension-free and consists of broadly based, well-vascularized soft tissue flaps over the intact bone. Successful closure of the oroantral fistula should be preceded by the complete elimination of any sinus pathology, the fistulous tract, sinus infection, degenerated mucosa, and diseased bone [27].

The most common flap procedures may be categorized into local flaps, distant flaps, and grafting. The flaps involving rotating or advancing soft tissues include buccal flap, palatal flap, submucosal tissue flap, and buccal fat pad and tongue flap [26]. The procedures utilizing buccal mucoperiosteal flap for closure include straight-advancement flap, rotation-advancement flap, transverse flap, and sliding flap techniques, and those utilizing palatal mucoperiosteum include straight-advancement flap, rotational advancement flap, hinged flap, and island flap procedures [26]. Double-layer closure utilizing local tissues includes the combination of inversion and rotational advancement flaps, double overlapping hinged flaps, double island flaps, and superimposition of reverse palatal and buccal flaps. However, the studies over the last 50 years point out the lack of consensus for a uniformly successful procedure [28].

Here we illustrate the most common flaps used for closure of oroantral communication/fistula: the buccal flap and the palatal pedicle flap techniques.

8.2 Buccal advancement flap

It has been described [14, 29] the use of a buccal flap with a thin layer of buccinator muscle to close an oroantral defect. Later, [30] reported a buccal sliding flap technique, which is still in use, as a tool to close small to medium size (<1 cm) lateral or mid-alveolar fistulas, located either laterally or in the middle of the alveolar process. Krompotie and Bagatin [13] reported the immediate closure of an oroantral communication by a rotating gingiva-vestibular flap. This technique can also be employed for closing oroantral fistulas. It is a modification of a vestibular flap in order to avoid lowering of the vestibular sulcus, an event that takes place normally when using vestibular flaps. Two vertical release incisions are made to provide a flap with dimensions suitable for closure of the antral communication (**Figure 34**).

Incision removal of the epithelial lining of the palatal mucosa behind the communication might also be required. The flap with a trapezoidal shape consists of both epithelium and connective tissues and is positioned over the defect using mattress sutures from the buccal flap to the palatal mucosa.

Advantage

- It is possibly utilized in cases of severly resorbed alvealr ridge, and the fistula is located in a more mesial area [31]

Limitation

- Loss of vestibular depth buccally

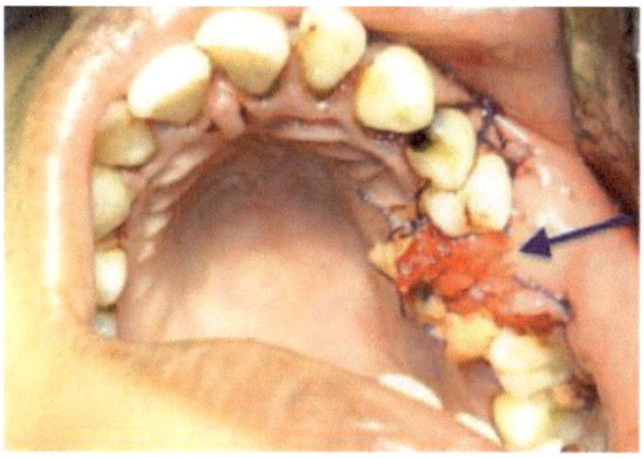

Figure 34.
The buccal advancement flap is used to close OAC (arrow).

8.3 Palatal pedicle flap technique

The first procedure for closing oroantral fistulas using a palatal full-thickness flap was described by Ashley [26, 32]. After excising the epithelium from its edges and cutting the palatal fibro-mucosa, the flap is created with an axial stack with a posterior base, supplied by the greater palatine artery. The palatal flap with its total thickness laterally rotated must have a large base to include the greater palatine artery at the site of its exit from the foramen (**Figure 35**) [33, 34]. The anterior extension of the flap must exceed the diameter of the bony defect and have a length sufficient to allow its lateral rotation and replacement, and the suture has no exerting tension on the vestibular mucosa [35]. Further improvement of the techniques was advocated [35, 36] by adding a flap of mucosa to the connective tissue island to cover the raw area of the palatal bone. The bone is covered, and the island flap retains excellent mobility without causing bunching of the mucosa of the hard palate and recipient site.

Advantages

- Good vascularization, adequate thickness, and optimal tissue quality
- The use of mucous membrane from the hard palate. In 1980, Ehrl demonstrated the possibility of employing this technique with wide fistulas 1 cm in diameter [37]
- This method allows replacement of the denture a short time after the wound healing

Limitation

- It is only indicated if the fistula is located at the area of the premolar to avoid excessive rotation of the flap
- The area of the palatal flap will heal by secondary epithelialization, which causes pain and discomfort
- Necrosis of the flap can happen if excessive rotation to the flap is performed

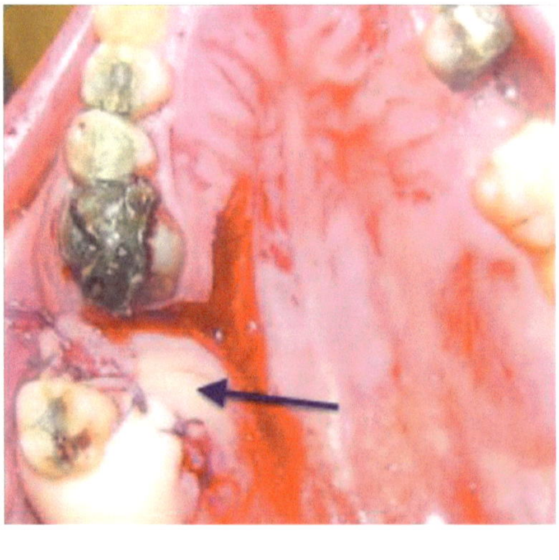

Figure 35.
The palatal rotation flap used to close OAC (arrow).

8.4 Buccal pad of flat flap (BPF)

Since Egyedi reported the BFP flap as a suitable method to close the OAC, oronasal communication, and maxillary postsurgery defects, the technique has been widely used. In addition, according to the study by Rapidis et al. [38], the BFP can be used as a free flap to close oral defects. Tideman et al. described the detailed anatomy, vascularization, and operative techniques of BFP [39]. The pedunculated BFP has been employed for the reconstruction of an oral defect of moderate size following surgical removal of a malignant lesion [38]. A gentle dissection with fine curved artery forceps exposes the yellowish-colored buccal fat. The buccal fat pad flap, especially the pedicled type, has been used most commonly for the closure of the OAF due to the location of the buccal fat pad, which is anatomically favorable, and due to the easy and minimal dissection, with which it can be harvested and mobilized.

Advantages

- Good rate of epithelialization [40]
- Low rate of failure [40]

Limitations

- Mild reduction in the vestibular height
- A second surgery is required in order to achieve closure if there is a low rate of recurrence of fistulas

8.5 Double-layer closure techniques

8.5.1 Palatal inversion flap and buccal advancement flap

This technique designs the palatal inversion flap on the basis of the greater palatine vessels after measuring the bone defect, but not the soft-tissue defect, as shown in **Figure 35**. Once the flap is raised, the residual palatal raw surface is left to heal by secondary intension with the formation of the granulation tissue. The horizontal palatal flap is then inverted so that the oral palatal epithelial surface covers the bone defect and faces the maxillary sinus. Subsequently, it will be covered by the buccal advancement flap that is released by extending the incision inside the cheek from the gingivolabial sulcus to have a wide base and ensure a good blood supply, as shown in **Figure 34**.

Advantages

- Indicated if there is an increased risk of wound breakdown and recuurant oroantrual defect
- It provides epithelial covering to both the superior and inferior surfaces
- Blood perfusion of the palatal flap is better than that of the single technique

Limitations

- It has a risk of subsequent pathology

- Perfusion of buccal flaps is poor
- Narrowing of the gingivobuccal sulcus may occur

8.5.2 Closure of oroantral fistula using a buccal fat pad (BFP)

BFP is anatomically favorable, and the easy and minimal dissection of the fat tissue from the buccal pad of fat and then harvesting and mobilization made it a popular technique (**Figure 36**). Furthermore, it has excellent blood supply. A quick surgical technique is preferred due to fact that BFP and the defects to be covered are located in the same surgical field, and a good rate of epithelialization allows for replacement of the mucoperiosteal flap without loss of vestibular depth.

Advantages

- Low rate of complications
- Minimal donor site morbidity
- Easy and versatile technique
- No loss of vestibular depth

Limitations

- While harvesting BFP, perforation or/and shrinkage may occur
- The amount of BFP is inadequate in some cases

8.5.3 Double-layer closure techniques

This technique combines BFP and buccal advancement or skin flaps. BFP can be covered by the partial thickness skin flap [41] or buccal advancement flap, especially for defects larger than $5 \times 1\ cm^2$. This technique can also be better managed with the use of BFP with buccal advancement flap than BFP alone [42] (**Figure 37**).

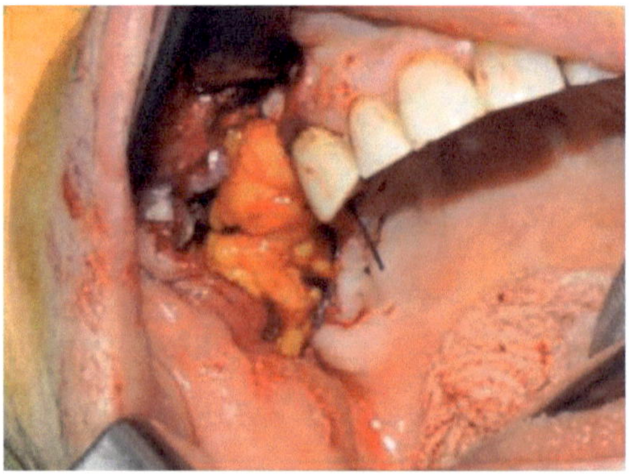

Figure 36.
Intraoral photograph shows the harvested buccal fat and is adapted to the defect in the molar and premolar/molar areas.

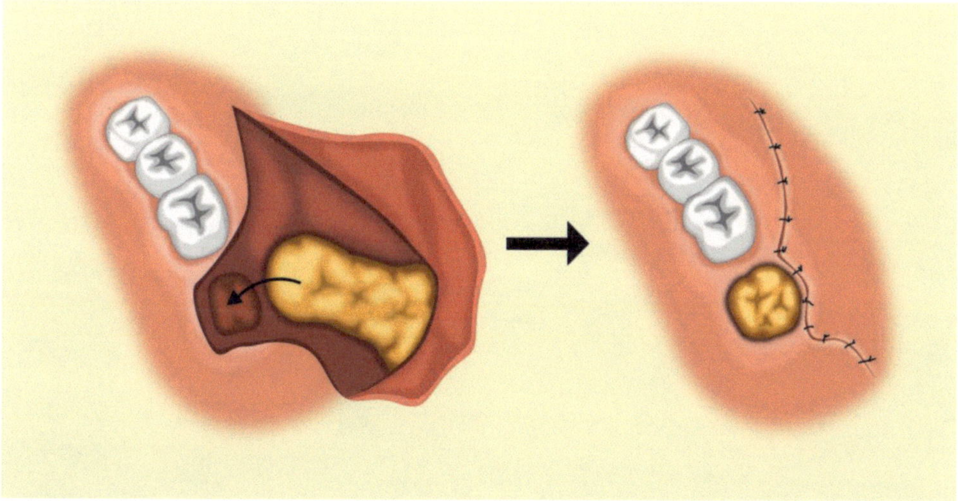

Figure 37.
Illustration shows harvesting BFP from the buccal tissue, and the buccal advancement flap is then sutured.

Advantages

- Provides more stability
- Can be used when there is a deficient BFP for closure
- Can be used in cases where a trapezoidal flap is raised for some reasons and in cases with perforation and shrinkage of BFP [43–45]
- Used to minimize the risk of shallow sulcus [42]

Limitations

- More time is needed to perform the surgery
- An experienced surgeon may be needed
- It requires high patient's compliance

9. Conclusions

A wide variety of intraoral flaps and their modifications have been reported in the literature. This chapter illustrates some familiar flap techniques, as well as their advantages and limitations. The application and design of each flap should be tailored to the patient's diagnosis and needs. Surgeons should be aware of patient diagnosis, the anatomical limitation, and the application of different flap's designs. Careful planning, implications, and selection of suitable flap designs would affect final aesthetic outcomes or postoperative morbidity, which may have important medical-legal and economic impacts.

Conflict of interest

The authors declare no conflict of interest.

Author details

Randa Abdulmoein AlFotawi
Oral and Maxillofacial Department, Dental Faculty, King Saud University, Kingdom of Saudia Arabia

*Address all correspondence to: ralfotawei@ksu.edu.sa

References

[1] Jakse N, Bankaoglu V, Wimmer G, Eskici A, Pertl C. Primary wound healing after lower third molar surgery: Evaluation of 2 different flap designs. Oral Surgery, Oral Medicine, Oral Pathology, Oral Radiology, and Endodontology. 2002;**93**(1):7-12. DOI: 10.1067/moe.2002.119519

[2] Ash MM, Costich ER, H. J. A study of periodontal hazards of third molars. Periodontology 2000. 1962;**33**:209-219

[3] Stephens RJ, App GR, Foreman DW. Periodontal evaluation of two mucoperiosteal flaps used in removing impacted mandibular third molars. Journal of Oral and Maxillofacial Surgery: Official Journal of the American Association of Oral and Maxillofacial Surgeons. 1983;**41**(11):719-724. DOI: 10.1016/0278-2391(83)90188-x

[4] Chin Quee TA, Gosselin D, Millar EP, Stamm JW. Surgical removal of the fully impacted mandibular third molar: The influence of flap design and alveolar bone height on the periodontal status of the second molar. Journal of Periodontology. 1985;**56**(10):625-630. DOI: 10.1902/jop.1985.56.10.625

[5] Kugelberg CF, Ahlström U, Ericson S, Hugoson A, Kvint S. Periodontal healing after impacted lower third molar surgery in adolescents and adults: A prospective study. International Journal of Oral and Maxillofacial Surgery. 1991;**20**(1):18-24. DOI: 10.1016/S0901-5027(05)80689-7

[6] Szmyd L. Impacted teeth. Dental Clinics of North America. 1971;**15**: 299-318

[7] Klatil L. Komplikationen bei der Entfernung von Weisheitszähnen. KF-University Graz; [PhD thesis] 1998

[8] Yolcu Ü, Acar AH. Comparison of a new flap design with the routinely used triangular flap design in third molar surgery. International Journal of Oral and Maxillofacial Surgery. 2015;**44**(11): 1390-1397. DOI: 10.1016/j.ijom.2015. 07.007

[9] Vermette ME, Kokich VG, Kennedy DB. Uncovering labially impacted teeth: Apically positioned flap and closed-eruption techniques. The Angle Orthodontist. 1995;**65**(1):23-32. DOI: 10.1043/0003-3219(1995)065< 0023:ULITAP>2.0.CO;2

[10] Johnston WD. Treatment of palatally impacted canine teeth. American Journal of Orthodontics. 1969; **56**(6):589-596. DOI: 10.1016/0002-9416 (69)90194-8

[11] Kokich VG, M.D. Surgical and orthodontic management of impacted teeth. Dental Clinics of North America. 1993;**37**:181-204

[12] Kokich VG. Surgical and orthodontic management of impacted maxillary canines. American Journal of Orthodontics and Dentofacial Orthopedics. 2004;**126**(3):278-283. DOI: 10.1016/j.ajodo.2004.06.009

[13] Huang Y-S, Lin Y-C, Hung C-Y, Lai Y-L. Surgical considerations and management of bilateral labially impacted canines. Journal of Dental Sciences. 2016;**11**(2):202-206. DOI: 10.1016/J.JDS.2013.02.027

[14] Ramfjord SR, Nissle RR. The modified Widman. Journal of Periodontology. 1974;**45**(8):601-607

[15] Prasanth T. Management of localized gingival recession by two-stage surgical procedure—Double pedicle flap with CTG and coronally advanced flap: A novel technique. Journal of Indian Society of Periodontology. 2009;**13**(1): 44-47. DOI: 10.4103/0972-124X.51895

[16] AL-Juboori, M.J. Flap designs for implant-related surgical procedures: A review. Implant Dentistry. 2016;**25**(6). Available from: https://journals.lww.com/implantdent/Fulltext/2016/12000/Flap_Designs_for_Implant_Related_Surgical.23.aspx

[17] Von Arx T, Salvi GE, Janner S, J. S. Gingival recession following apicalsurgery in the esthetic zone: A clinical study with 70 cases. The European Journal of Esthetic Dentistry. 2009;**4**(1):28-45

[18] Von Arx T, Vinzens-Majaniemi T, Bürgin W, Jensen SS. Changes of periodontal parameters following apical surgery: A prospective clinical study of three incision techniques. International Endodontic Journal. 2007;**40**(12): 959-969. DOI: 10.1111/j.1365-2591.2007.01306.x

[19] Kreisler M, Gockel R, Schmidt I, Kühl S, d'Hoedt B. Clinical evaluation of a modified marginal sulcular incision technique in endodontic surgery. Oral Surgery, Oral Medicine, Oral Pathology, Oral Radiology, and Endodontology. 2009;**108**(6):e22-e28. DOI: 10.1016/j.tripleo.2009.08.005

[20] Vreeland DL, Tidwell E. Flap design for surgical endodontics. Oral Surgery, Oral Medicine, Oral Pathology. 1982; **54**(4):461-465. DOI: 10.1016/0030-4220(82)90396-6

[21] Peñarrocha M. Técnica quirúrgica. In: Cirugía Periapical. Barcelona: Ars Medica; 2004

[22] Velvart P, Peters CI. Soft tissue management in endodontic surgery. Journal of Endodontics. 2005;**31**(1): 4-16. DOI: 10.1097/01.DON.000014532.08454.5C

[23] Velvart P, Ebner-Zimmermann U, Ebner JP. Comparison of papilla healing following sulcular full-thickness flap and papilla base flap in endodontic surgery. International Endodontic Journal. 2003;**36**(10):653-659. DOI: 10.1046/j.1365-2591.2003. 00693.x

[24] Peñarrocha-Diago M, Peñarrocha-Diago M. Atlas de cirugía periapical. In: Atlas de cirugía periapical. Madrid: Ergon; 2013. pp. 47-97

[25] Hassan O, Shoukry T, Raouf AA, W. H. Combined palatal and buccal flaps in oroantral fistula repair. Egyptian Journal of Ear, Nose, Throat and Allied Sciences. 2012;**13**:77-81

[26] Scattarella A, Ballini A, Grassi FR, Carbonara A, Ciccolella F, Dituri A, et al. Treatment of oroantral fistula with autologous bone graft and application of a non-reabsorbable membrane. International Journal of Medical Sciences. 2010;**7**(5):267-271. DOI: 10.7150/ijms.7.267

[27] Awang MN. Closure of oroantral fistula. International Journal of Oral and Maxillofacial Surgery. 1988;**17**(2): 110-115. DOI: 10.1016/s0901-5027(88)80162-0

[28] Lazow SK. Surgical management of the oroantral fistula flap procedures. Operative Techniques in Otolaryngology-Head and Neck Surgery. 1999;**10**(2):148-152

[29] Fickling BW. Oral surgery involving the maxillary sinus. Annals of the Royal College of Surgeons of England. 1957;**20**: 3-35

[30] Berger A. Oroantral openings and their surgical corrections. Arch Otolaryngology. 1939;**130**:400-402

[31] Amaratunga NA. Oro-antral fistulae —A study of clinical, radiological and treatment aspects. The British Journal of Oral & Maxillofacial Surgery. 1986;**24**: 433-437

[32] McGregor IA, M.F. Reconstructive techniques ini ntraoral surgery. In:

Mcgregor FM, editor. Cancer of the Faceand Mouth. 1st ed. London: Churchill Livingst; 1986. pp. 412-419

[33] Baxhausen G. Closure of oroantral fistulae. Les Annales d'Oto-Laryngologie. 1939;**48**:632-638

[34] Sokler K, Vuksan V, L.T. Treatment of oroantral fistula. Acta stomatologica Croatica. 2002;**36**:135-140

[35] Rintala A. A double overlapping hinge flap to close palatal fistula. Scandinavian Journal of Plastic and Reconstructive Surgery. 1971;**5**:91-95

[36] Salins PC, Kishore SK. Anteriorly based palatal flap for closure of large oroantral fistula. Oral Surgery, Oral Medicine, Oral Pathology, Oral Radiology, and Endodontology. 1996; **82**(3):253-256. DOI: 10.1016/S1079-2104(96)80348-9

[37] Chonkas NC. Modified palatal flap technique for closure of oroantral fistulas. Journal of Oral Surgery. 1974; **32**:112-113

[38] Rapidis AD, Alexandridis CA, Eleftheriadis E, Angelopoulos AP. The use of the buccal fat pad for reconstruction of oral defects: Review of the literature and report of 15 cases. Journal of Oral and Maxillofacial Surgery: Official Journal of the American Association of Oral and Maxillofacial Surgeons. 2000;**58**(2): 158-163. DOI: 10.1016/s0278-2391(00)90330-6

[39] Tideman H, Bosdnquet A, S.J. Use of the buccal fat pad as a pedicled graft. Journal of Oral and Maxillofacial Surgery. 1986;**44**:435-440

[40] Ferrari S, Ferri A, Bianchi B, Copelli C, Magri AS, Sesenna E. A novel technique for cheek mucosa defect reconstruction using a pedicled buccal fat pad and buccinator myomucosal island flap. Oral Oncology. 2009;**45**(1): 59-62. DOI: 10.1016/J.ORALONCOLOGY.2008.03.018

[41] Egyedi P. Utilization of the buccal fat pad for closure of oro-antral and/or oro-nasal communications. Journal of Maxillofacial Surgery. 1977;**5**:241-244. DOI: 10.1016/S0301-0503(77)80117-3

[42] Candamourty R, Jain MK, Sankar K, Babu MRR. Double-layered closure of oroantral fistula using buccal fat pad and buccal advancement flap. Journal of Natural Science, Biology, and Medicine. 2012;**3**(2):203-205. DOI: 10.4103/0976-9668.101930

[43] Fujimura N, Nagura H, Enomoto S. Grafting of the buccal fat pad into palatal defects. Journal of Cranio-Maxillofacial Surgery. 1990;**18**(5): 219-222. DOI: 10.1016/S1010-5182(05)80415-9

[44] Batra Hemantand Jindal G, K. S. Evaluation of different treatment modalities for closure of oro-antral communications and formulation of a rational approach. Journal of Maxillofacial and Oral Surgery. 2010; **9**(1):13-18. DOI: 10.1007/s12663-010-0006-y

[45] Pandolfi PJ, Yavuzer R, Jackson IT. Three-layer closure of an oroantral-cutaneous defect. International Journal of Oral and Maxillofacial Surgery. 2000; **29**(1):24-26. DOI: 10.1016/S0901-5027(00)80118-6